Emergency Cardiac Care 2012: From the ED to the CCU

Editors

AMAL MATTU
MANDEEP R. MEHRA

CARDIOLOGY CLINICS

www.cardiology.theclinics.com

Consulting Editor
MICHAEL H. CRAWFORD

November 2012 • Volume 30 • Number 4

ELSEVIER

1600 John F. Kennedy Blvd. • Suite 1800 • Philadelphia, PA 19103-2899

http://www.theclinics.com

CARDIOLOGY CLINICS Volume 30, Number 4

November 2012 ISSN 0733-8651, ISBN-13: 978-1-4557-4891-4

Editor: Barbara Cohen-Kligerman

Cardiology Clinics (ISSN 0733-8651) is published quarterly by Elsevier Inc., 360 Park Avenue South, New York, NY 10010-1710. Months of issue are February, May, August, and November. Business and Editorial Offices: 1600 John F. Kennedy Blvd., Ste. 1800, Philadelphia, PA 19103-2899. Customer Service Office: 3251 Riverport Lane, Maryland Heights, MO 63043. Periodicals postage paid at New York, NY and additional mailing offices. Subscription prices are $305.00 per year for US individuals, $508.00 per year for US institutions, $149.00 per year for US students and residents, $373.00 per year for Canadian individuals, $630.00 per year for Canadian institutions, $432.00 per year for international individuals, $630.00 per year for international institutions and $211.00 per year for Canadian and international students/residents. To receive student/resident rate, orders must be accompanied by name of affiliated institution, data of term, and the *signature* of program/residency coordinator on institution letterhead. Orders will be billed at individual rate until proof of status is received. Foreign air speed delivery is included in all *Clinics* subscription prices. All prices are subject to change without notice. **POSTMASTER:** Send address changes to *Cardiology Clinics*, Elsevier Health Sciences Division, Subscription Customer Service, 3251 Riverport Lane, Maryland Heights, MO 63043. **Customer Service: 1-800-654-2452 (U.S. and Canada); 314-447-8871 (outside U.S. and Canada). Fax: 314-447-8029. E-mail: journalscustomerservice-usa@ elsevier.com (for print support); journalsonlinesupport-usa@elsevier.com (for online support).**

Reprints. For copies of 100 or more, of articles in this publication, please contact the Commercial Reprints Department, Elsevier Inc., 360 Park Avenue South, New York, NY 10010-1710. Tel.: 212-633-3812; Fax: 212-462-1935; E-mail: reprints@elsevier.com.

Cardiology Clinics is also published in Spanish by McGraw-Hill Interamericana Editores S. A., P.O. Box 5-237, 06500, Mexico D. F., Mexico; in Portuguese by Reichmann and Alfonso Editores Rio de Janeiro, Brazil; and in Greek by Dimitrios P. Lagos, 8 Pondon Street, GR115-28 Ilissia, Greece.

Cardiology Clinics is covered in *MEDLINE/PubMed (Index Medicus), Excerpta Medica, The Cumulative Index to Nursing and Allied Health Literature* (CINAHL).

Printed and bound by CPI Group (UK) Ltd, Croydon, CR0 4YY

Transferred to digital print 2012

Contributors

CONSULTING EDITOR

MICHAEL H. CRAWFORD, MD
Professor of Medicine, University of California,
San Francisco; Lucie Stern Chair in Cardiology
and Chief of Clinical Cardiology, University of
California, San Francisco Medical Center,
San Francisco, California

GUEST EDITORS

AMAL MATTU, MD
Professor and Vice Chair; Director, Emergency
Cardiology Fellowship, Department of
Emergency Medicine, University of Maryland
School of Medicine, Baltimore, Maryland

MANDEEP R. MEHRA, MBBS
Professor of Medicine, Harvard Medical
School; Department of Medicine, Brigham
and Women's Hospital, Boston,
Massachusetts

AUTHORS

HIROKO BECK, MD
Fellow, Cardiac Electrophysiology Section,
Division of Cardiology, Department of
Medicine, University of Maryland School of
Medicine, University of Maryland Medical
Center, Baltimore, Maryland

R. MICHAEL BENITEZ, MD
Division of Cardiology, University of Maryland
School of Medicine, Baltimore, Maryland

JEREMY S. BOCK, MD
Division of Cardiology, University of Maryland
School of Medicine, Baltimore, Maryland

WILLIAM BRADY, MD
Professor, Departments of Emergency
Medicine and Medicine, University of Virginia
School of Medicine, Charlottesville, Virginia

JENNIFER R. BROWN, MD
Associate Professor of Medicine,
Division of Cardiology, Department of
Medicine, Emory University School of
Medicine, Atlanta, Georgia

ANNA MARIE CHANG, MD
Emergency Cardiac Care Research Fellow,
Department of Emergency Medicine, University
of Pennsylvania, Philadelphia, Pennsylvania

TAPAN GODIWALA, MD
Department of Cardiology, University of
Maryland, Baltimore, Maryland

STEPHEN S. GOTTLIEB, MD
Professor of Medicine and Director, Clinical
Research Program in Cardiology, Division of
Cardiology, Department of Medicine,
University of Maryland School of Medicine,
Baltimore, Maryland

ANUJ GUPTA, MD, FACC
Department of Cardiology, University of
Maryland, Baltimore, Maryland

ERIK P. HESS, MD, MSc
Assistant Professor of Emergency Medicine,
Division of Emergency Medicine Research,
Department of Emergency Medicine, Mayo
Clinic College of Medicine; Knowledge and
Evaluation Research Unit, Mayo Clinic,
Rochester, Minnesota

JUDD E. HOLLANDER, MD
Professor and Clinical Research Director,
Department of Emergency Medicine,
University of Pennsylvania, Philadelphia,
Pennsylvania

AYMAN A. HUSSEIN, MD
Cardiac Arrhythmia and Electrophysiology,
University of Maryland, Baltimore, Maryland

MIRIAM S. JACOB, MD
Assistant Professor of Medicine, Division of
Cardiology, Department of Medicine,
University of Maryland School of Medicine,
University of Maryland, Baltimore, Maryland

WALLACE JOHNSON, MD, FASH
Hypertension Section, Division of Cardiology,
University of Maryland School of Medicine,
Baltimore, Maryland

THOMAS KLEIN, MD
Fellow, Division of Cardiology, University of
Maryland School of Medicine, Baltimore,
Maryland

BENJAMIN J. LAWNER, DO, EMT-P
Assistant Professor, Department of Emergency
Medicine, University of Maryland School of
Medicine; Deputy Medical Director, Baltimore
City Fire Department, Baltimore, Maryland

AMAL MATTU, MD
Professor and Vice Chair; Director, Emergency
Cardiology Fellowship, Department of
Emergency Medicine, University of Maryland
School of Medicine, Baltimore, Maryland

NEVILLE F. MISTRY, MD
Cardiology Fellow, Division of Cardiology,
Department of Medicine, University of
Maryland School of Medicine, Baltimore,
Maryland

JOSE V. NABLE, MD, NREMT-P
Clinical Instructor and Emergency Medical
Services Fellow, Department of Emergency
Medicine, University of Maryland School of
Medicine, Baltimore, Maryland

DAVID M. NESTLER, MD, MS
Assistant Professor of Emergency Medicine,
Division of Emergency Medicine Research,
Department of Emergency Medicine, Mayo
Clinic College of Medicine, Rochester,
Minnesota

MY-LE NGUYEN, MD
Division of Cardiology, University of Maryland
School of Medicine, Baltimore, Maryland

RONAK PATEL, MD
Division of Cardiology, University of Maryland
School of Medicine, Baltimore, Maryland

PETER POLLAK, MD
Senior Cardiology Fellow, Division of
Cardiovascular Medicine, Department of
Medicine, University of Virginia School of
Medicine, Charlottesville, Virginia

GAUTAM V. RAMANI, MD
Assistant Professor of Medicine, Division of
Cardiology, University of Maryland School of
Medicine, Baltimore, Maryland

ANASTASIOS SALIARIS, MD
Assistant Professor of Medicine, Cardiac
Arrhythmia and Electrophysiology, University
of Maryland, Baltimore, Maryland

VINCENT Y. SEE, MD
Assistant Professor of Medicine, Cardiac
Electrophysiology Section, Division of
Cardiology, Department of Medicine,
University of Maryland School of Medicine,
University of Maryland Medical Center,
Baltimore, Maryland

MUKTA SRIVASTAVA, MD
Department of Cardiology, University of
Maryland, Baltimore, Maryland

SEMHAR Z. TEWELDE, MD
Clinical Instructor of Emergency Medicine and
Emergency Cardiology Fellow, Department of
Emergency Medicine, University of Maryland
Medical Center, Baltimore, Maryland

MARK R. VESELY, MD, FACC, FSCAI
Assistant Professor of Medicine, Division of
Cardiology, Department of Medicine,
University of Maryland School of Medicine,
Baltimore, Maryland

MICHAEL E. WINTERS, MD, FACEP, FAAEM
Associate Professor of Emergency Medicine
and Medicine; Co-Director, Emergency
Medicine/Internal Medicine/Critical Care
Program, University of Maryland School of
Medicine, Baltimore, Maryland

Contents

Many institutions have developed outpatient observation units as an alternative to short-stay inpatient admissions. In this article, we highlight evidence to support the efficacy of EDOU care for chest pain and identify areas in which additional research is needed. Evidence-based protocols and collaborative approaches to care have potential to achieve similar clinical and improved economic outcomes compared with hospital admission. The potential for the EDOU to provide the right care for the right patient at the right time is only beginning to be realized, with significant advances in health care delivery anticipated in the near future.

Reducing hospital admissions through improved risk stratification of patients with potential acute coronary syndrome represents a critical focus for reducing health care expenditure. Coronary computed tomographic angiography (CTA) has been used with increasing frequency as part of the evaluation of chest pain in the Emergency Department. In the appropriate group of patients at low to intermediate risk CTA appears to be an excellent evaluation strategy, safely and efficiently allowing for the rapid discharge of patients home.

Hypertensive crises, which include hypertensive emergencies and urgencies, are frequently encountered in the emergency department, and require immediate attention as they can lead to irreversible end-organ damage. Normal blood pressure (BP) regulation is altered during acute rises in BP, leading to end-organ damage. Multiple organs can be injured. Special considerations should be given to hypertensive pregnant patients and patients with postoperative hypertension. Treatment should be individualized to each patient based on the type and extent of end-organ damage, degree of BP elevation, and the specific side effects that each medication could have on a patient's preexisting comorbidities.

Blunt chest trauma represents a spectrum of injuries to the heart and aorta that vary markedly in character and severity. The setting, signs, and symptoms of chest trauma are often nonspecific, which represents a challenge to emergency providers. Individuals with suspected blunt chest trauma who have only mild or no symptoms, a normal electrocardiogram (ECG), and are hemodynamically stable typically have a benign course and rarely require further diagnostic testing or long periods of close observation. Individuals with pain, ECG abnormalities, or hemodynamic instability may require rapid evaluation of the heart by echocardiography and the great vessels by advanced imaging.

Syncope is the transient loss of consciousness and postural tone caused by transient cerebral hypoperfusion. It is a common problem that is often alarming to patients and their families. The differential diagnosis of the patient with transient loss of consciousness is broad and workup may be expensive. It is important to identify patients with life-threatening conditions and those with red flags indicating an increased risk of sudden death. An initial approach consisting of a careful history, physical examination, and electrocardiograms is essential. This review covers the general diagnostic approach to the patient with syncope.

Atrial fibrillation (AF) is the most common tachyarrhythmia encountered in clinical practice. One-third of hospitalizations in the United States are attributed to AF, with increasing rates in the past decade. Significant morbidity and mortality, including ~15% to 20% of all ischemic strokes, result from AF. AF is associated with many causes and comorbidities. Hallmarks of acute AF management are accurate diagnosis, clinical stabilization, symptom relief through rate or rhythm control, thromboembolic stroke risk modification, and treatment of underlying causes. Meticulous and individualized acute evaluation based on these goals facilitates successful transition to long-term collaborative optimization of outcomes.

Diagnosis of ST-segment elevation myocardial infarction has long been considered time sensitive. Several other electrocardiogram abnormalities, sometimes referred to as "STEMI-equivalents", should also alert the clinician to conditions similarly requiring aggressive intervention. The de Winter/ST/T complex, ST-segment elevation in lead aVR, Wellens' phenomenon, posterior wall myocardial infarction, and pathologic ST changes in the presence of left bundle branch block and pacemakers are all discussed in this article.

The 12-lead electrocardiogram (ECG) remains the cornerstone of prompt diagnosis of STEMI; Furthermore, the 12-lead ECG provides the primary indication for emergent reperfuison therapy in the STEMI patient. In certain cases, a patient's ECG can resemble STEMI yet manifest ST-segment elevation from a non-coronary-based syndrome; these entities are termed the STEMI mimics and include benign early re-polarization, acute pericarditis, and left ventricular aneurysm, to name only a few. In other situations, the patient's ECG makes it difficult or impossible to determine whether STEMI is present, the so-called STEMI confounders and include left bundle branch block pattern, left ventricular hypertrophypattern, and the ventricular paced pattern. The goal with STEMI mimics and confounders is to maximize rapid, accurate diagnosis while avoiding delays in treatment of alternative causes of ST-segment elevation.

Acute coronary syndromes result in a significant burden of morbidity and mortality in the United States. This spectrum of acute coronary thrombosis (including unstable angina, non-ST-segment elevation myocardial infarction, and ST-elevation myocardial infarction) has been well studied in large clinical trials. This review details the initial management of patients presenting with possible acute coronary syndromes in the context of care from the emergency department to the cardiac care unit. The importance of a rapid and focused evaluation, risk stratification, and appropriate therapies are discussed.

Approximately 330,000 ST-elevation myocardial infarctions (STEMI) occur yearly in the United States. Emergent reperfusion is the cornerstone of STEMI therapy and the key to restoration of coronary blood flow in an infarct-related vessel. Reperfusion methods include thrombolysis, primary percutaneous coronary intervention, or both methods combined. Selection of the appropriate reperfusion strategy is essential, along with having an efficient system of care capable of delivering these therapies. Timely reperfusion is highly dependent on a well-structured care system designed to meet the needs of each individual community. This article reviews the data behind different reperfusion strategies and introduces successful systems-of-care models.

Care of the patient with return of spontaneous circulation following sudden cardiac death is complex and challenging. A systematic and comprehensive approach can increase the chances of meaningful recovery of the postarrest patient. This article focuses on a systematic approach to the postarrest patient, which includes optimizing oxygenation and ventilation, maintaining adequate perfusion pressure, monitoring oxygen delivery, initiating and maintaining therapeutic hypothermia, and identifying patients appropriate for emergent cardiac catheterization. Using this approach, providers treating the postarrest patient can maximize the chance that a patient walks out of the hospital neurologically intact.

Cardiogenic shock remains a major cause of morbidity and mortality in patients hospitalized with myocardial infarction, severe valvular disease, and other causes of cardiomyopathy. Emergency physicians play a pivotal role in the initial management of these patients, as they are most often the point of first contact with the medical system. This review discusses the initial assessment and management of cardiogenic shock, emphasizing the importance and role of the emergency physician.

Acute decompensated heart failure (ADHF) is the most common cause of cardiovascular hospital admission; 1 in 4 patients with heart failure is readmitted within 30 days of being discharged, and ADHF consumes 1% to 2% of the total health care resources. The most effective approach for preventing heart failure hospitalizations is a combination of improvement in management of patients while they are in the hospital and comprehensive post hospitalization care. Decreasing the length of hospitalization can increase readmission rate, so optimization of inpatient and outpatient care is essential.

As the prevalence of systolic heart failure increases, the population of patients in need of advanced therapies becomes larger. As the number of transplants performed each year plateaus, the prevalence of community-dwelling patients with ventricular assist devices (VADs) increases. A broad range of physicians, including emergency physicians, general cardiologists, and generalists, will be exposed to these patients, and must be informed on the disease processes and complications specific to these devices. With an understanding of up-front evaluation and management, these patients may be triaged and stabilized, and will benefit before referral for definitive care by a VAD specialist.

CARDIOLOGY CLINICS

NOW AVAILABLE FOR YOUR iPhone and iPad

Foreword
Emergency Cardiovascular Care

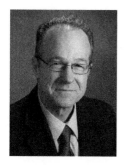

Michael H. Crawford, MD
Consulting Editor

For most of the latter half of the twentieth century, Emergency Department (ED) and Cardiology Department care of acute cardiovascular disease patients moved in parallel but separate paths. Perhaps because for a long time we didn't have much to offer such patients, coordination of services was not a priority. Several advances in cardiovascular diagnosis and treatment changed this dynamic. On the diagnostic side, we had troponin levels, which made diagnosing acute cardiac damage more feasible. In fact, troponin is now the central feature for diagnosing acute myocardial infarction. Also, the enhancement of CT scanning and the deployment of CT scanners in most EDs have greatly improved the rapid diagnosis of aortic dissection, pulmonary embolus, and, more recently, significant coronary artery lesions. Treatment advances include safer, more effective surgical approaches to aortic dissection, percutaneous coronary interventions, and advanced circulatory support devices. Finally, the demand for quality-of-care metrics by health care funding agencies has spawned "door-to-balloon" times and other treatment outcome measures. All these forces and more have made it imperative that the Emergency and Cardiology Departments work together more closely in the care of acute cardiovascular diseases.

Most hospitals and medical centers have worked largely in isolation to develop protocols, care pathways, and special teams to solve coordination issues in emergency care. More recently, national organizations have fostered sharing of these approaches with variable success. Although some national standards have been developed for things such as door-to-balloon times and certification programs have been promulgated for things such as chest pain centers, finding the best practices for all cardiovascular emergency conditions is not easy. Hence, the origin of this issue of *Cardiology Clinics*. Drs Mattu and Mehra have brought together an outstanding group of experts in Emergency Medicine and Cardiology to lay out the issues and present best practices for the care of these patients, who have a high mortality if not treated expeditiously. This issue should be required reading for anyone who practices in an ED or an acute care hospital.

Michael H. Crawford, MD
University of California
San Francisco Medical Center
505 Parnassus Avenue, Box 0124
San Francisco, CA 94143-0124, USA

E-mail address:
crawfordm@medicine.ucsf.edu

Cardiol Clin 30 (2012) xi
http://dx.doi.org/10.1016/j.ccl.2012.09.005
0733-8651/12/$ – see front matter © 2012 Elsevier Inc. All rights reserved.

cardiology.theclinics.com

Preface

Emergency Cardiovascular Care: From ED to CCU and Beyond

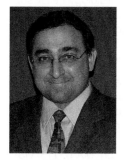
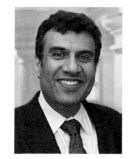

| Amal Mattu, MD | Mandeep R. Mehra, MBBS |

Guest Editors

Cardiac disease accounts for more deaths in the United States and many other first-world countries than any other cause. Many advances in preventive medicine, diagnostics, and therapeutics have marked improvements in health status and outcome from cardiovascular diseases. Most of these salutary benefits accrue from efforts at controlling risk markers with high attributable risk penetrance, such as hypertension, or in other cases, strides in our understanding of the pathophysiology of myocardial infarction and recognition that "time is muscle." Yet, in other instances, we continue to struggle. One vivid example is the syndrome of acute decompensated heart failure, wherein the science had critically lagged behind the art of medicine. Many illnesses present to us in such a crisis and in that regard a confluence of practice thought in emergency medicine and cardiovascular medicine is a timely need.

These two specialties, although philosophically different in their approach to many other types of patients, are very similar in their approach to acute cardiovascular patients. Practitioners in both specialties work under significant time constraints, are forced to make life-and-death decisions, often with minimal objective data, and are often held to high expectations in outcome by society. Although traveling in the same boat, we don't always row in synchrony and this can lead to a gap in optimal patient care delivery and outcomes.

The goal of this issue of *Cardiology Clinics* is to bridge these critical gaps between our two specialties of emergency medicine and cardiovascular medicine. To accomplish this, we've brought together a confluence of experts in both specialties to collaborate and create a repository of what are identified as the best practices for emergency cardiac conditions. We believe that we've been able to formulate approaches to workup and management that will help these two specialties work in greater unison and optimize patient care.

Although this issue of *Cardiology Clinics* is certainly not comprehensive with regards to emergency cardiac care, we've been able to address many of the most common emergency cardiac conditions, as well as some conditions that are rising in import around the world. Acute coronary syndrome (ACS) is addressed in depth, including articles focusing on systems of care, recognition, and management, and the most recent "hot topic"—coronary CT angiography. Two additional articles focus on electrocardiography of ACS, including discussions of novel electrocardiography patterns as well as mimics of ACS. Decompensated heart failure and cardiogenic shock are also addressed. A separate article is devoted to recent advances in cardiac arrest, with an emphasis on post-arrest care. Additional articles address hypertensive emergencies, blunt chest trauma and commotio cordis, atrial fibrillation, syncope, and complications of implanted cardiac devices. Finally an article is provided that addresses the true interface between emergency department and in-patient practice—the use of observation units for emergency cardiac conditions.

Cardiol Clin 30 (2012) xiii–xiv
http://dx.doi.org/10.1016/j.ccl.2012.09.001

cardiology.theclinics.com

In overseeing the development of this issue of *Cardiology Clinics*, we have tried to maintain both an emergency medicine as well as a cardiology perspective on the content of the articles. The reader, therefore, should find a coordinated approach to the evaluation and initial management of patients presenting with these cardiac emergencies. We believe not only that physicians from the two represented specialties will benefit from this compendium but also that this issue of the *Cardiology Clinics* will be of relevance to other subspecialists who wish to acquire a more keen understanding of these "hot" topics. It is our sincere hope that this issue will help to bridge the gap between our specialties so that we may row in unison toward our common goal—optimization of patient care.

We would like to thank the dedicated authors of this issue of *Cardiology Clinics* for their time and effort in writing outstanding articles. We would also like to thank Barbara Cohen-Kligerman and Elsevier for their support of this work. Finally, on behalf of our authors as well, we thank our families for their support, encouragement, and patience throughout the production of this issue.

Amal Mattu, MD
Emergency Cardiology Fellowship
Department of Emergency Medicine
University of Maryland School of Medicine
110 S. Paca Street, Sixth Floor, Suite 200
Baltimore, MD 21201, USA

Mandeep R. Mehra, MBBS
Harvard Medical School
Department of Medicine
Brigham and Women's Hospital
75 Francis Street
Boston, MA 02115, USA

E-mail addresses:
amattu@smail.umaryland.edu (A. Mattu)
mmehra@partners.org (M.R. Mehra)

Transforming the Emergency Department Observation Unit
A Look Into the Future

Erik P. Hess, MD, MSc[a,b],*, David M. Nestler, MD, MS[a]

KEYWORDS

- Chest pain • Syncope • Cardiac arrhythmias • Heart failure • Atrial fibrillation
- Emergency medical services

KEY POINTS

- Because of the rising volume of emergency department visits, hospital overcrowding, and greater attention to the cost-effectiveness of health care, observation unit care has become an attractive alternative to inpatient admission.
- There are varying levels of evidence and growing interest in managing patients with chest pain potentially caused by acute coronary syndrome, syncope, atrial fibrillation, and acute decompensated heart failure at low to intermediate short-term risk for adverse outcomes in an emergency department observation unit setting.
- Evidence-based protocols and collaborative approaches to care have the potential to achieve similar clinical and improved economic outcomes compared with hospital admission.

INTRODUCTION

Since the mid 1990s, the proportion of inpatient admissions originating from the emergency department (ED) has increased from approximately one-third to one-half of all hospital admissions.[1] This trend has been accompanied by a progressively rising number of ED visits. Data from the National Ambulatory Healthcare Survey estimate nearly 120 million annual ED visits, and this number has increased by 23% since 1997.[2] This increasing volume of patients has put greater demand for acute care services than can be provided, contributing to overcrowding in both the hospital and ED settings. In 2006, the Centers for Medicare and Medicaid Services, the largest insurer in the United States, began the Recovery Audit Contractor (RAC) program to identify waste in the Medicare program. One area of charge recovery identified by the RAC program was short-stay admissions, which were considered an inappropriate use of inpatient services.[3]

Many institutions have developed outpatient observation units as an alternative to short-stay inpatient admissions, with 36% of US EDs reporting having observation units in 2007.[3,4] Several single-center studies have demonstrated equivalent clinical and improved economic outcomes when ED observation units (EDOU) are used as an alternative to inpatient admission for select conditions.[5–8] EDOU care, as currently delivered, is provided for select patients by means of streamlined evidence-based protocols before safe discharge from the ED.

In this article, we highlight evidence to support the efficacy of EDOU care for select cardiac conditions, as well as identify areas in which additional research is needed to develop and evaluate optimized approaches to health care delivery. The

[a] Division of Emergency Medicine Research, Department of Emergency Medicine, Mayo Clinic College of Medicine, 200 First Street Southwest, Mayo Clinic, Rochester, MN 55905, USA; [b] Knowledge and Evaluation Research Unit, Mayo Clinic, Rochester, MN, USA
* Corresponding author. Division of Emergency Medicine Research, Department of Emergency Medicine, Mayo Clinic College of Medicine, 200 First Street Southwest, Rochester, MN 55905.
E-mail address: hess.erik@mayo.edu

Cardiol Clin 30 (2012) 501–521
http://dx.doi.org/10.1016/j.ccl.2012.07.013
0733-8651/12/$ – see front matter © 2012 Elsevier Inc. All rights reserved.

cardiac conditions discussed include the following: chest pain potentially caused by acute coronary syndrome (ACS), syncope, atrial fibrillation, and acute decompensated heart failure.

CHEST PAIN POTENTIALLY CAUSED BY ACS

Chest pain is the second most common reason patients present to US EDs, accounting for more than 8 million visits annually.[2] Given the frequency with which patients present for evaluation of chest pain, the amount of time needed to reach a diagnosis, and established research on the subject, it is not surprising that it currently accounts for 84% of EDOU visits.[4] Quickly identifying and treating patients with ACS and other life-threatening etiologies of chest pain and risk stratifying the remaining into those safe for discharge and those who require further investigation is an ongoing challenge for clinicians, especially given the morbidity and mortality associated with missing a diagnosis of ACS. Observation unit care has arisen as an

attractive alternative to hospital admission for patients with symptoms suggestive of ACS without objective evidence of ischemia.

Patient Selection for Observation Unit Care

When patients present to the ED with chest pain, the initial evaluation focuses on the identification and exclusion of potential life-threatening etiologies. If the initial evaluation is unrevealing, the focus of the evaluation shifts to determining the likelihood of ACS (**Fig. 1**).[9] Patients with objective evidence of ACS or hemodynamic or electrical instability are admitted to the hospital for urgent therapy. Patients recognized as having a noncardiac etiology of chest pain are treated as appropriate for the alternative diagnosis. Patients with chronic stable angina are referred for outpatient follow-up and management according to American College of Cardiology/American Heart Association (ACC/AHA) guidelines for chronic stable angina.[10] Hemodynamically stable patients with no objective evidence of ischemia on

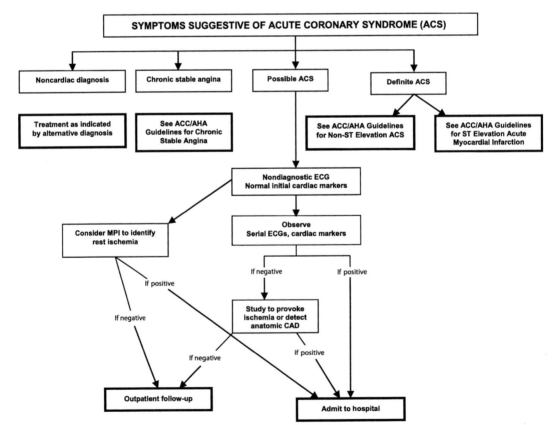

Fig. 1. Evaluation of patients presenting with symptoms suggestive of ACS. (*Reproduced from* Amsterdam EA, Kirk JD, Bluemke DA, et al, on behalf of the American Heart Association Exercise, Cardiac Rehabilitation, and Prevention Committee of the Council on Clinical Cardiology Council on Cardiovascular Nursing, and Interdisciplinary Council on Quality of Care and Outcomes Research. Testing of low-risk patients presenting to the emergency department with chest pain. Circulation 2010;122:1756–76; with permission.)

electrocardiogram (ECG) and negative initial cardiac troponin with ongoing concern for possible ACS are considered for further evaluation in an EDOU.

Evidence to Support the Efficacy of Observation Unit Care

Seminal research conducted in the mid-1990s demonstrated equivalent clinical outcomes and improved economic efficiency when patients at intermediate short-term risk for cardiac events were evaluated in an EDOU compared with hospital admission.[11] Patients randomized to the EDOU underwent a 6-hour observation period during which continuous ECG monitoring, serial cardiac biomarkers, and serial ECGs were performed. Patients who "passed" the 6-hour observation period underwent functional cardiac stress testing. Those with negative stress tests were discharged from the EDOU, and those with equivocal or positive stress tests were admitted to the hospital. No significant difference in the rate of cardiac events between groups was observed, and there were no cardiac events within 6 months in those who were randomized to the EDOU and eventually discharged home. Resource use was greater in the group randomized to hospital admission. Several single-center studies[5,8,12] provided additional evidence to support the safety and economic efficiency of EDOU care for patients with chest pain possibly caused by ACS. Goodacre and colleagues[8] conducted a single-center trial in the UK to assess the effect of EDOU care in patients with undifferentiated chest pain. This study, which included 972 patients who were treated in the EDOU or according to standard care, observed a lower rate of hospital admission and a lower rate of inappropriate discharge of patients with ACS in those who received care in the EDOU. These investigators subsequently conducted the ESCAPE trial, a multicenter cluster randomized trial to evaluate the effectiveness and safety of chest pain unit care in 14 hospitals in the United Kingdom.[13] This study reported no difference in the proportion of patients with chest pain who were admitted to the hospital between the intervention and control hospitals and a small increase in the proportion of patients presenting to the ED and in the number returning to the ED for evaluation within 30 days. Between hospital differences in staffing levels and hours of operation, degree of multidisciplinary buy-in and staff enthusiasm, and inherent differences between the US and UK health systems are potential explanations for the findings observed.[14] This study also did not rigorously risk stratify patients to identify those who would likely benefit from EDOU admission, potentially diluting the effect of the intervention. With the exception of the ESCAPE trial, the weight of evidence largely supports the efficacy of EDOU care as an efficient, safe, and cost-effective approach to evaluating ED patients at low to intermediate risk for ACS.

Future Directions

The rationale for incorporating routine stress testing as part of an EDOU evaluation for chest pain is that a negative result substantially reduces the likelihood of ACS and is helpful prognostically in identifying patients at very low short-term risk for a cardiac event.[15–21] However, the converse is not the case; a positive stress test is not synonymous with the presence of unstable coronary disease. In one study with 1194 patients who were evaluated in an EDOU and underwent cardiac stress testing, the probability of having a positive or indeterminate stress test resulting in subsequent negative catheterization was double the probability of having a positive or indeterminate stress test resulting in catheterization that detected significant coronary artery disease (CAD).[22] Although routine stress testing has a high sensitivity for the detection of CAD, the value of a positive test in directing subsequent management is variable[18,21]; if the pre-test probability of disease is low, the yield of coronary angiography is also low.[23] A number of investigations have reported the limited utility of stress testing in patients younger than 40 in whom ECG and troponin testing have not identified ACS.[24–28] Future work is needed to develop approaches to selecting patients for stress testing in which a positive result is likely to identify significant CAD requiring intervention. In our institution, we have incorporated cardiology consultation in EDOU patients with positive stress tests and in selected cases even before stress testing. This provides an opportunity to minimize or clarify false-positive tests and to potentially avoid hospital admission if the probability of ACS is felt to be low. An approach such as this requires close collaboration between cardiologists and emergency physicians and, in our estimation, has potential to increase the appropriateness and yield of stress testing and decrease unnecessary hospital admissions. The safety and cost-effectiveness of this approach is a promising area for further investigation.

Another area of controversy is whether stress testing is necessary before ED discharge or whether it can be obtained in the outpatient setting within 24 to 72 hours.[9] Some investigators have found that arranging outpatient testing is unreliable, as patients often do not comply with outpatient follow-up,[29,30] whereas others have observed follow-up rates as high as 92%.[31] One study reported higher rates of follow-up when stress tests were scheduled before ED discharge compared with asking patients to contact their primary care physician to arrange a stress test.[32] Process-specific, patient-specific, and health-system–specific characteristics may contribute to the fidelity of follow-up. Additional investigation is needed to more clearly define the factors that affect compliance with outpatient follow-up, as such an approach could help decrease the length of stay in the ED and alleviate overcrowding. In our institution, we have established an EDOU protocol that includes the ability to obtain immediate stress testing if a patient's troponin evaluation is completed during business hours, or have a patient follow up with an outpatient appointment if troponins are completed after hours. An EDOU management diagram with this strategy is noted in **Fig. 2**.

Finally, new diagnostics for ACS such as high-sensitivity troponins,[33,34] coronary computed tomography (CT),[35] and cardiac magnetic resonance imaging[36] have potential to identify patients safe for discharge without the need for EDOU admission and to improve the diagnostic yield among those who undergo EDOU evaluation.

SYNCOPE

Syncope is a symptom of cerebral hypoperfusion and is defined as a sudden, transient loss of consciousness with inability to maintain postural tone that terminates spontaneously.[37,38] Syncope accounts for 1% to 3% of all ED visits and up to 6% of hospital admissions.[39–41] A number of insults can lead to transient cerebral hypoperfusion, resulting in a myriad of diagnostic possibilities for clinicians to consider. The first task is to differentiate syncope from other conditions that can present similarly, such as seizure or narcolepsy. Once the presentation has been confirmed as syncope, the next task for the clinician is to identify the few patients with a serious underlying etiology, such as cardiac arrhythmia, ACS, pulmonary embolism, aortic dissection, or subarachnoid hemorrhage. Because patients with syncope are often asymptomatic on arrival to the hospital, concerns about the possibility of a serious underlying cause drive a largely conservative approach to evaluation. Up to 86% of patients are admitted to the hospital[42] despite a lack of evidence to suggest that hospitalization improves outcome. This results in substantial economic burden to the US health care system, with estimated costs

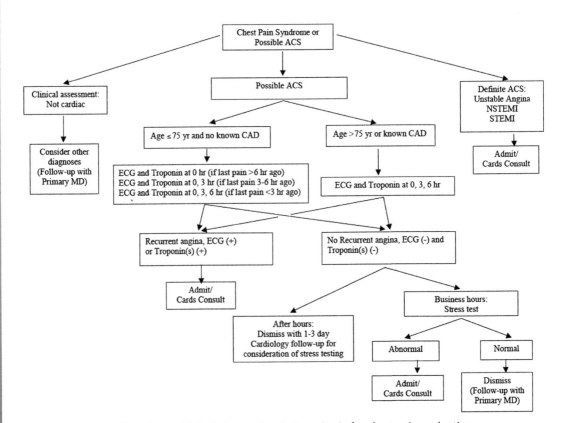

Fig. 2. Sample EDOU flow chart with inclusion and exclusion criteria for chest pain evaluation.

of $2 billion spent on hospitalization of patients with syncope annually.[43]

Evidence to Support the Efficacy of Observation Unit Care

Table 1 summarizes the relevant literature examining ED and hospital-based syncope units for evaluation of patients with syncope. The only clinical trial demonstrating the potential utility of EDOU care for patients with syncope, SEEDS (Syncope Evaluation in the Emergency Department Study), was conducted in Rochester, MN.[7] In this trial, the investigators developed a risk stratification scheme from the literature and position papers from the American College of Physicians[44,45] and the American College of Emergency Physicians,[46] which stratified patients with syncope into low risk, intermediate risk, and high risk. High-risk patients were admitted to the hospital, low-risk patients were treated as appropriate for the etiology of syncope and dismissed home, and intermediate-risk patients were randomized to standard care or EDOU admission. Patients randomized to EDOU admission underwent 6 hours of cardiac monitoring, orthostatic blood pressure checks, a carotid sinus massage test, tilt table testing, transthoracic echocardiography, and cardiology consultation by an electrophysiologist. Compared with intermediate-risk patients with standard care (n = 52), intermediate-risk patients with EDOU protocolized care (n = 51) had a lower frequency of hospital admission (43% vs 98%, P<.001), a higher rate of presumptive diagnosis of syncope etiology (67% vs 10%, P<.001), and similar all-cause mortality and recurrent syncope event rates. Suggestions for risk stratification are shown in **Table 2** and a patient management flow diagram for EDOU management used in the SEEDS trial is noted in **Fig. 3**.

Additional studies have assessed the clinical performance of hospital-based syncope units. Kenny and colleagues[47] established a syncope and falls facility in Newcastle, UK, at the Royal Victoria Infirmary. This facility received referrals for hospital inpatients and EDs that were evaluated within 1 week, outpatient referrals that were evaluated within 1 to 3 weeks, and nonurgent outpatient referrals that were evaluated within 6 weeks. Health care use was compared between adults older than 65 years admitted to the syncope unit and similar patients admitted to 13 peer hospitals. A shorter length of stay was observed in hospitalized patients at the Royal Victoria Infirmary, and fewer cases of syncope and falls were evaluated on an emergency basis. Numeroso and colleagues[48] evaluated the efficacy of a short-stay ward for patients with syncope in Parma, Italy. Although this observational study had no control group, they reported a 79% discharge rate from the syncope ward and a mean length of stay of 3.5 days, with 21% requiring transfer to another hospital service. Ammirati and colleagues[49] retrospectively analyzed 102 patients referred to their specialized syncope unit. Patients admitted to the syncope unit had a greater frequency of diagnosis (82% vs 75%) and 85% lower hospital costs in follow-up. Brignole and colleagues[50] recently conducted a multicenter prospective observational study in 9 Italian hospitals with hospital-based syncope units that met certification requirements by the European Society of Cardiology and the Associazione Italiana di Aritmologia e Cardiostimolazione. Of the 891 patients included in the analysis, 60% were referred from clinicians in the outpatient setting or self-referred, 24% were referrals from the ED, and the remaining 16% were hospitalized patients. Eighty-two percent of patients admitted to the syncope unit received a diagnosis; 21% of diagnoses were made during the initial evaluation, 61% within 45 days, and in 18% the cause remained undetermined. Overall, preliminary evidence suggests increased diagnostic yield and lower rates of hospital admission for patients evaluated in an EDOU or hospital-based syncope unit.

Future Directions

One of the limitations of the SEEDS study[7] was that the investigators used a consensus-based risk stratification scheme that had not been previously validated. Moreover, there were only 263 patients enrolled in the study, 5 of whom died and 9 of whom had recurrent syncope, which is an insufficient number of outcomes to robustly assess the prognostic accuracy of the risk-stratification scheme. Since publication of this trial, 5 different risk-stratification tools for ED patients with syncope have been published, including the San Francisco syncope rule,[39,40,51] the Boston Syncope Rule,[52] the syncope risk score,[53] the STePS (short-term prognosis of syncope) study,[54] and the ROSE study.[55,56] Although these studies successfully identified risk factors for short-term serious outcomes (**Table 3**), they are of limited methodological quality and prognostic accuracy[57] and have not been shown to increase diagnostic sensitivity or specificity or reduce health care costs when implemented in practice.[58] Additional research is needed to develop a robust, reliable risk score for ED patients with syncope to guide disposition and to facilitate clinical decision making. Current prospective studies are under

Table 1
Summary of relevant studies examining the efficacy of syncope units

Authors, Country	Study Design, Sample Size and Setting	Study Aim or Objectives	Main Findings
Ammirati et al,[49] 2008 Italy	Single-center observational cohort study (n = 102) Hospital-based syncope unit	To evaluate the clinical performance of a syncope unit to determine its impact on syncope management	A higher frequency of diagnosis (82% vs 75%) and an 85% reduction in hospital costs were observed in follow-up
Brignole et al,[50] 2010 Italy	Multicenter observational cohort study (n = 941) Hospital-based syncope unit	To document the organizational model of syncope units in Italy and their effectiveness in clinical practice	60% of referrals were from physicians in the outpatient setting or self-referred, 24% were from the ED, and 16% were hospitalized patients; 82% received a diagnosis during their syncope unit stay (21% were made during the initial evaluation, 61% within 45 d, and in 18% the diagnosis was undetermined
Kenny et al,[47] 2002 UK	Single-center observational cohort study using administrative data to compare health care delivery between the Royal Victory Infirmary hospital and 13 peer hospitals. Hospital-based syncope and falls facility		A shorter length of stay was observed for hospitalized patients (2.4 d vs 8.6 d), and fewer cases of syncope and falls were evaluated on an emergency basis (35% vs 97%)
Numeroso et al,[48] 2010 Italy	Single-center observational cohort study (n = 200) Hospital-based syncope ward	To evaluate the efficacy of a short-stay hospital-based syncope ward	There was a 79% discharge rate and a mean length of stay of 3.5 d for patients with syncope admitted to the ward, with 21% requiring transfer to another hospital service. The mean length of hospitalization among transfers was 6 d
Shen et al,[7] 2004 USA	Single-center randomized controlled trial (n = 103) EDOU	To determine whether an emergency department observation unit ("syncope unit") could affect diagnostic yield and the rate of hospital admission for patients with intermediate-risk syncope	Patients randomized to EDOU had a higher rate of syncope diagnosis (67% vs 10%, $P<.001$) and a lower rate of hospital admission (43% vs 98%, $P<.001$)

Abbreviation: EDOU, emergency department observation unit.

Table 2
Inclusion and exclusion criteria for syncope

High-Risk Group	Intermediate-Risk Group	Low-Risk Group
Chest pain compatible with acute coronary syndrome	Age ≥50 y	Age <50 y
Signs of congestive heart failure	Previous history of coronary artery disease, myocardial infarction, heart failure, cardiomyopathy without active symptoms or signs on cardiac medications	With no previous history of cardiovascular disease
Moderate/severe valvular disease	Bundle branch block or Q-wave without acute changes on ECG	Symptoms consistent with reflex-mediated or vasovagal syncope
History of ventricular arrhythmia	Family history of premature unexplained sudden death (<50 y)	Normal cardiovascular examination
ECG/cardiac monitor findings of ischemia	Symptoms not consistent with reflex-mediated or vasovagal cause	Normal ECG findings
Prolonged QTC (>500 ms)	Cardiac devices without evidence of dysfunction	
Trifasicular block or pauses between 2 and 3 s	Physician's judgement that a cardiac syncope is possible	
Third-degree atrioventricular block		
Persistent sinus bradycardia between 40 and 60 beats per minute atrial fibrillation or nonsustained ventricular tachycardia without symptoms		
Cardiac devices (pacemaker or defibrillator with dysfunction)		

Abbreviation: ECG, electrocardiogram.

Adapted from Smars PA, Decker WW, Shen WK. Syncope evaluation in the emergency department. Curr Opin Cardiol 2007;22:44–8; with permission.

way to develop such a score, both in Canada and the United States. As such scores are developed it will be important to carefully consider how they can be integrated into clinical pathways of care rather than developed solely to aid individual clinicians' decision making at the bedside. Such an approach has the potential to assist clinicians in determining which patients with syncope require hospital admission, which can be considered for evaluation in an EDOU or discharged for urgent follow-up in a syncope specialty clinic (in settings in which these models of care exist), and which can be safely discharged for routine follow-up with a primary care physician.

Additional areas for future research include designing and testing the impact of different models of health care delivery for patients with syncope, such as EDOUs, hospital-based syncope units, and the potential role of outpatient syncope specialty clinics. The evolving role of new diagnostics for syncope, such as serum markers (eg, N-terminal [NT]-pro-brain natriuretic peptide [BNP],[59] serum neuron-specific enolase[60]) and

the yield of specific diagnostic modalities in relation to the pretest probability for serious outcomes are also promising areas for further research.

ATRIAL FIBRILLATION

Atrial fibrillation is a common condition, affecting 6% of the population older than 65.[61] The prevalence is expected to double by 2020.[62] Atrial fibrillation is the most common arrhythmia treated in the ED and accounts for 1% of all ED visits[63,64]; 65% of ED visits result in hospital admission, costing $6.65 billion.[64,65] Atrial fibrillation accounts for one-third of all hospitalizations for cardiac rhythm disturbances, and the frequency of atrial fibrillation hospitalizations is increasing over time.[66,67]

Treatment of atrial fibrillation is aimed at controlling the symptoms that disrupt quality of life for the patient and reducing the chance of ischemic stroke, which, without anticoagulation, averages 5% per year or 2 to 7 times that of a matched population.[68–70] Atrial flutter is a similar condition that occurs less frequently but often coexists with atrial

Syncope unit in emergency department

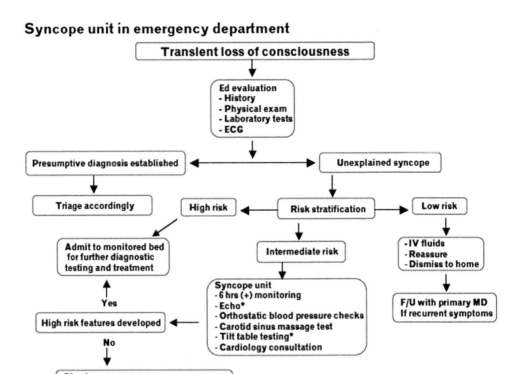

Fig. 3. Sample EDOU flow chart for syncope. * Obtained on a case by case basis as indicated through consultation with a cardiologist. (*Adapted from* Smars PA, Decker WW, Shen WK. Syncope evaluation in the emergency department. Curr Opin Cardiol 2007;22:44–8; with permission.)

Table 3
Risk factors for short-term outcomes in patients with syncope

Major risk factors (Should have urgent cardiac assessment)	
Abnormal ECG	Any bradyarrhythmia, tachyarrhythmia, or conduction disease
	New ischemic or old infarct
History of cardiac disease	Ischemic, arrhythmic, obstructive, valvular
Hypotension	Systolic blood pressure <90 mm Hg
Heart failure	Either past history or current state
Minor risk factors (could have urgent cardiac assessment)	
Age >60 y	
Dyspnea	
Anemia	Hematocrit <0.30
Hypertension	
Cerebrovascular disease	
Family history of early sudden death	Age <50 y
Specific situations	Syncope while supine, during exercise, or with no prodromal symptoms

We defined major risk factors as those independently derived in more than 1 study; minor risk factors were derived in only 1 study. Patients with syncope should have an urgent cardiac assessment in the presence of a single major risk factor, and consideration could be given to obtaining an urgent specialist assessment with 1 or more minor risk factors. Urgent cardiac assessment should take place within 2 weeks, as either an inpatient or outpatient.
Reproduced from Sheldon RS, Morillo CA, Krahn AD, et al. Standardized approaches to the investigation of syncope: Canadian Cardiovascular Society position paper. Can J Cardiol 2011;27:246–53; with permission.

fibrillation. Because of its similar pathophysiology, treatment goals, and anticoagulation recommendations, atrial flutter and atrial fibrillation are often grouped together when discussing approaches to management.[71,72]

Evidence to Support the Efficacy of Observation Unit Care

Because of the frequency of atrial fibrillation–related complaints in the ED and the associated costs of hospitalization, there is growing interest in the desire to manage patients initially in the ED setting and transition them to the outpatient setting, possibly after a stay in an EDOU. In particular, there is a growing body of literature regarding the management of recent-onset atrial fibrillation/atrial flutter (RAFF), defined as symptoms starting less than 48 hours before evaluation. Discussions focus on RAFF because of the lack of need for transesophageal echocardiography, along with the higher likelihood of patients responding to rhythm control during the first 48 hours of symptoms.[6]

Despite the frequency of RAFF visits to the ED, significant debate persists regarding the optimal management strategy.[71–74] Two competing strategies exist: rate control versus rhythm control. With the rate control strategy, the heart rate is controlled and need for anticoagulation is determined based on the patient's risk factor profile for stroke. With the rhythm control strategy, the patient is either pharmacologically or electrically cardioverted in the ED, with outpatient recommendations for anticoagulation as appropriate. Large national studies comparing the 2 treatment strategies observed little difference in outcomes, but most patients in these studies had permanent atrial fibrillation, with relatively few having RAFF.[75,76] Although the debate of rate versus rhythm control continues, the desire to manage patients without inpatient admission continues to evolve.

Even before EDOUs came on the scene, studies evaluating the safety and efficacy of managing stable patients with RAFF in the ED were conducted (**Table 4**). In 1999, Michael and colleagues[77] administered chemical and/or electrical cardioversion with subsequent discharge in hemodynamically stable patients with RAFF without other significant comorbidities and were able to discharge 97% of patients directly from the ED. Domanovits and colleagues[78] evaluated the efficacy of ibutilide, a Class III antiarrhythmic, for pharmacologic conversion in stable patients with RAFF. Eighty-five percent of patients were chemically cardioverted, and the remaining nonresponders were electrically cardioverted, with

92% of patients discharged from the ED. These authors concluded that cardioversion in the ED was safe and effective and could lead to reduced admissions.

Two additional studies assessed outcomes in patients who were electrically cardioverted in the ED. Burton and colleagues,[79] using primarily monophasic defibrillators, reported an 86% success rate of electrical cardioversion, with only 6% of patients returning to the ED with recurrent atrial fibrillation within 1 week. Two years later, Lo and colleagues,[80] using biphasic defibrillators, showed a 91% success rate of electrical cardioversion, with a 22% recurrence rate at 3 months. Both studies concluded that electrical cardioversion in the ED with subsequent discharge was successful for the vast majority of patients and could potentially avoid hospital admission.

Zimetbaum and colleagues[81] examined the safety and cost-effectiveness of an ED protocol designed to decrease hospital admissions. Their protocol recommended immediate inpatient management for atrial fibrillation patients with concomitant heart failure, hypotension, or myocardial ischemia, as well as for those who were not anticoagulated and had a history of stroke or transient ischemic attack, rheumatic disease, or congestive heart failure. Otherwise, they encouraged oral rate-controlling medications, standard criteria for ED cardioversion, and specialty clinic follow-up within 48 hours. These investigators observed a lower rate of hospital admission after implementation of the protocol, with similar rates of 30-day return visits, readmission, and adverse events with the new protocol compared with standard management. They also reported an average cost savings of approximately $1400 per patient.

These studies suggested that ED management without admission might be safe and efficient and led to a desire to explore using the EDOU for short-term management of RAFF. Two articles from William Beaumont Hospital examined the feasibility of an EDOU management plan for stable RAFF and the integration of this EDOU management plan into a hospital-wide care plan.[82,83] To be eligible for observation in the EDOU, patients had to be symptomatic for less than 48 hours, have a ventricular rate less than 110 before transfer to the EDOU, and could not be receiving ongoing medication infusions for rate control. The EDOU was presented as an option to providers with suggestions about possible treatment options while there, but management decisions were left to the discretion of the providers. They concluded that EDOU management was safe and effective for avoiding inpatient admission in certain patients.

Table 4
Summary of relevant literature examining EDOU use for atrial fibrillation

Authors, Country	Study Design, Sample Size and Setting	Study Aim or Objectives	Main Findings
Michael et al,[77] 1999 Canada	Single-center observational cohort study (n = 289) Emergency Department	To evaluate the safety and efficacy of ED chemical and/or electrical cardioversion with subsequent discharge	62% of patients had chemical cardioversion (50% success rate), 28% had electrical cardioversion (89% success rate); overall, 6% complication rate with 97% discharge rate
Domanovits et al,[78] 2000 Austria	Single-center observational cohort study (n = 51) Emergency Department	To evaluate safety and efficacy of ibutilide for conversion of RAFF, with electrical cardioversion for nonresponders, in the ED	38/51 patients converted with ibutilide; remaining 13/51 patients were electrically cardioverted; 100% of patients successfully converted, and 92% were discharged from ED with median stay of 9 h
Koenig et al,[83] 2002 USA	Single-center observational cohort study (n = 67) EDOU	To evaluate the feasibility of an EDOU protocol for RAFF management	82% of EDOU patients converted to sinus rhythm; 5 (7%) EDOU patients were admitted for positive diagnostic test results and further care; 81% of EDOU patients were discharged (mean stay 11.8 h); 3 discharged EDOU patients returned within 1 wk; no major complications attributed to EDOU management
Zimetbaum et al,[81] 2003 USA	Single-center observational cohort study (n = 446) Emergency Department	To evaluate a RAFF protocol focused on ED cardioversion and expedited outpatient referral, examining cost-effectiveness and 30-d adverse events	Protocol management led to decreased hospitalizations (38%, down from 74%), no difference in 30-day ED return visits or hospital readmissions, and an estimated $1400/patient lower 30-day total direct health care costs, when compared with pre-intervention group
Burton et al,[79] 2004 USA	Single-center observational cohort study (n = 388) Emergency Department	To evaluate efficacy, outcomes, and complications of ED electrical cardioversion	ED electrical cardioversion was successful in 332 (86%) patients; 28 complications (22 owing to sedation, and 6 owing to cardioversion) were noted; 86% of patients were discharged from the ED, with 6% of successfully cardioverted patients returning within 7 days because of relapse

Zahir and Lheureux,[85] 2005 Belgium	Single-center observational cohort study (n = 67) Emergency Department	To identify factors that correlate with early conversion and to identify patients that may be ideal for EDOU care	Factors associated with early conversion including patients <65 y, symptoms <48 h, and no signs of heart failure
Deasy et al,[84] 2006 Ireland	Single-center observational cohort study (n = 111) Emergency Department	To retrospectively apply the criteria used by Koenig et al to evaluate potential candidates for EDOU management	Of the retrospective cohort examined, 8% of RAFF patients would likely have been eligible to be managed in an EDOU setting
Lo et al,[80] 2006 Australia	Single-center observational cohort study (n = 34) Emergency Department	To evaluate efficacy and outcomes of biphasic electrical cardioversion in the ED	Biphasic electrical cardioversion was successful in 31 (91%) of attempts. There were 3 complications, all related to sedation; 31 (97%) of patients were satisfied on telephone follow-up, and 7 (22%) of patients had recurrence at 3 mo.
Decker et al,[6] 2008 USA	Single-center prospective randomized controlled study (n = 154) EDOU	To evaluate feasibility and efficacy of EDOU protocol (initial rate control followed by electrical cardioversion after 6 h) vs routine inpatient care for RAFF	85% of EDOU patients, compared with 73% of inpatients, converted ($P = .06$), with median stay of 10.1 vs 25.2 h ($P<.001$); 9 EDOU patients required subsequent admission. During the following 6 mo, 11% of EDOU patients and 10% of inpatients had recurrence ($p=0.93$), with similar hospitalization and adverse events
Cristoni et al,[87] 2011 Italy	Single-center observational cohort study (n = 322) EDOU	To compare EDOU electrical vs pharmacologic cardioversion strategies for RAFF patients	159/171 (93%) of electrical cardioversion patients were discharged, compared with 77/151 (51%) of pharmacologic cardioversion patients ($P<.001$), with similar lengths of stay, admission rates, and short term complications

Abbreviations: EDOU, emergency department observation unit; RAFF, recent-onset atrial fibrillation and flutter.

A similar study was conducted in Ireland.[84] This retrospective study applied the same criteria used by Koenig and colleagues[83] to their practice setting. They estimated that 8% of their patients had stable RAFF, were in atrial fibrillation after initial ED management, and yet were admitted to the hospital as part of their standard management. They hypothesized that this group of patients would be ideal for EDOU management, potentially avoiding hospital admissions.

To further identify patients appropriate for EDOU admission, Zahir and Lheureux[85] retrospectively analyzed all patients with atrial fibrillation presenting to the ED at their hospital in Belgium to examine predictors of early conversion to sinus rhythm. These investigators found that age younger than 65 years, symptoms for less than 48 hours, and absence of signs of heart failure were associated with early conversion to sinus rhythm. They proposed that these criteria might be used to identify patients for EDOU evaluation.

In 2009, Decker and colleagues[6] published a study in which patients were randomized to EDOU care or routine inpatient care for RAFF. They noted a trend to increased conversion to sinus rhythm, a significantly shorter length of stay, and equivalent 6-month recurrence rates for EDOU patients compared with inpatients. A sample patient management flow chart summarizing the EDOU protocol used in this study is included in **Fig. 4**.[86]

Despite data to suggest the safety and efficiency of cardioversion for RAFF and the potential to avoid inpatient admissions, there is limited work regarding optimal protocols for EDOU management. To evaluate how providers are currently managing RAFF, Stiell and colleagues[71] surveyed several hospitals in Canada, where inpatient admission occurs less frequently than in the United States. Investigators identified wide variation in the management of these patients. Treatment options included rhythm control using electrical or pharmacologic cardioversion, and rate control, with the choice of medications varying widely. These investigators note, however, that 83% of the patients managed at these Canadian centers were dismissed without hospital admission and felt that avoiding hospital admission was reasonable despite the variation in management strategies during the patient's time in the ED.

To better understand the safety and efficacy of different EDOU treatment strategies, a recent study from Italy compared an electrical cardioversion strategy at one affiliated hospital with a pharmacologic cardioversion strategy at another.[87] These investigators found that, compared with pharmacologic cardioversion, patients undergoing electrical cardioversion were discharged in sinus rhythm more often and admitted to the hospital less frequently. Both groups had similar ED lengths of stay and rates of short-term complications.

Despite the growing body of literature discussing EDOU management of RAFF, adoption into national guidelines has been slow. Neither the 2006 ACC/AHA/European Society of Cardiology Guidelines for the Management of Patients with Atrial Fibrillation nor their 2010 and 2011 updates discuss EDOU management.[72,74,88] The 2010 Canadian Cardiovascular Society Atrial Fibrillation Guidelines, however, have a dedicated section on ED management of RAFF.[89] The recommendations are that, for hemodynamically stable patients with RAFF, rate-slowing agents are acceptable and cardioversion may be used in the ED. They recommend hospital admission only for highly symptomatic patients with heart failure, myocardial ischemia, or in whom adequate rate control cannot be achieved.

Future Directions

Although ED and EDOU management protocols have been discussed in the literature, they lack rigorous design and implementation.[6,71,81,82] There is also a dearth of evidence on rate control versus rhythm control in patients with RAFF and limited data to guide decisions about medication or cardioversion choice. This may explain the relative lack of implementation of ED management strategies into national guideline recommendations. Risk stratification data are limited as well. Near-term adverse events for patients who present with RAFF are poorly described in the literature. Most ED studies have little or no follow-up data on patients once they are discharged from the ED.

Finally, only one cost analysis has been performed on management of RAFF, and this is now more than 10 years old.[81] Future robust, large-scale studies with high-fidelity follow-up have potential to improve risk stratification for patients with RAFF and to lead to increased acceptance and generalizability of RAFF management on an international scale.

ACUTE HEART FAILURE SYNDROME

Heart failure (HF) poses a significant health burden on Americans with a prevalence of 5.7 million adults and nearly 1 in 100 adults older than 65 years receiving a new diagnosis each year.[90] HF is the most common diagnosis-related group for Medicare patient hospitalizations and, in total, the most expensive.[91] Hospitalizations for HF have

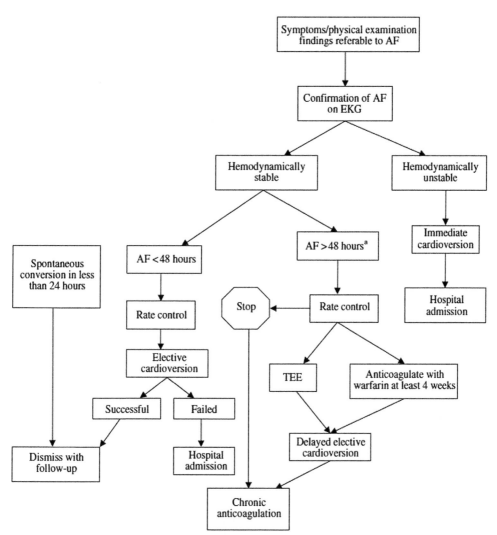

Fig. 4. Sample EDOU flow chart with inclusion and exclusion criteria for atrial fibrillation. [a] AF of greater than 48 hours often requires hospital admission in most settings to initiate rate control and anticoagulation. TEE, transesophageal echocardiogram. (*Adapted from* Raghavan AV, Decker WW, Meloy TD. Management of atrial fibrillation in the emergency department. Emerg Med Clin North Am 2005;23:1127–39; with permission.)

tripled over 3 decades and will likely continue to increase because of the aging of the population, improved survival from myocardial infarction, and better prevention of sudden cardiac death.[92,93] In 2009 there were 668,000 ED visits for heart failure, where emergent visits for symptomatic heart failure are termed acute decompensated heart failure (ADHF).[90] The vast majority of patients presenting to an ED with ADHF are admitted, with 80% of heart failure hospitalizations originating from the ED.[94]

Evidence to Support the Efficacy of Observation Unit Care

Because of the ADHF population's high prevalence and cost of management, there is growing interest in the ED management and disposition of these patients. Because nearly all patients with ADHF are admitted, studies have assessed the feasibility and safety of initial management in an EDOU as an alternative to hospital admission **Table 5**.

Initial work focused on the feasibility of initiating protocolized care for ADHF in an EDOU setting. Because the focus of initial care for the hemodynamically stable ADHF patient focuses on diagnostics and diuresis, multidisciplinary protocols were developed to guide immediate and efficient initiation of care. Peacock and colleagues[95,96] developed a comprehensive EDOU management protocol for stable patients with ADHF that included the following: cardiac monitoring, strict input and output measurement, weight measurement,

Table 5
Summary of relevant original research studies examining EDOU use for acute decompensated heart failure

Authors, Country	Study Design, Sample Size and Setting	Study Aim or Objectives	Main Findings
Peacock and Albert,[95] 1999 USA	Single-center observational cohort study (n = not reported) EDOU	To evaluate whether treatment protocol started in EDOU setting led to decreased admission rates, inpatient length of stay, and costs	EDOU protocol led to 9% fewer hospital admissions (p=0.008), 40% shorter median hospital stay if hospitalized from EDOU ($P = .15$), and $37,217 per patient costs savings over 5 mo
Peacock et al,[96] 2002 USA	Single-center observational cohort study (n = 154) EDOU	To evaluate ADHF patient outcomes before and after EDOU protocol implementation	90 d after EDOU management, patients had 56% fewer return visits ($P<.0001$), 64% fewer rehospitalizations ($P = .007$), death rate declined from 4% to 1% ($P = .096$), and HF readmission declined from 18% to 11% ($P = .099$)
Storrow et al,[97] 2005 USA	Single-center observational cohort study (n = 64) EDOU	To evaluate outcomes of patients with ADHF, using risk-matched patients in EDOU vs directly admitted to hospital	EDOU patients had no difference in outcomes, shorter total length of stay (26 vs 59 h, $P<.001$), and less total cost of care $4203 vs $7824, $P = .001$) compared with directly admitted patients
Diercks et al,[98] 2006 USA	Single-center observational cohort study (n = 499) Emergency Department	To evaluate all patients with ADHF to identify predictors of those with hospital stay <24 h and no serious adverse events within 30 d	27% of patients with ADHF stayed <24 h with no 30 d adverse events; independent predictors were SBP>160 (OR 1.8, 95% CI 1.15–2.7) and normal troponin I (OR 14.7, 95% CI 1.9–105)
Collins et al,[100] 2009 USA	Cost-effective modeling study (n = 3 scenarios) No clinical setting	To use a decision analytic model to evaluate cost-effectiveness of different ADHF management strategies	If postdischarge readmission rates exceed 36% within 5 d and 74% within 30 d of ED discharge, EDOU becomes less costly and more effective than ED discharge. Similarly, as postdischarge event rates increase in those discharged from EDOU, hospital admission becomes more effective

(continued on next page)

Table 5
(continued)

Authors, Country	Study Design, Sample Size and Setting	Study Aim or Objectives	Main Findings
Collins et al,[100] 2009 USA	Retrospective validation of Society of Chest Pain Center's risk stratification (n = 201) Emergency Department	To validate the Society of Chest Pain Center's risk stratification recommendations against prior HEARD-IT trial ADHF registry	Patients meeting Society of Chest Pain Center EDOU inclusion criteria had only 25 (12.4%) 30 d events, including 1 (0.5%) death, validating this risk stratification

Abbreviations: ADHF, acute decompensated heart failure; CI, confidence interval; EDOU, emergency department observation unit; OR, odds ratio; SBP, systolic blood pressure.

angiotensin-converting enzyme inhibitor and furosemide dosing recommendations, echocardiogram testing if not done within the past year, cardiac biomarker testing, a 15-minute patient education video, heart failure specialist consultation, and social work, home health care, and dietary consultations as needed. They noted that initiating EDOU-protocolized management led to decreased hospital admission rates, hospital length of stay, costs, and 90-day ED return visits and rehospitalizations. Similarly, Storrow and colleagues[97] found decreased inpatient bed hours and fewer total charges, with similar safety outcomes, in risk-matched patients with ADHF who were initially managed in the EDOU as compared with those who were admitted.

Further studies developed approaches to risk stratification, attempting to identify a cohort of patients ideal for EDOU management rather than hospital admission. This has been a challenge because most risk stratification research for ADHF has focused on high-risk features. As EDOU management has emerged as an alternative to hospital admission, interest has grown in defining low-risk criteria, or criteria that are correlated with relatively short lengths of stay in the hospital. Diercks and colleagues[98] looked at several hundred patients with ADHF who were managed in a large academic hospital and examined the length of stay for all patients. They analyzed clinical variables in patients who were discharged within 24 hours and compared these with patients with longer durations of hospitalization in an effort to identify patients appropriate for EDOU care. Their analysis suggested that normal troponin testing combined with elevated initial blood pressures might identify a cohort of patients with shorter hospital length of stay, suggesting that this population may be good candidates for EDOU management.

As evidence mounted for the use of EDOUs for patients with ADHF, national societies began

---

Box 1
Criteria to identify patients with ADHF for observation stay

Recommended

- Stable hemodynamic and respiratory status
- Systolic blood pressure (SBP) ≥100 mm Hg on presentation
- Blood urea nitrogen <40 mg/dL
- Creatinine <3.0 mg/dL
- Absence of ischemic ECG changes and/or elevated cardiac troponin levels
- Preexisting heart failure
- No intravenous vasoactive infusions being actively titrated
- No significant comorbidities requiring acute interventions
- Respiratory rate <32 breaths/min and not requiring noninvasive ventilation at the time of OU entry
- No signs of poor perfusion
- At least partial response to initial therapy with increased urine output and/or improvement in vital signs

Consider

- SBP >120 mm Hg
- Adequate social support
- Adequate follow-up
- BNP <1000 pg/mL or NT-BNP <5000 pg/mL

From Heart Failure Executive Committee, Peacock WF, Fonarow GC, et al. Society of chest pain centers recommendations for the evaluation and management of the observation stay acute heart failure patient: a report from the society of chest pain centers acute heart failure committee. Crit Pathw Cardiol 2008;7:83–6; with permission.

acknowledging this as a reasonable treatment strategy. In 2008, the Society of Chest Pain Centers created a document outlining recommendations for EDOU management of ADHF.[99] The aim of this publication was to discuss patients who may be best served by initial management in an EDOU. This document expanded on the risk stratification discussion, performing a systematic review of all high-risk features for ADHF. The investigators acknowledge that a lack of high-risk criteria for near-term adverse events does not reliably identify a low-risk patient; however, they developed inclusion criteria for those who may be suitable for EDOU care, excluding patients with high-risk features. The suggested inclusion criteria are shown in **Box 1** and patient management recommendations for EDOU care are noted in **Fig. 5**.[99]

To further evaluate these selection criteria Collins and colleagues[100] applied them to an existing ADHF patient registry. These investigators identified 201 patients who met these criteria in their database. Of these, only 1 (0.5%) had near-term death attributed to ADHF. The investigators concluded that the selection criteria proposed by the Society of Chest Pain Centers accurately predict an ADHF population that may be at low risk for near-term mortality and potentially suitable for EDOU management.

A 2010 Scientific Statement on ED disposition of patients with ADHF from the AHA also supports EDOU care.[101] Although this document acknowledges the limited ability to define low-risk patients and the challenge of appropriate disposition of patients with ADHF from the ED, it offers support

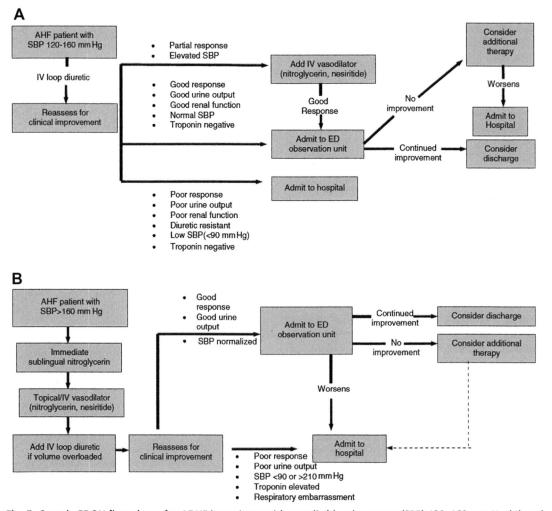

Fig. 5. Sample EDOU flow charts for ADHF in patients with systolic blood pressure (SBP) 120–160 mm Hg (*A*) and in patients with SBP >160 mm Hg (*B*) at presentation. (*From* Heart Failure Executive Committee, Peacock WF, Fonarow GC, et al. Society of chest pain centers recommendations for the evaluation and management of the observation stay acute heart failure patient: a report from the society of chest pain centers acute heart failure committee. Crit Pathw Cardiol 2008;7:83–6; with permission.)

for EDOU use, noting that "because most patients with ADHF are admitted for decongestion as a result of worsening chronic HF, a brief period of management in the ED or an ED-based observation unit may be a reasonable alternative to hospitalization in those patients without high-risk features. Such approaches have proved feasible and have been shown to conserve hospital resources."

Future Directions

The ultimate goal of EDOUs for ADHF management is rapid stabilization, early initiation of treatment, patient education, and successful transition to the outpatient setting with low near-term adverse events or recidivism. To successfully create EDOU programs that can achieve these goals routinely and efficiently, additional research is needed. Goals should include prospective multicenter trials examining the optimal patient selection and protocol design. Repeatedly, literature on the topic emphasizes that the lack of high-risk features does not define a low-risk patient. What patients can be dismissed immediately from the ED with outpatient follow-up? What patients require a short stay in an EDOU, versus those who require full inpatient management? Also, what are the optimum treatment and patient education protocols that lead to successful transition to the outpatient setting with low near-term adverse events? As additional data addressing these questions accumulate, it is likely that increasing numbers of patients with ADHF will be managed in EDOUs.

SUMMARY

Because of the rising volume of ED visits, hospital overcrowding, and greater attention to the cost-effectiveness of health care, observation unit care has become an attractive alternative to inpatient admission. There are varying levels of evidence and growing interest in managing patients with chest pain potentially caused by ACS, syncope, atrial fibrillation, and ADHF at low to intermediate short-term risk for adverse outcomes in an EDOU setting. Evidence-based protocols and collaborative approaches to care have potential to achieve similar clinical and improved economic outcomes compared with hospital admission. The potential for the EDOU to provide the right care for the right patient at the right time is only beginning to be realized, with significant advances in health care delivery anticipated in the near future.

ACKNOWLEDGMENTS

The authors give special thanks to Sue L. Kirk for her administrative assistance in preparing this article and Dr Allan S. Jaffe for reviewing the article and providing meaningful intellectual contribution to increase the quality of the work.

REFERENCES

1. Baugh CW, Venkatesh AK, Bohan JS. Emergency department observation units: a clinical and financial benefit for hospitals. Health Care Manage Rev 2011;36:28–37.
2. Niska R, Bhuiya F, Xu J. National hospital ambulatory medical care survey: 2007 emergency department summary. Natl Health Stat Report 2010;(26):1–31.
3. Venkatesh AK, Geisler BP, Gibson Chambers JJ, et al. Use of observation care in US emergency departments, 2001 to 2008. PLoS One 2011;6:e24326.
4. Wiler JL, Ross MA, Ginde AA. National study of emergency department observation services. Acad Emerg Med 2011;18:959–65.
5. Roberts RR, Zalenski RJ, Mensah EK, et al. Costs of an emergency department-based accelerated diagnostic protocol vs hospitalization in patients with chest pain: a randomized controlled trial. JAMA 1997;278:1670–6.
6. Decker WW, Smars PA, Vaidyanathan L, et al. A prospective, randomized trial of an emergency department observation unit for acute onset atrial fibrillation. Ann Emerg Med 2008;52:322–8.
7. Shen WK, Decker WW, Smars PA, et al. Syncope evaluation in the emergency department study (SEEDS): a multidisciplinary approach to syncope management. Circulation 2004;110:3636–45.
8. Goodacre S, Nicholl J, Dixon S, et al. Randomised controlled trial and economic evaluation of a chest pain observation unit compared with routine care. BMJ 2004;328:254.
9. Amsterdam EA, Kirk JD, Bluemke DA, et al, American Heart Association Exercise, Cardiac Rehabilitation, and Prevention Committee of the Council on Clinical Cardiology, Council on Cardiovascular Nursing, and Interdisciplinary Council on Quality of Care and Outcomes Research. Testing of low-risk patients presenting to the emergency department with chest pain. Circulation 2010;122:1756–76.
10. Fraker TD Jr, Fihn SD, Chronic Stable Angina Writing Committee. 2007 chronic angina focused update of the ACC/AHA 2002 guidelines for the management of patients with chronic stable angina: a report of the American College of Cardiology/American Heart Association task force on practice guidelines writing group to develop the focused update of the 2002 guidelines for the management of patients with chronic stable angina. J Am Coll Cardiol 2007;50:2264–74.

11. Farkouh ME, Smars PA, Reeder GS, et al. A clinical trial of a chest-pain observation unit for patients with unstable angina. Chest pain evaluation in the emergency room (CHEER) investigators. N Engl J Med 1998;339:1882–8.

12. Gomez MA, Anderson JL, Karagounis LA, et al. An emergency department-based protocol for rapidly ruling out myocardial ischemia reduces hospital time and expense: results of a randomized study (ROMIO). J Am Coll Cardiol 1996;28:25–33.

13. Goodacre S, Cross E, Lewis C, et al. Effectiveness and safety of chest pain assessment to prevent emergency admissions: escape cluster randomised trial. BMJ 2007;335:659.

14. Clancy M. Effectiveness of chest pain units. BMJ 2007;335:623–4.

15. Polanczyk CA, Johnson PA, Hartley LH, et al. Clinical correlates and prognostic significance of early negative exercise tolerance test in patients with acute chest pain seen in the hospital emergency department. Am J Cardiol 1998;81:288–92.

16. Gibler WB, Runyon JP, Levy RC, et al. A rapid diagnostic and treatment center for patients with chest pain in the emergency department. Ann Emerg Med 1995;25:1–8.

17. Zalenski RJ, McCarren M, Roberts R, et al. An evaluation of a chest pain diagnostic protocol to exclude acute cardiac ischemia in the emergency department. Arch Intern Med 1997;157:1085–91.

18. Kirk JD, Turnipseed S, Lewis WR, et al. Evaluation of chest pain in low-risk patients presenting to the emergency department: the role of immediate exercise testing. Ann Emerg Med 1998;32:1–7.

19. Diercks DB, Gibler WB, Liu T, et al. Identification of patients at risk by graded exercise testing in an emergency department chest pain center. Am J Cardiol 2000;86:289–92.

20. Ramakrishna G, Milavetz JJ, Zinsmeister AR, et al. Effect of exercise treadmill testing and stress imaging on the triage of patients with chest pain: CHEER substudy. Mayo Clin Proc 2005;80:322–9.

21. Amsterdam EA, Kirk JD, Diercks DB, et al. Immediate exercise testing to evaluate low-risk patients presenting to the emergency department with chest pain. J Am Coll Cardiol 2002;40:251–6.

22. Khare RK, Powell ES, Venkatesh AK, et al. Diagnostic uncertainty and costs associated with current emergency department evaluation of low risk chest pain. Crit Pathw Cardiol 2008;7:191–6.

23. Patel MR, Peterson ED, Dai D, et al. Low diagnostic yield of elective coronary angiography. N Engl J Med 2010;362:886–95.

24. Hermann LK, Weingart SD, Duvall WL, et al. The limited utility of routine cardiac stress testing in emergency department chest pain patients younger than 40 years. Ann Emerg Med 2009;54:12–6.

25. Dawson M, Youngquist S, Bledsoe J, et al. Low-risk young adult patients with chest pain may not benefit from routine cardiac stress testing: a Bayesian analysis. Crit Pathw Cardiol 2010;9:170–3.

26. Hess EP, Brison RJ, Perry JJ, et al. Development of a clinical prediction rule for 30-day cardiac events in emergency department patients with chest pain and possible acute coronary syndrome. Ann Emerg Med 2012;59(2):115–125.e1.

27. Marsan RJ Jr, Shaver KJ, Sease KL, et al. Evaluation of a clinical decision rule for young adult patients with chest pain. Acad Emerg Med 2005;12:26–31.

28. Collin MJ, Weisenthal B, Walsh KM, et al. Young patients with chest pain: 1-year outcomes. Am J Emerg Med 2011;29:265–70.

29. Madsen T, Mallin M, Bledsoe J, et al. Utility of the emergency department observation unit in ensuring stress testing in low-risk chest pain patients. Crit Pathw Cardiol 2009;8:122–4.

30. Milano P, Carden DL, Jackman KM, et al. Compliance with outpatient stress testing in low-risk patients presenting to the emergency department with chest pain. Crit Pathw Cardiol 2011;10:35–40.

31. Meyer MC, Mooney RP, Sekera AK. A critical pathway for patients with acute chest pain and low risk for short-term adverse cardiac events: role of outpatient stress testing. Ann Emerg Med 2006;47(435):e431–3.

32. Richards D, Meshkat N, Chu J, et al. Emergency department patient compliance with follow-up for outpatient exercise stress testing: a randomized controlled trial. CJEM 2007;9:435–40.

33. Body R, Carley S, McDowell G, et al. Rapid exclusion of acute myocardial infarction in patients with undetectable troponin using a high-sensitivity assay. J Am Coll Cardiol 2011;58:1332–9.

34. Jaffe AS. The 10 commandments of troponin, with special reference to high sensitivity assays. Heart 2011;97:940–6.

35. Hollander JE, Chang AM, Shofer FS, et al. Coronary computed tomographic angiography for rapid discharge of low-risk patients with potential acute coronary syndromes. Ann Emerg Med 2009;53:295–304.

36. Miller CD, Hwang W, Hoekstra JW, et al. Stress cardiac magnetic resonance imaging with observation unit care reduces cost for patients with emergent chest pain: a randomized trial. Ann Emerg Med 2010;56:209–19.e202.

37. Moya A, Sutton R, Ammirati F, et al. Guidelines for the diagnosis and management of syncope (version 2009). Eur Heart J 2009;30:2631–71.

38. Huff JS, Decker WW, Quinn JV, et al. Clinical policy: critical issues in the evaluation and management of adult patients presenting to the emergency department with syncope. Ann Emerg Med 2007;49:431–44.

39. Quinn JV, Stiell IG, McDermott DA, et al. Derivation of the San Francisco syncope rule to predict patients with short-term serious outcomes. Ann Emerg Med 2004;43:224–32.

40. Quinn J, McDermott D, Stiell I, et al. Prospective validation of the San Francisco syncope rule to predict patients with serious outcomes. Ann Emerg Med 2006;47:448–54.

41. Olde Nordkamp LR, van Dijk N, Ganzeboom KS, et al. Syncope prevalence in the ED compared to general practice and population: a strong selection process. Am J Emerg Med 2009;27:271–9.

42. Birnbaum A, Esses D, Bijur P, et al. Failure to validate the San Francisco syncope rule in an independent emergency department population. Ann Emerg Med 2008;52:151–9.

43. Sun BC, Emond JA, Camargo CA Jr. Direct medical costs of syncope-related hospitalizations in the United States. Am J Cardiol 2005;95:668–71.

44. Linzer M, Yang EH, Estes NA 3rd, et al. Diagnosing syncope. Part 1: value of history, physical examination, and electrocardiography. Clinical efficacy assessment project of the American College of Physicians. Ann Intern Med 1997;126:989–96.

45. Linzer M, Yang EH, Estes NA 3rd, et al. Diagnosing syncope. Part 2: unexplained syncope. Clinical efficacy assessment project of the American College of Physicians. Ann Intern Med 1997;127:76–86.

46. American College of Emergency Physicians. Clinical policy: critical issues in the evaluation and management of patients presenting with syncope. Ann Emerg Med 2001;37:771–6.

47. Kenny RA, O'Shea D, Walker HF. Impact of a dedicated syncope and falls facility for older adults on emergency beds. Age Ageing 2002;31:272–5.

48. Numeroso F, Mossini G, Spaggiari E, et al. Syncope in the emergency department of a large northern Italian hospital: incidence, efficacy of a short-stay observation ward and validation of the OESIL risk score. Emerg Med J 2010;27: 653–8.

49. Ammirati F, Colaceci R, Cesario A, et al. Management of syncope: clinical and economic impact of a syncope unit. Europace 2008;10:471–6.

50. Brignole M, Ungar A, Casagranda I, et al. Prospective multicentre systematic guideline-based management of patients referred to the syncope units of general hospitals. Europace 2010;12:109–18.

51. Thiruganasambandamoorthy V, Hess EP, Alreesi A, et al. External validation of the San Francisco syncope rule in the Canadian setting. Ann Emerg Med 2010;55:464–72.

52. Grossman SA, Fischer C, Lipsitz LA, et al. Predicting adverse outcomes in syncope. J Emerg Med 2007;33:233–9.

53. Sun BC, Derose SF, Liang LJ, et al. Predictors of 30-day serious events in older patients with syncope. Ann Emerg Med 2009;54:769–78, e761–765.

54. Costantino G, Perego F, Dipaola F, et al. Short- and long-term prognosis of syncope, risk factors, and role of hospital admission: results from the steps (short-term prognosis of syncope) study. J Am Coll Cardiol 2008;51:276–83.

55. Reed MJ, Newby DE, Coull AJ, et al. The risk stratification of syncope in the emergency department (ROSE) pilot study: a comparison of existing syncope guidelines. Emerg Med J 2007;24:270–5.

56. Reed MJ, Newby DE, Coull AJ, et al. The ROSE (risk stratification of syncope in the emergency department) study. J Am Coll Cardiol 2010;55: 713–21.

57. Serrano LA, Hess EP, Bellolio MF, et al. Accuracy and quality of clinical decision rules for syncope in the emergency department: a systematic review and meta-analysis. Ann Emerg Med 2010;56:362–73. e361.

58. Sheldon RS, Morillo CA, Krahn AD, et al. Standardized approaches to the investigation of syncope: Canadian cardiovascular society position paper. Can J Cardiol 2011;27:246–53.

59. Pfister R, Diedrichs H, Larbig R, et al. NTt-pro-BNP for differential diagnosis in patients with syncope. Int J Cardiol 2009;133:51–4.

60. Lee SY, Choi YC, Kim JH, et al. Serum neuron-specific enolase level as a biomarker in differential diagnosis of seizure and syncope. J Neurol 2010; 257:1708–12.

61. Lakshminarayan K, Solid CA, Collins AJ, et al. Atrial fibrillation and stroke in the general Medicare population: a 10-year perspective (1992 to 2002). Stroke 2006;37:1969–74.

62. Go AS, Hylek EM, Phillips KA, et al. Prevalence of diagnosed atrial fibrillation in adults: national implications for rhythm management and stroke prevention: the anticoagulation and risk factors in atrial fibrillation (ATRIA) study. JAMA 2001;285:2370–5.

63. Li H, Easley A, Barrington W, et al. Evaluation and management of atrial fibrillation in the emergency department. Emerg Med Clin North Am 1998;16: 389–403.

64. McDonald AJ, Pelletier AJ, Ellinor PT, et al. Increasing US emergency department visit rates and subsequent hospital admissions for atrial fibrillation from 1993 to 2004. Ann Emerg Med 2008;51: 58–65.

65. Coyne KS, Paramore C, Grandy S, et al. Assessing the direct costs of treating nonvalvular atrial fibrillation in the united states. Value Health 2006;9:348–56.

66. Friberg J, Buch P, Scharling H, et al. Rising rates of hospital admissions for atrial fibrillation. Epidemiology 2003;14:666–72.

67. Wattigney WA, Mensah GA, Croft JB. Increasing trends in hospitalization for atrial fibrillation in the

United States, 1985 through 1999: implications for primary prevention. Circulation 2003;108:711–6.

68. Flegel KM, Shipley MJ, Rose G. Risk of stroke in non-rheumatic atrial fibrillation. Lancet 1987;1:526–9.

69. Wolf PA, Abbott RD, Kannel WB. Atrial fibrillation as an independent risk factor for stroke: the Framingham study. Stroke 1991;22:983–8.

70. Krahn AD, Manfreda J, Tate RB, et al. The natural history of atrial fibrillation: incidence, risk factors, and prognosis in the Manitoba follow-up study. Am J Med 1995;98:476–84.

71. Stiell IG, Clement CM, Brison RJ, et al. Variation in management of recent-onset atrial fibrillation and flutter among academic hospital emergency departments. Ann Emerg Med 2011;57(1):13–21.

72. European Heart Rhythm Association, European Association for Cardio-Thoracic Surgery, Camm AJ, et al. Guidelines for the management of atrial fibrillation: the task force for the management of atrial fibrillation of the European Society of Cardiology (ESC). Eur Heart J 2010;31:2369–429.

73. Hiatt WR. Acute pharmacological conversion of atrial fibrillation to sinus rhythm: is short-term symptomatic therapy worth it? A report from the December 2007 meeting of the cardiovascular and renal drugs advisory committee of the Food and Drug Administration. Circulation 2008;117:2956–7.

74. Fuster V, Rydén LE, Cannom DS, et al, American College of Cardiology/American Heart Association Task Force on Practice Guidelines, European Society of Cardiology Committee for Practice Guidelines, European Heart Rhythm Association, Heart Rhythm Society. ACC/AHA/ESC 2006 guidelines for the management of patients with atrial fibrillation: a report of the American College of Cardiology/American Heart Association task force on practice guidelines and the European Society of Cardiology Committee for Practice Guidelines (writing committee to revise the 2001 guidelines for the management of patients with atrial fibrillation): developed in collaboration with the European Heart Rhythm Association and the Heart Rhythm Society. Circulation 2006;114:e257–354.

75. Wyse DG, Waldo AL, DiMarco JP, et al, Atrial Fibrillation Follow-up Investigation of Rhythm Management (AFFIRM) Investigators. A comparison of rate control and rhythm control in patients with atrial fibrillation. N Engl J Med 2002;347:1825–33.

76. Roy D, Talajic M, Nattel S, et al, Atrial Fibrillation and Congestive Heart Failure Investigators. Rhythm control versus rate control for atrial fibrillation and heart failure. N Engl J Med 2008;358:2667–77.

77. Michael JA, Stiell IG, Agarwal S, et al. Cardioversion of paroxysmal atrial fibrillation in the emergency department. Ann Emerg Med 1999;33:379–87.

78. Domanovits H, Schillinger M, Thoennissen J, et al. Termination of recent-onset atrial fibrillation/flutter in the emergency department: a sequential approach with intravenous ibutilide and external electrical cardioversion. Resuscitation 2000;45:181–7.

79. Burton JH, Vinson DR, Drummond K, et al. Electrical cardioversion of emergency department patients with atrial fibrillation. Ann Emerg Med 2004;44:20–30.

80. Lo GK, Fatovich DM, Haig AD. Biphasic cardioversion of acute atrial fibrillation in the emergency department. Emerg Med J 2006;23:51–3.

81. Zimetbaum P, Reynolds MR, Ho KK, et al. Impact of a practice guideline for patients with atrial fibrillation on medical resource utilization and costs. Am J Cardiol 2003;92:677–81.

82. Ross MA, Davis B, Dresselhouse A. The role of an emergency department observation unit in a clinical pathway for atrial fibrillation. Crit Pathw Cardiol 2004;3:8–12.

83. Koenig BO, Ross MA, Jackson RE. An emergency department observation unit protocol for acute-onset atrial fibrillation is feasible. Ann Emerg Med 2002;39:374–81.

84. Deasy C, Wakai A, Mc Mahon GC. Emergency department protocolised management of acute atrial fibrillation: how many patients in a tertiary hospital are eligible? Ir Med J 2006;99:272–3.

85. Zahir S, Lheureux P. Management of new-onset atrial fibrillation in the emergency department: is there any predictive factor for early successful cardioversion? Eur J Emerg Med 2005;12:52–6.

86. Raghavan AV, Decker WW, Meloy TD. Management of atrial fibrillation in the emergency department. Emerg Med Clin North Am 2005;23:1127–39.

87. Cristoni L, Tampieri A, Mucci F, et al. Cardioversion of acute atrial fibrillation in the short observation unit: comparison of a protocol focused on electrical cardioversion with simple antiarrhythmic treatment. Emerg Med J 2011;28:932–7.

88. Wann LS, Curtis AB, January CT, et al. 2011 ACCF/AHA/HRS focused update on the management of patients with atrial fibrillation (updating the 2006 guideline). J Am Coll Cardiol 2011;57:223–42.

89. Stiell IG, Macle L, Committeec CA. Canadian Cardiovascular Society atrial fibrillation guidelines 2010: management of recent-onset atrial fibrillation and flutter in the emergency department. CJCA 2011;27:38–46.

90. Members WG, Roger VL, Go AS, et al, American Heart Association Statistics Committee and Stroke Statistics Subcommittee. Heart disease and stroke statistics—2012 update: a report from the American Heart Association. Circulation 2012;125:e2–220.

91. Massie BM, Shah NB. Evolving trends in the epidemiologic factors of heart failure: rationale for preventive strategies and comprehensive disease management. Am Heart J 1997;133:703–12.

92. Fang J, Mensah GA, Croft JB, et al. Heart failure-related hospitalization in the US, 1979 to 2004. J Am Coll Cardiol 2008;52:428–34.

93. Hugli O, Braun JE, Kim S, et al. United States emergency department visits for acute decompensated heart failure, 1992 to 2001. Am J Cardiol 2005;96: 1537–42.

94. Peacock WF, Braunwald E, Abraham W, et al. National Heart, Lung, and Blood Institute working group on emergency department management of acute heart failure. J Am Coll Cardiol 2010;56: 343–51.

95. Peacock W, Albert N. Patient outcome and costs following an acute heart failure (HF) management program in an emergency department (ED) observation unit (OU). J Heart Lung Transplant 1999;18:1–1.

96. Peacock WF, Remer EE, Aponte J, et al. Effective observation unit treatment of decompensated heart failure. Congest Heart Fail 2002;8:68–73.

97. Storrow AB, Collins SP, Lyons MS, et al. Emergency department observation of heart failure: preliminary analysis of safety and cost. Congest Heart Fail 2005;11:68–72.

98. Diercks DB, Peacock WF, Kirk JD, et al. ED patients with heart failure: identification of an observational unit-appropriate cohort. Am J Emerg Med 2006;24: 319–24.

99. Committee HF, Peacock WF, Fonarow GC, et al. Society of Chest Pain Centers recommendations for the evaluation and management of the observation stay acute heart failure patient: a report from the Society of Chest Pain Centers Acute Heart Failure Committee. Crit Pathw Cardiol 2008;7:83–6.

100. Collins SP, Lindsell CJ, Naftilan AJ, et al. Low-risk acute heart failure patients: external validation of the Society of Chest Pain Center's recommendations. Crit Pathw Cardiol 2009;8:99–103.

101. Weintraub NL, Collins SP, Pang PS, et al, American Heart Association Council on Clinical Cardiology and Council on Cardiopulmonary CC, Perioperative and Resuscitation. Acute heart failure syndromes: emergency department presentation, treatment, and disposition: current approaches and future aims: a scientific statement from the American Heart Association. Circulation 2010; 122:1975–96.

Is it Prime Time for "Rapid Comprehensive Cardiopulmonary Imaging" in the Emergency Department?

Anna Marie Chang, MD, Judd E. Hollander, MD*

KEYWORDS

- Coronary CT angiography • Emergency Department risk stratification • Diagnostic accuracy

KEY POINTS

- Coronary computed tomographic angiography (CTA) has been used with increasing frequency as part of the evaluation of patients with chest pain or other signs and symptoms consistent with potential acute coronary syndrome in the Emergency Department.
- Studies have shown that it has a high negative predictive value in the low to intermediate risk cohort, and those without coronary artery disease can be discharged home.
- Technological advances have significantly decreased the radiation risk with respect to CTA.

INTRODUCTION

Nature of the Problem

More than 5 million patients are evaluated in the Emergency Department (ED) annually for chest pain, most of whom (up to 85%) are found to have a noncardiac cause for their symptoms.[1,2] At an estimated cost of $10 billion a year,[3,4] reducing hospital admissions through improved risk stratification of patients with potential acute coronary syndrome represents a critical focus for saving on health care expenditure.

Patient History and Physical Examination

The tools most readily available to guide disposition of the patient with chest pain are the patient's age and sex, history of coronary artery disease (CAD) or its risk factors, and the characteristics of the chest pain. Usually an initial 12-lead electrocardiogram (ECG) is added as well. Despite the fact that cardiac risk factors have prognostic value in population-based studies of asymptomatic patients, they are poor predictors of acute myocardial infarction (AMI), acute coronary syndrome (ACS), and 30-day cardiovascular events in symptomatic patients. The initial 12-lead ECG has low sensitivity for AMI,[5] and a single set of biochemical markers also has poor sensitivity.[1,6] Because none of these tools used alone is a reliable predictor of ACS and "low risk is not no risk," observation-unit strategies incorporate serial ECGs and cardiac markers over a 6- to 12-hour period. A negative evaluation consistent with no evidence of myocardial infarction (MI) or ischemia is followed by a confirmatory study to exclude inducible ischemia, the absence of which permits patient discharge.[7] Given the concerns nationwide of crowding in EDs, protocols that reduce length of stay and eliminate potentially avoidable admissions are widely needed.

CORONARY CTA

In recent years, coronary computed tomographic angiography (CTA) has been shown to identify ED patients with potential ACS who are at low

Department of Emergency Medicine, University of Pennsylvania, Ground Floor, Ravdin Building, 3400 Spruce Street, Philadelphia, PA 19104-4283, USA
* Corresponding author.

Cardiol Clin 30 (2012) 523–532
http://dx.doi.org/10.1016/j.ccl.2012.07.009
0733-8651/12/$ – see front matter © 2012 Elsevier Inc. All rights reserved.

risk for cardiovascular events, thereby safely allowing early discharge.

In most institutions, a low-dose noncontrast ECG-triggered acquisition is performed through the entire chest for the purpose of calcium scoring and evaluation of lung abnormalities. This procedure is followed by a weight-based intravenous injection of 80 to 120 mL of nonionic iodinated contrast with bolus tracking in the descending aorta. After a scan delay, an ECG-gated acquisition from the pulmonary artery bifurcation through the inferior heart border is performed. Studies are usually interpreted by radiologists or cardiologists with subspecialty training in cardiovascular imaging (American College of Cardiology/American Heart Association level 3 training) on dedicated 3-dimensional workstations using axial, multiplanar reformatted, and thin-slab maximum-intensity projection images on an interactive display. Image data are reconstructed at multiple phases of the cardiac cycle, postprocessed, and analyzed on independent workstations. The degree of any observed stenosis can be measured with an electronic caliper by comparing the lumen diameter with the diameter of a proximal reference segment.

Diagnostic Accuracy

Large studies and meta-analyses have established the diagnostic accuracy of coronary CTA, and it has been found to be comparable with invasive angiography. Technological improvement has increased sensitivity of detection of coronary artery stenosis from 84% for 4-slice computed tomography (CT) to 83% for 16-slice CT to 93% for 64-slice CT, with concurrent specificities from 93% to 96% to 96%, respectively.[8] A systematic review of 41 studies totaling 2515 patients indicated sensitivity of 95% and specificity of 85% for detection of CAD in all types of scanners combined.[9] A report by the European Society of Cardiology and the European Council of Nuclear Cardiology reporting on a pooled analysis of 800 patients found a sensitivity of 89% (95% confidence interval [CI] 87–90) with a specificity of 96% (95% CI 96–97) in 64-slice CT.[10]

Budoff and colleagues[11] compared the diagnostic accuracy of coronary CTA with that of invasive coronary angiography (ICA) in 230 patients. On a per-patient basis, the sensitivity, specificity, and positive and negative predictive values to detect stenosis of 50% or more were 95%, 83%, 64%, and 99%, respectively. Miller and colleagues[12] also compared the accuracy of coronary CTA with that of ICA in 291 patients and found similar results. Further examples of large studies comparing 64-slice coronary CTA with ICA are shown in **Table 1**. These sensitivities and specificities translate to a high negative predictive value for the low- to intermediate-risk patient in the ED.

Meijboom and colleagues[13] evaluated the diagnostic utility of those found at high, intermediate, and low pretest risk of CAD. The investigators found that in the low pretest probability group, a negative coronary CTA was present in 75% of the patients. The negative predictive value of coronary CTA to exclude significant CAD was excellent in these patients, reducing the estimated posttest probability to zero, and concluded that these patients would not need further downstream diagnostic tests. Coronary CTA was found to be of limited clinical value in the evaluation of the high estimated pretest probability group.

Calcium score

The role of calcium score (CACS) has been debated. The American College of Cardiology

Table 1
Studies of 64-slice coronary CTA diagnostic properties

Authors,[Ref.] Year	No. of Patients	Sensitivity	Specificity	PPV	NPV
Pugliese et al,[51] 2006	35	100	90	96	100
Leschka et al,[52] 2005	67	94	97	87	99
Raff et al,[53] 2005	70	95	90	93	93
Nikolaou et al,[54] 2006	72	97	79	96	NR
Ropers et al,[55] 2006	84	96	91	98	83
Maffei et al,[56] 2010	177	100	98	92	100
Miller et al,[12] 2008	291	83	91	92	81
Meijboom et al,[57] 2008	360	99	64	86	97
Hoffman et al,[58] 2009	368	100	54	17	100

Abbreviations: NPV, negative predictive value; NR, not reported; PPV, positive predictive value.

foundation/American Heart Association 2007 Clinical Expert Consensus Document on Coronary Artery Calcium Scoring by Computed Tomography evaluated 6 published reports on 27,622 patients, none of whom were symptomatic ED patients.[14] The relative risk for MI or death was 4.3 for any measurable calcium as compared with a CACS = 0. These data imply that the 3- to 5-year risk of any detectable calcium elevates a patient's CHD risk of events by nearly 4-fold. It was reported that patients without detectable calcium (or a CAC score = 0) have a very low rate of death from CHD or MI (0.4%) within this time frame. However, Gottlieb and colleagues[15] evaluated 291 patients who were undergoing coronary CTA and ICA, of whom most (95%) were at intermediate to high probability of obstructive CAD. A total of 72 patients had CACS = 0, among whom 14 (19%) had at least 1 stenosis of 50% or more. This finding holds true among the low-risk population as well. Chang and colleagues[16] found that in patients with a CACS = 0, 23.5% of patients still had CAD (4 of 17). Within the CONFIRM registry, more than 5000 patients had a CACS = 0, yet 16% of these patients still had evidence of CAD on coronary CTA. Those with CAD despite a CACS = 0 had higher rates of MI and revascularization at 90 days.[17] Therefore, freedom from CACS does not provide enough information to effectively risk-stratify patients in the ED for acute events.

30-Day Events

There is a fair amount of literature proving that negative coronary CTA (defined as maximal stenosis <50% in all vessels) is useful in the prediction of freedom from 30-day cardiovascular events of MI, coronary revascularization, or death. **Table 2** summarizes studies that used coronary CTA in the ED for decision making and patient disposition. In a recent meta-analysis of studies of 1559 patients with symptoms suggestive of ACS that presented to the ED, sensitivity was 93.3%, specificity 89.9%, positive predictive value 48.1%, and negative predictive value 99.3% for 30-day cardiovascular events.[18]

The American College of Radiology Imaging Network (ACRIN) 4005 trial randomized 1370 patients to either coronary CTA or traditional care. Patients with a negative CTA (less than 50% maximal stenosis) were free from cardiac death or MI at 30 days (the upper limit of 95% CI was 0.57%). In addition, a coronary CTA-based strategy resulted in double the discharge rate (50% vs 23%) and considerably shorter length of stay (18 vs 25 hours) while identifying more patients with coronary disease (9% vs 3%). Although there was some worry that testing with CTA might lead to more testing, this trial found that the likelihood of receiving a negative invasive angiogram was decreased in the CTA group relative to those managed traditionally.[19]

In the authors' experience, patients without any stenosis beyond 50% in any vessel can be safely discharged home from the ED (**Fig. 1**).

Longer-Term Events

Hollander and colleagues[20] evaluated 588 low-risk patients who received coronary CTA in the ED. Of those, 481 patients had less than 50% stenosis in any vessel without depressed left ventricular function. Over the ensuing year 53 patients (11%) were rehospitalized, and 51 patients (11%) received further diagnostic testing (stress or catheterization) over the subsequent year. There was 1 death (0.2%), no AMI (0%), and no revascularization procedures (0%) during this time period. Hadamitzky and colleagues[21] enrolled 1256 consecutive patients with suspected CAD undergoing 64-slice coronary CTA and observed them prospectively

Table 2
Studies of 64-slice coronary CTA used in the ED disposition of patients based on their results

Authors,[Ref.] Year	No. of Patients	Follow-Up Time (mo)	No. Discharged	Event Rate (%) in Those with Maximal Stenosis <50%
Gallagher et al,[59] 2007	99	6	88	0
Rubinshtein et al,[60] 2007	58	12	32	0
Takakuwa and Halpern,[43] 2008	197	1	133	0
Hollander et al,[29] 2009	568	1	476	0

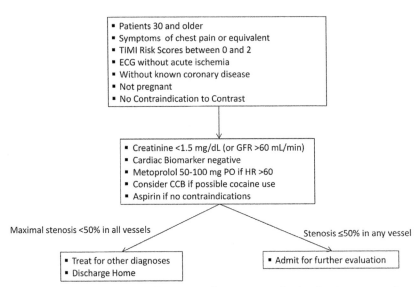

Fig. 1. The authors' protocol for computed tomographic angiography in the Emergency Department. CCB, calcium-channel blocker; ECG, electrocardiogram; GFR, glomerular filtration rate; HR, heart rate; PO, by mouth; TIMI, Thrombolysis in Myocardial Infarction.

for the occurrence of cardiac death, MI, or unstable angina requiring hospitalization. Of the 802 patients without at least 50% stenosis, only 1 case of unstable angina occurred during the initial 90 days. Within a median of 18 months there were 4 events in patients, whereas in 348 patients with obstructive CAD there were 17 cardiac events.

Two other studies focused on low- to intermediate-risk patients with chest pain. The ROMICAT (Rule Out Myocardial Infarction using Computer-Assisted Tomography) trial recently published 2-year outcomes for their cohort. Of 368 patients who presented to the ED with acute chest pain, negative initial troponin, and a nonischemic ECG, 333 patients (90.5%) had a median follow-up period of 23 months. Contrast-enhanced 64-slice CT was obtained during index hospitalization. At the end of the follow-up period, 25 patients (6.8%) experienced 35 events (no cardiac deaths, 12 MIs, and 23 revascularizations). Cumulative probability of 2-year events increased across CT strata for CAD (no CAD 0%; nonobstructive CAD 4.6%; obstructive CAD 30.3%).[22]

In a cohort of 227 patients, 172 patients were without CAD ($n = 96$) or nonobstructive CAD ($n = 76$) on coronary CTA. At 2.3-year follow-up, there were no cardiovascular events in the no-CAD group and 2 events in the mild-CAD group. On the other hand, in the 55 patients with disease, 11 (20%) patients had a cardiovascular event during the time interval.[23] Abdulla and colleagues[24] conducted a meta-analysis that included 5675 patients who were mostly intermediate to high risk in 10 studies with mean follow-up of 21 months. Of these patients, 2045 (36%) had normal CTA, 2068 (36%) had nonobstructive CAD, and 1562 (28%) had obstructive CAD. Overall, 331 (5.8%) had cardiac death, nonfatal MI, and revascularization. The event rate was 0.5% in patients with normal CTA, 3.5% in patients with nonobstructive CAD, and 16% in patients with obstructive CAD.

Large, multicenter studies are also being completed to further research into coronary CTA. The CONFIRM (COroNary computed tomography angiography evaluation For clinical outcomes: an InteRnational Multicenter) registry screened 27,125 coronary CTA patients at 12 participating centers. Clinical information was available for more than 14,000 patients, with 13,966 (99.3%) patients with a mean follow-up of 22.5 months. All-cause mortality (271 deaths) occurred in 0.6% of patients without coronary atherosclerosis, 1.9% of patients with nonobstructive CAD, 2.9% of patients with non–high-risk CAD, and 4.9% of patients with high-risk CAD.[25,26] There are also several trials that are currently ongoing. The Multicenter Study to Rule Out Myocardial Infarction by Cardiac Computed Tomography (ROMICAT-II) states its goal as determining whether length of hospital stay is significantly reduced in the CT arm compared with standard of care at 6 months.[27] At the time of writing, the data are not yet available. The PROspective Multicenter Imaging Study for Evaluation of Chest Pain (PROMISE) trial

(ClinicalTrials.gov identifier NCT 01174550) is multicenter, randomized clinical trial sponsored by the National Institutes of Health that will enroll 10,000 patients to evaluate the 2-year incidence of death, MI, major complications from cardiovascular procedures or testing, and unstable angina hospitalizations, comparing coronary CTA with stress testing. It hopes to answer the question as to whether anatomic imaging from coronary CTA versus functional imaging will be more useful for the diagnosis of CAD and its complications.[28] From 2010 to date, the trial has enrolled 3500 patients.

Do We Even Need Serial Biomarkers/ Observation?

Hollander and colleagues[29] examined 568 low-risk (Thrombolysis in Myocardial Infarction[30] score 0–2) patients with chest pain in the ED; of these, 285 received coronary CTA without serial cardiac biomarkers, of whom 214 (75%) were discharged home after testing. Those who had immediate coronary CTA in the ED had a median length of stay of 7.1 hours compared with 20.8 hours for those who had serial marker testing in the observation unit. Of those with a negative evaluation, no patient suffered an adverse cardiovascular event at 30 days. Although this is a small cohort, the results suggest that serial cardiac biomarker testing is not necessary for the evaluation of these patients with chest pain, further reducing the length of stay.

Cost

Coronary CTA has been associated with decreased length of stay as well as decreased costs for patients. Khare and colleagues[31] used computer-based modeling and found that an evaluation using coronary CTA dominated (ie, less costly and more effective) both observation unit plus stress echocardiography and observation unit plus stress ECG strategies. Chang and colleagues[32] compared 4 strategies in the evaluation of chest pain in the ED: immediate coronary CTA, observation unit, coronary CTA versus observation unit, and stress test versus usual care. Median costs were less, and length of stay was shorter. Diagnosis of CAD was similar, but fewer patients had 30-day death, MI, or readmissions in the coronary CTA groups. Goldstein and colleagues[33] conducted a randomized trial of patients allocated to coronary CTA (n = 361) or myocardial perfusion imaging (n = 338) as the index noninvasive test. The coronary CTA resulted in a 54% reduction in time to diagnosis in comparison with stress tests. Costs of care were 38% lower compared with standard (median $2137 vs $3458). The diagnostic strategies showed no difference in major adverse cardiac events after normal index testing.

One study found higher costs associated with coronary CTA. Shreibati and colleagues[34] used a 20% sample of Medicare beneficiaries and compared functional imaging to coronary CTA in costs and subsequent use of the health service. Coronary CTA was associated with an increased likelihood of subsequent cardiac catheterization (22.9% vs 12.1%), percutaneous coronary intervention (7.8% vs 3.4%), and coronary artery bypass graft surgery (3.7% vs 1.3%). Coronary CTA was also associated with higher total health care spending ($4200) but no difference in all-cause mortality. However, this study only focused on outpatient claims and not on ED or inpatient tests. Furthermore, this study only evaluated patients older than 66 years (median age, 73.6 years), and thus may not be applicable to the ED population of low-risk patients with chest pain.

Areas Unknown

Although it is established that patients with CAD on coronary CTA are at increased risk for cardiovascular events at 30 days and up to 2 years, there are no clear guidelines for the evaluation of patients with detected CAD, especially those with greater than 50% stenosis in any vessel. Weustink and colleagues[35] recommend that in patients with a low (<20%) pretest probability of disease, negative stress test or coronary CTA results suggest no need for further testing. In patients with an intermediate (20%–80%) pretest probability, a positive coronary CTA result suggests the need to proceed with ICA and a negative result suggests no need for further testing. Physicians could proceed directly with ICA in patients with a high (>80%) pretest probability. However, most patients in this study had a stress test if diagnosed with obstructive CAD, so it is unclear how this would translate to clinical practice.

Furthermore, it is unclear as to what the downstream medical management of these patients with nonobstructive disease on coronary CTA should be. Thus far, only 2 published studies have examined the use of cardiovascular medications after coronary CTA. Both studies found an increased use of antiplatelet and lipid-lowering agents in those found to have both nonobstructive and obstructive disease.[36,37] However, the study had variable effects on blood-pressure control and medications for such. It is also unclear whether these patients would benefit from early aggressive management of their CAD.

RADIATION

When 64-slice coronary CTA was first used, retrospectively gated techniques were used with high doses of radiation. Using then-current dose protocols, Einstein and colleagues[38] calculated the relative risk of cancer for men and women evaluated with coronary CTA, and considered that there was a 4-fold increase in the lifetime attributable risk of cancer incidence associated with radiation exposure. Synchronization to the ECG can be performed in 3 ways: (a) retrospective gating, whereby the x-ray tube is at full current throughout a spiral scan, resulting in increased radiation exposure; (b) a dose-modulated spiral scan, whereby the tube current is reduced outside the diastolic window during which cardiac motion is reduced; (c) a prospective gating ("step-and-shoot") axial scan, whereby slices are acquired only in diastole and summed together to form a volume of data. Prospective gating is becoming more frequently used, as it results in high-quality images at the lowest possible radiation dose, but requires adequate patient preparation and heart-rate control to avoid artifacts.[39] New studies and techniques now report that radiation using the prospective gating method can decrease the radiation dose to 2 to 4 mSv.[40] This radiation dose is much lower than the estimated dose of between 7 mSv for a rest-only technetium-99m myocardial perfusion imaging or 24 mSv for a dual-isotope study.[41]

Furthermore, in those with a negative coronary CTA, there may be less downstream testing. At a single academic institution during a 10-year period, 1097 patient records were evaluated. A total of 344 patients (31.4%) received cumulative estimated effective dose from all medical sources of more than 100 mSv, and multiple myocardial perfusion imaging studies were performed in 424 patients (38.6%), for whom the cumulative estimated effective dose was 121 mSv.[42] Thus, if coronary CTA can decrease future testing as indicated by some studies, and given that the overall cumulative radiation dose is of concern, coronary CTA may be beneficial.

OTHER IMAGING MODALITIES
Triple Rule-Out

Coronary CTA has a limited capacity to diagnose noncardiac causes of chest pain arising from sources outside the anatomic window it interrogates. Technical advances in cardiac CT and intravenous contrast injection protocols have made a "triple rule-out" protocol feasible, which can effectively image the coronary, aortic, and pulmonary arterial beds to exclude CAD, aortic dissection, and pulmonary embolism as causes of acute chest pain. Takakuwa and Halpern[43] evaluated 197 patients who had a triple rule-out protocol performed. No further diagnostic testing was performed in 133 (76%) of 175 of patients with no to mild coronary disease within 30 days. Three cases of pulmonary embolism and one case of aortic dissection were found. Rogers and colleagues[44] randomized patients to receive a comprehensive cardiothoracic CT or a coronary CTA in 59 patients. No significant difference was found in the median length of stay, rate of hospital discharge without additional imaging, costs of care, and the number of revisits between the dedicated and comprehensive arms, respectively. Furthermore, radiation dosages were similar between the 2 arms. Madder and colleagues[45] identified patients who underwent triple rule-out or coronary CTA at 2 hospitals in Michigan; 272 patients had triple rule-out and 1796 patients underwent coronary CTA. Pulmonary embolism was identified in only 1.1% of triple rule-out and 0.2% of cardiac CT examinations, and there were no aortic dissections. At 90 days, there were no differences in death, ACS, pulmonary embolism, or aortic dissection diagnosis, or major differences in use of downstream resources. Given that the radiation dose and intravenous contrast dose is higher[45] in these triple rule-out scans, it does not seem to provide enough additional information to warrant the examination in the majority of patients.

Coronary CTA with Perfusion Stress

One of the major critiques of coronary CTA is that it does not provide information on the physiologic significance of coronary luminal stenosis. Multiple prior studies have shown that a coronary luminal stenosis of at least 50% identified by CTA is a poor predictor of ACS. Thus, the best noninvasive diagnostic test for evaluating chest pain in the ED would be a test that can measure the presence of both CAD and myocardial ischemia in patients. Bezerra and colleagues[46] conducted a subset analysis from the ROMICAT trial of 35 subjects who had chest pain and underwent ICA; 22 of the patients were diagnosed with ACS. The sensitivity and specificity of myocardial perfusion defects (MPD) for ACS were 86% (95% CI 64%–96%) and 62% (95% CI 32%–85%). Adding MPD and abnormality of regional wall motion to the assessment for significant stenosis (>50%) resulted in a higher sensitivity of 91% (95% CI 69%–98%) and specificity of 85% (95% CI 54%–97%), and a significantly increased overall diagnostic accuracy, when compared with assessment for stenosis.

A recent review of the literature shows sensitivity ranges from 79% to 97% and specificity from 72% to 98% depending on the scanner type, reference standard, and studied population, and whether analysis is per patient, segment, or territory. Most studies have been completed on intermediate- to high-risk patients.[47] However, given that none of these studies had more than 47 patients, more data are needed regarding this technology. CORE-320 is a currently ongoing international multicenter trial that will compare the diagnostic capability of the combination of quantitative 320-row multidetector CTA and quantitative perfusion imaging with the combination of conventional coronary angiography and single-positron emission CT (SPECT) myocardial perfusion imaging at the patient level. A positive patient will be defined as having at least one vessel with a stenosis diameter of at least 50% defined by quantitative coronary angiography and a corresponding positive SPECT territorial myocardial perfusion defect. The group intends to enroll 450 patients in this phase III trial.[48]

Cardiovascular Magnetic Resonance Imaging

A full discussion of cardiovascular magnetic resonance (CMR) is beyond the scope of this article. CMR allows a comprehensive evaluation of myocardial function, perfusion, and morphology in patients with CAD. In a recent meta-analysis that compared CT with CMR, the investigators found that for ruling out CAD, CT was more accurate than CMR. In a total of 19 studies, the mean sensitivity of CMR was 87% and specificity was 70% for the detection of CAD.[49] In cardiovascular disease, MR imaging has been proved to be a reliable and well-tolerated tool, and is useful post-ACS to focus on remodeling or for diagnoses of diseases such as myocarditis. However, in the setting of acute chest pain in the ED rapid diagnosis is required to ensure instant therapy, and thus CMR may not be the examination of choice.[50]

SUMMARY

CTA has been used with increasing frequency as part of the evaluation of chest pain in the ED. In the appropriate group of patients at low to intermediate risk CTA appears to be an excellent evaluation strategy, safely and efficiently allowing for the rapid discharge of patients home.

REFERENCES

1. Fesmire FM, Hughes AD, Fody EP, et al. The Erlanger chest pain evaluation protocol: a one-year experience with serial 12-lead ECG monitoring, two-hour delta serum marker measurements, and selective nuclear stress testing to identify and exclude acute coronary syndromes. Ann Emerg Med 2002;40(6):584–94.

2. Blomkalns AL, Gibler WB. Chest pain unit concept: rationale and diagnostic strategies. Cardiol Clin 2005;23(4):411–21, v.

3. Gibler WB, Runyon JP, Levy RC, et al. A rapid diagnostic and treatment center for patients with chest pain in the emergency department. Ann Emerg Med 1995;25(1):1–8.

4. Roberts RR, Zalenski RJ, Mensah EK, et al. Costs of an emergency department-based accelerated diagnostic protocol vs hospitalization in patients with chest pain. JAMA 1997;278(20):1670–6.

5. Fesmire FM, Percy RF, Wears RL, et al. Initial ECG in Q wave and non-Q wave myocardial infarction. Ann Emerg Med 1989;18(7):741–6.

6. Fesmire FM, Christenson RH, Fody EP, et al. Delta creatine kinase-MB outperforms myoglobin at two hours during the emergency department identification and exclusion of troponin positive non-ST-segment elevation acute coronary syndromes. Ann Emerg Med 2004;44(1):12–9.

7. Amsterdam EA, Kirk JD, Bluemke DA, et al. Testing of low-risk patients presenting to the emergency department with chest pain. A scientific statement from the American Heart Association. Circulation 2010;122(17):1756–76. Available at: http://www.ncbi.nlm.nih.gov/pubmed/20660809. Accessed October 21, 2010.

8. Vanhoenacker PK, Heijenbrok-Kal MH, Van Heste R, et al. Diagnostic performance of multidetector CT angiography for assessment of coronary artery disease: meta-analysis1. Radiology 2007;244(2):419–28.

9. Janne d'Othée B, Siebert U, Cury R, et al. A systematic review on diagnostic accuracy of CT-based detection of significant coronary artery disease. Eur J Radiol 2008;65(3):449–61.

10. Schroeder S, Achenbach S, Bengel F, et al. Cardiac computed tomography: indications, applications, limitations, and training requirements. Eur Heart J 2008;29(4):531–56.

11. Budoff MJ, Dowe D, Jollis JG, et al. Diagnostic performance of 64-multidetector row coronary computed tomographic angiography for evaluation of coronary artery stenosis in individuals without known coronary artery disease: results from the prospective multicenter ACCURACY (Assessment by Coronary Computed Tomographic Angiography of Individuals Undergoing Invasive Coronary Angiography) trial. J Am Coll Cardiol 2008;52(21):1724–32.

12. Miller JM, Rochitte CE, Dewey M, et al. Diagnostic performance of coronary angiography by 64-row CT. N Engl J Med 2008;359(22):2324–36.

13. Meijboom WB, van Mieghem CA, Mollet NR, et al. 64-Slice computed tomography coronary angiography in patients with high, intermediate, or low pretest probability of significant coronary artery disease. J Am Coll Cardiol 2007;50(15):1469–75.

14. Greenland P, Bonow RO, Brundage BH, et al. ACCF/AHA 2007 clinical expert consensus document on coronary artery calcium scoring by computed tomography in global cardiovascular risk assessment and in evaluation of patients with chest pain. Circulation 2007;115(3):402–26.

15. Gottlieb I, Miller JM, Arbab-Zadeh A, et al. The absence of coronary calcification does not exclude obstructive coronary artery disease or the need for revascularization in patients referred for conventional coronary angiography. J Am Coll Cardiol 2010;55(7):627–34.

16. Chang AM, Le J, Matsuura AC, et al. Does coronary artery calcium scoring add to the predictive value of coronary computed tomography angiography for adverse cardiovascular events in low-risk chest pain patients? Acad Emerg Med 2011;18(10):1065–71.

17. Villines TC, Hulten EA, Shaw LJ, et al. Prevalence and severity of coronary artery disease and adverse events among symptomatic patients with coronary artery calcification scores of zero undergoing coronary computed tomography angiography: results from the CONFIRM (Coronary CT Angiography Evaluation for Clinical Outcomes: an International Multicenter) registry. J Am Coll Cardiol 2011;58(24):2533–40.

18. Takakuwa KM, Keith SW, Estepa AT, et al. A meta-analysis of 64-section coronary CT angiography findings for predicting 30-day major adverse cardiac events in patients presenting with symptoms suggestive of acute coronary syndrome. Acad Radiol 2011;18(12):1522–8.

19. Litt HI, Gatsonis C, Snyder B, et al. CT angiography for safe discharge of patients with possible acute coronary syndromes. N Engl J Med 2012;366(15):1393–403.

20. Hollander JE, Chang AM, Shofer FS, et al. One-year outcomes following coronary computerized tomographic angiography for evaluation of emergency department patients with potential acute coronary syndrome. Acad Emerg Med 2009;16(8):693–8.

21. Hadamitzky M, Distler R, Meyer T, et al. Prognostic value of coronary computed tomographic angiography in comparison with calcium scoring and clinical risk scores/clinical perspective. Circ Cardiovasc Imaging 2011;4(1):16–23.

22. Schlett CL, Banerji D, Siegel E, et al. Prognostic value of CT angiography for major adverse cardiac events in patients with acute chest pain from the emergency department: 2-year outcomes of the RO-MICAT trial. JACC Cardiovasc Imaging 2011;4(5):481–91.

23. Carrigan TP, Nair D, Schoenhagen P, et al. Prognostic utility of 64-slice computed tomography in patients with suspected but no documented coronary artery disease. Eur Heart J 2009;30(3):362–71.

24. Abdulla J, Asferg C, Kofoed KF. Prognostic value of absence or presence of coronary artery disease determined by 64-slice computed tomography coronary angiography a systematic review and meta-analysis. Int J Cardiovasc Imaging 2011;27(3):413–20. Available at: http://www.ncbi.nlm.nih.gov/pubmed/20549366. Accessed December 21, 2010.

25. Min JK, Dunning A, Lin FY, et al. Rationale and design of the CONFIRM (COronary CT Angiography EvaluatioN For Clinical Outcomes: An InteRnational Multicenter) Registry. J Cardiovasc Comput Tomogr 2011;5(2):84–92.

26. Chow BJ, Small G, Yam Y, et al. Incremental prognostic value of cardiac computed tomography in coronary artery disease using CONFIRM/clinical perspective. Circ Cardiovasc Imaging 2011;4(5):463–72.

27. Multicenter study to rule out myocardial infarction by cardiac computed tomography. Full text view—ClinicalTrials.gov. Available at: http://clinicaltrials.gov/ct2/show/NCT01084239. Accessed January 30, 2012.

28. PROspective Multicenter Imaging Study for Evaluation of Chest Pain. Full text view—ClinicalTrials.gov. Available at: http://www.clinicaltrials.gov/ct2/show/NCT01174550?term=promise+trial&rank=1. Accessed December 27, 2011.

29. Hollander JE, Chang AM, Shofer FS, et al. Coronary computed tomographic angiography for rapid discharge of low-risk patients with potential acute coronary syndromes. Ann Emerg Med 2009;53(3):295–304.

30. Pollack CV, Sites FD, Shofer FS, et al. Application of the TIMI risk score for unstable angina and non-ST elevation acute coronary syndrome to an unselected emergency department chest pain population. Acad Emerg Med 2006;13(1):13–8.

31. Khare RK, Courtney DM, Powell ES, et al. Sixty-four-slice computed tomography of the coronary arteries: cost-effectiveness analysis of patients presenting to the emergency department with low-risk chest pain. Acad Emerg Med 2008;15(7):623–32.

32. Chang AM, Shofer FS, Weiner MG, et al. Actual financial comparison of four strategies to evaluate patients with potential acute coronary syndromes. Acad Emerg Med 2008;15(7):649–55.

33. Goldstein JA, Chinnaiyan KM, Abidov A, et al. The CT-STAT (Coronary Computed Tomographic Angiography for Systematic Triage of Acute Chest Pain Patients to Treatment) trial. J Am Coll Cardiol 2011;58(14):1414–22.

34. Shreibati JB, Baker LC, Hlatky MA. Association of coronary ct angiography or stress testing with subsequent utilization and spending among Medicare beneficiaries. JAMA 2011;306(19):2128–36.

35. Weustink AC, Mollet NR, Neefjes LA, et al. Diagnostic accuracy and clinical utility of noninvasive testing for coronary artery disease. Ann Intern Med 2010;152(10):630–9.

36. Ovrehus KA, Bøtker HE, Jensen JM, et al. Influence of coronary computed tomographic angiography on patient treatment and prognosis in patients with suspected stable angina pectoris. Am J Cardiol 2011; 107(10):1473–9.

37. LaBounty TM, Devereux RB, Lin FY, et al. Impact of coronary computed tomographic angiography findings on the medical treatment and control of coronary artery disease and its risk factors. Am J Cardiol 2009;104(7):873–7.

38. Einstein AJ, Henzlova MJ, Rajagopalan S. Estimating risk of cancer associated with radiation exposure from 64-slice computed tomography coronary angiography. JAMA 2007;298(3):317–23.

39. Earls JP. How to use a prospective gated technique for cardiac CT. J Cardiovasc Comput Tomogr 2009; 3(1):45–51.

40. Fink C, Krissak R, Henzler T, et al. Radiation dose at coronary CT angiography: second-generation dual-source CT versus single-source 64-MDCT and first-generation dual-source CT. AJR Am J Roentgenol 2011;196(5):W550–7.

41. Einstein AJ. Radiation risk from coronary artery disease imaging: how do different diagnostic tests compare? Heart 2008;94(12):1519–21.

42. Einstein AJ, Weiner SD, Bernheim A, et al. Multiple testing, cumulative radiation dose, and clinical indications in patients undergoing myocardial perfusion imaging. JAMA 2010;304(19):2137–44.

43. Takakuwa KM, Halpern EJ. Evaluation of a "triple rule-out" coronary CT angiography protocol: use of 64-Section CT in low-to-moderate risk emergency department patients suspected of having acute coronary syndrome. Radiology 2008;248(2): 438–46.

44. Rogers IS, Banerji D, Siegel EL, et al. Usefulness of comprehensive cardiothoracic computed tomography in the evaluation of acute undifferentiated chest discomfort in the emergency department (CAPTURE). Am J Cardiol 2011;107(5):643–50.

45. Madder RD, Raff GL, Hickman L, et al. Comparative diagnostic yield and 3-month outcomes of "triple rule-out" and standard protocol coronary CT angiography in the evaluation of acute chest pain. J Cardiovasc Comput Tomogr 2011;5(3): 165–71.

46. Bezerra HG, Loureiro R, Irlbeck T, et al. Incremental value of myocardial perfusion over regional left ventricular function and coronary stenosis by cardiac CT for the detection of acute coronary syndromes in high-risk patients: a subgroup analysis of the ROMICAT trial. J Cardiovasc Comput Tomogr 2011;5(6):382–91.

47. Ko BS, Cameron JD, DeFrance T, et al. CT stress myocardial perfusion imaging using multidetector CT—a review. J Cardiovasc Comput Tomogr 2011; 5(6):345–56.

48. Combined Non-invasive Coronary Angiography and Myocardial Perfusion Imaging Using 320 Detector Computed Tomography. Full text view—Clinical Trials.gov. Available at: http://clinicaltrials.gov/ct2/show/NCT00934037?term=core320&rank=1. Accessed January 2, 2012.

49. Schuetz GM, Zacharopoulou NM, Schlattmann P, et al. Meta-analysis: noninvasive coronary angiography using computed tomography versus magnetic resonance imaging. Ann Intern Med 2010;152(3):167–77.

50. Hunold P, Bischoff P, Barkhausen J, et al. Acute chest pain: The role of MR imaging and MR angiography. Eur J Radiol 2011. Epub ahead of print. Available at: http://www.ncbi.nlm.nih.gov/pubmed/21543179. Accessed January 10, 2012.

51. Pugliese F, Mollet NR, Runza G, et al. Diagnostic accuracy of non-invasive 64-slice CT coronary angiography in patients with stable angina pectoris. Eur Radiol 2006;16(3):575–82.

52. Leschka S, Alkadhi H, Plass A, et al. Accuracy of MSCT coronary angiography with 64-slice technology: first experience. Eur Heart J 2005;26(15): 1482–7.

53. Raff GL, Gallagher MJ, O'Neill WW, et al. Diagnostic accuracy of noninvasive coronary angiography using 64-slice spiral computed tomography. J Am Coll Cardiol 2005;46(3):552–7.

54. Nikolaou K, Knez A, Rist C, et al. Accuracy of 64-MDCT in the diagnosis of ischemic heart disease. AJR Am J Roentgenol 2006;187(1):111–7.

55. Ropers D, Rixe J, Anders K, et al. Usefulness of multidetector row spiral computed tomography with 64- x 0.6-mm collimation and 330-ms rotation for the noninvasive detection of significant coronary artery stenoses. Am J Cardiol 2006;97(3): 343–8.

56. Maffei E, Seitun S, Martini C, et al. CT coronary angiography and exercise ECG in a population with chest pain and low-to-intermediate pre-test likelihood of coronary artery disease. Heart 2010; 96(24):1973–9.

57. Meijboom WB, Meijs MFL, Schuijf JD, et al. Diagnostic accuracy of 64-slice computed tomography coronary angiography: a prospective, multicenter, multivendor study. J Am Coll Cardiol 2008;52(25): 2135–44.

58. Hoffmann U, Bamberg F, Chae CU, et al. Coronary computed tomography angiography for early triage

of patients with acute chest pain: the ROMICAT (Rule Out Myocardial Infarction using Computer Assisted Tomography) trial. J Am Coll Cardiol 2009; 53(18):1642–50.

59. Gallagher MJ, Ross MA, Raff GL, et al. The diagnostic accuracy of 64-slice computed tomography coronary angiography compared with stress nuclear imaging in emergency department low-risk chest pain patients. Ann Emerg Med 2007;49(2): 125–36.

60. Rubinshtein R, Halon DA, Gaspar T, et al. Impact of 64-slice cardiac computed tomographic angiography on clinical decision-making in emergency department patients with chest pain of possible myocardial ischemic origin. Am J Cardiol 2007; 100(10):1522–6.

Hypertension Crisis in the Emergency Department

Wallace Johnson, MD[a,*], My-Le Nguyen, MD[b],
Ronak Patel, MD[b]

KEYWORDS

- Hypertension crisis • Hypertensive urgency • Hypertensive emergency • Malignant hypertension
- Guidelines • Management • Treatment

KEY POINTS

- An elevated blood pressure (BP) reading in the emergency department should be confirmed in more than one anatomic location based on JNC 7 guidelines and reassessed multiple times before and during therapy.
- Patients with severely (>180/120 mm Hg) or moderately (140–179/90–119 mm Hg) elevated BP suspected of having end-organ damage should undergo appropriate testing to determine if they have hypertensive urgency versus emergency. Absolute BP cutoffs are not as important as the presence or absence of target end-organ damage.
- In general, patients with hypertensive emergency should have their mean arterial pressure (MAP) reduced by 20% to 25% in the first hour of this diagnosis. Exceptions are patients with ischemic stroke, in whom MAP should be reduced by 15% to 20%, and patients with aortic dissection that requires more aggressive BP reduction.
- Hypertensive patients with nausea/vomiting, headache, visual complaints, confusion, stupor, papilledema, or seizures may have hypertensive encephalopathy from cerebral edema. BP reduction should be gradual, and cerebral perfusion pressure should not be decreased too rapidly.
- Patients with evidence of myocardial ischemia attributable to hypertensive emergency should receive nitrates to reduce preload and improve coronary perfusion as well as β-blockers, which can reduce cardiac oxygen demand by lowering heart rate and afterload. β-Blockers should not be given if there is evidence of acute heart failure or an unstable bradyarrhythmia.
- In pregnant patients with hypertensive emergencies, consider the effects of antihypertensive medications on the fetus.

INTRODUCTION

Hypertension is a chronic, modifiable risk factor for cardiovascular disease; however, approximately 1% to 2% of patients with hypertension will present with a hypertensive emergency at some time in their lives.[1] Hypertension is defined as a systolic blood pressure (BP) of 140 mm Hg or higher and/or a diastolic BP of 90 mm Hg or higher (**Box 1**).[2] Prehypertension is defined as a systolic BP of 120 to 139 mm Hg and/or a diastolic BP of 80 to 89 mm Hg. This definition reflects the fact that patients with prehypertension have a tendency to develop full-blown hypertension over time. As BP increases there is a continuous, graded relationship between BP and cardiovascular risk, but as levels exceed 180/120 mm Hg, a hypertensive crisis may emerge.

The terms malignant hypertension and accelerated hypertension were used in the past, but

[a] Division of Cardiology, Hypertension Section, University of Maryland School of Medicine, 419 W. Redwood St, Suite 620, Baltimore, MD 21201, USA; [b] Division of Cardiology, University of Maryland School of Medicine, 419 W. Redwood St, Suite 620, Baltimore, MD 21201, USA
* Corresponding author.
E-mail address: WJohnson@medicine.umaryland.edu

Cardiol Clin 30 (2012) 533–543
http://dx.doi.org/10.1016/j.ccl.2012.07.011
0733-8651/12/$ – see front matter © 2012 Elsevier Inc. All rights reserved.

Box 1
Hypertension definitions

Term	Definition
Hypertensive crisis	
A. Hypertensive urgency	Abrupt rise in BP with no signs of end-organ damage; diastolic BP usually >120 mm Hg
B. Hypertensive emergency	Abrupt rise in BP with acute end-organ damage; diastolic BP usually >120 mm Hg
Prehypertension	Systolic BP 120–139 mm Hg and/or diastolic BP 80–89 mm Hg
Hypertension	Systolic BP >140 mm Hg and/or diastolic BP >90 mm Hg

now the term hypertensive crisis can refer to either a hypertensive emergency or hypertensive urgency. In the years since the term malignant hypertension was initially coined in 1914, a large number of both oral and intravenous medications have been developed for the treatment of hypertensive emergencies as well as chronic essential hypertension.[3–5] Malignant hypertension was initially named as such because the 1-year mortality rate after a hypertensive emergency in 1928 was 80% (similar to a malignant cancer prognosis); later, advances in medical therapy reduced the 1-year mortality to 10% by 1998.[6]

The significant reduction in the mortality related to hypertensive emergencies is undeniably associated with the development of both parental and oral antihypertensive agents, but increased awareness and published clinical guidelines have also contributed to better management of hypertensive emergencies. A recent publication found that although hospitalizations for hypertensive emergencies increased in 2007 when compared with the year 2000, the all-cause in-hospital mortality rate decreased.[1] Deshmukh and colleagues[1] believe the reduction in mortality is at least partly due to the release of the Seventh Joint National Committee[2] report on the prevention, detection, evaluation, and treatment of hypertension in 2003.

One of the first tasks in the emergency department (ED) evaluation is to determine whether the patient's condition represents a hypertensive emergency or urgency. A hypertensive emergency is defined as acute target end-organ damage typically associated with a severely elevated BP (systolic BP >180 mm Hg and/or diastolic BP >120 mm Hg) versus a hypertensive urgency, which is characterized by a similarly elevated BP and no target end-organ damage (see Box 1).[7]

The management of hypertensive emergencies in the ED is challenging because of the lack of evidence-based guidelines from large clinical trials. Hypertensive urgencies, in contrast to emergencies, can be treated with an oral regimen in an outpatient setting. Initiating treatment for hypertensive urgencies in the ED remains controversial because there is no consensus on whether it is cost-effective and improves long-term patient care.

Causes of hypertensive emergency and urgency are shown in Box 2.

NORMAL BLOOD PRESSURE REGULATION

In persons with normal BP regulation there is an appropriate balance between normal vital organ perfusion, hypoperfusion, and hyperperfusion. BP is dependent on cardiac output and peripheral vascular resistance. The balance between cardiac output and peripheral vascular resistance depends on a complex set of integrated actions between the cardiovascular, neural, renal, and endocrine systems, which is not totally understood. A multisystem approach to BP regulation allows the body to respond to internal and external demands such as dehydration, thirst, infection, trauma, and rapid changes in position or volume. The renin-angiotensin-aldosterone system is one of the key systems involved in the regulation of BP.[3,4]

The sympathetic nervous system also plays a major role, particularly during times of physical stress, psychological stress, and heavy exertion. The sympathetic nervous system can increase cardiac output and arterial vasoconstriction. Lastly, endothelial function is also involved in BP regulation. The endothelium found on the vascular wall acts a regulator of BP by secreting vasodilators and/or vasoconstrictors in response to various stimuli.[3]

ALTERED BLOOD PRESSURE REGULATION IN HYPERTENSIVE CRISES

The mechanisms underlying both primary (essential) hypertension and hypertensive crises are not totally understood. There seem to be several mechanisms that are found in both chronic primary hypertension and hypertensive crises. The initial event appears to be an abrupt rise in BP from a known or unknown stimulus followed by compensatory mechanisms arising from the vascular endothelium. Initially the endothelium releases the vasodilator nitric oxide in an attempt to compensate for the change in vasoreactivity. The arterioles sense a rise in BP and, in turn, arterial smooth muscle contracts in an effort to reduce the rise in BP and to limit the effect of the BP at the

Box 2
Causes of hypertensive emergency and urgency

Essential hypertension

Renovascular disease

    Renal artery stenosis: atheroma or fibromuscular dysplasia

    Polyarteritis nodosa

    Takayasu arteritis

Renal parenchymal disease

    Glomerulonephritis

    Tubulointerstitial nephritis

    Systemic sclerosis

    Hemolytic uremic syndrome

    Thrombotic thrombocytopenic purpura

    Diabetes mellitus

    Systemic lupus erythematosus

    Renal aplasia

    Renal cell carcinoma

Endocrine

    Pheochromocytoma

    Cushing syndrome

    Primary hyperaldosteronism

    Renin-secreting tumor

Drugs

    Cocaine, phencyclidine, sympathomimetics, erythropoietin, cyclosporine

    Antihypertensive medication withdrawal

    Amphetamines

    Lead intoxication

    Interactions with monoamine oxidase inhibitors

Autonomic hyperreactivity

    Guillain-Barré syndrome

    Acute intermittent porphyria

Pregnancy related

    Preeclampsia

    Eclampsia

Central nervous system disorders

    Head injury

    Cerebral infarction

    Cerebral hemorrhage

    Brain tumor

    Spinal cord injury

Coarctation of the aorta

Burns

Postoperative pain and/or anesthesia complications

cellular level. A vicious cycle occurs, with prolonged arterial smooth muscle contraction leading to more endothelial dysfunction and an inability to release more nitric oxide, only resulting in a further increase in BP.

Inflammation is also a part of the pathophysiology of endothelial dysfunction. The mechanical shear forces on the vascular wall result in endothelial damage and dysfunction. Endothelial dysfunction results in the expression of inflammatory markers such as endothelin-1, endothelial adhesion molecules, and cytokines.[3,8,9] The inflammatory component of hypertension is believed to promote coagulation, platelet aggregation, endothelial layer permeability, and vasoconstriction. Thus, "hypertension begets hypertension," and there appears to be a complex interaction of the renin-angiotensin-aldosterone system, sympathetic nervous system, and endothelial dysfunction regardless of the initial stimulus. There is also evidence that angiotensin II activates the expression of genes for proinflammatory cytokines and activation of transcription factor NF-κB, causing a direct toxic effect to the vessel wall.[10] An increased level of von Willebrand factor, von Willebrand factor prepeptide, plasmin-antiplasmin complexes, and reduced levels of ADAMTS13 are seen in patients with hypertensive crisis, suggesting that thrombotic microangiopathy may play a role.[11]

Hypertensive crisis appears to have a similar pathophysiology to primary chronic hypertension, but the difference seems to be that the abrupt rise in BP promotes acute target end-organ damage. The target end-organ damage may actually accelerate the rise in the BP, leading to organ tissue hyperperfusion and endothelial damage owing to blunted or inadequate compensatory mechanisms. This hypertensive emergency BP threshold can occur at markedly different levels in individual patients. Patients with chronic hypertension have more smooth muscle hypertrophy because of a sustained elevation in BP, allowing temporary and incomplete end-organ protection at the capillary level. By contrast, normotensive patients who undergo an abrupt increase in BP do not have the same degree of smooth muscle hypertrophy. Thus, even small abrupt rises in BP can induce a hypertensive crisis in normotensives, partly due to the capillary damage that occurs.[3] At present, there is not enough evidence to support a treatment approach based on the potential underlying pathophysiology of hypertensive crisis, so clinicians should achieve disease-specific BP targets in these patients using whatever agents necessary, as long as there are no contraindications (**Tables 1** and **2**).

CLINICAL MANIFESTATIONS OF HYPERTENSIVE CRISIS

The central nervous system is particularly susceptible to high BP and its associated hyperperfusion and shear mechanical forces. In one

Table 1
Parenteral medications used for treatment of hypertensive crisis

	Dosing	Onset of Action	Preload	Afterload	Cardiac Output
Sodium nitroprusside	0.25–10 µg/kg/min IV infusion	Within seconds to minutes	↓	↓↓	No effect
Nitroglycerin	5–100 µg/min IV infusion	1–5 min	↓↓	↓	No effect
Labetalol	20–80 mg bolus every 10 min, or 0.5–2 mg/min IV infusion	5–10 min	No effect	↓	↓
Esmolol	80 mg bolus over 30 secs then 150 µg/kg/min IV infusion	1–2 min	No effect	No effect	↓
Hydralazine	10–20 mg IV bolus	10–20 min	No effect	↓	↑
Phentolamine	5–15 mg IV bolus	1–2 min	No effect	↓	↑
Nicardipine	2–15 mg/h IV infusion	5–10 min	No effect	↓	↑
Clevidipine	1–2 mg/h then titrate to maximum 16 mg/h IV infusion	1–4 min	No effect	↓	↑
Fenoldopam	0.1–0.6 µg/kg/min IV infusion	5–10 min	No effect	↓	↑
Enalaprilat	1.25–5 mg every 6 h IV bolus	15–30 min	No effect	↓	↑

Abbreviation: IV, intravenous.
Data from Refs.[2–4]

Table 2
Special indications and warnings for parenteral medications

	Special Indications	Warnings
Sodium nitroprusside	Most hypertensive emergencies	Caution with renal insufficiency; can develop cyanide toxicity, acidosis, methemoglobinemia, increased intracranial pressure, nausea, vomiting, muscle twitching, theoretical "coronary steal" (shunting of blood from diseased vessels to well-perfused vessels may produce coronary ischemia)
Nitroglycerin	Most hypertensive emergencies, coronary ischemia	Headache; can develop tolerance, tachycardia, vomiting, methemoglobinemia, flushing
Labetalol	Most hypertensive emergencies, aortic dissection	Avoid in acute heart failure, bradycardia, and bronchoconstrictive disease
Esmolol	Aortic dissection	Avoid in acute heart failure, bronchoconstrictive disease, and heart block
Hydralazine	Eclampsia[a]	Can cause reflex tachycardia, headache
Phentolamine	Catecholamine excess	Flushing, headache, tachycardia
Nicardipine	Most hypertensive emergencies	Avoid in acute heart failure and coronary ischemia; causes reflex tachycardia, nausea, vomiting, headache, increased intracranial pressure
Clevidipine	Most hypertensive emergencies	Atrial fibrillation; avoid in soy allergy
Fenoldopam	Most hypertensive emergencies, acute renal impairment, and/or hematuria	Caution with glaucoma; can cause headache, flushing, tachycardia, local phlebitis
Enalaprilat	Acute left ventricular failure	Avoid in acute myocardial ischemia

[a] Labetalol is safer during pregnancy.
Data from Aggarwal M, Khan I. Hypertensive crisis: hypertensive emergencies and urgencies. Cardiol Clin 2006;24:135–46; and Acelajado MC, Calhoun DA. Resistant hypertension, secondary hypertension, and hypertensive crises: diagnostic evaluation and treatment. Cardiol Clin 2010;28:639–54.

representative study of the prevalence of end-organ complications, cerebral infarctions were noted in 24%, intracerebral or subarachnoid hemorrhage in 4%, and hypertensive encephalopathy in 16% of patients. Cardiovascular complications in the same study included acute heart failure in 36% of patients and acute myocardial infarction and/or unstable angina in 12%. Aortic dissection was noted in 2% of patients and eclampsia of pregnancy in 4.5%.[12] In the ED, clinicians need to be aware that substance abuse, medical noncompliance, and secondary hypertension are major causes of hypertensive crisis. Initial evaluation of hypertensive crisis should be focused on assessment of potential cardiovascular, cerebrovascular, and renal damage.

CLINICAL EVALUATION OF HYPERTENSIVE CRISIS IN THE ED

The usefulness of routine testing for patients with severely elevated BP is controversial. However,

the authors believe that patients presenting to the ED with hypertensive crisis should undergo electrocardiography (ECG), chest radiography, computed tomography (CT) of the brain if neurologic symptoms are present, urinalysis, electrolytes/creatinine, complete blood count, and cardiac enzymes if acute coronary syndrome is suspected. This guideline is based on expert opinion and not on data from large randomized clinical trials. As always, sound clinical judgment should be used in the ED setting for each individual patient.

Neurologic Syndromes

The brain relies on a fairly constant cerebral BP to function properly. The cerebral vasculature must help maintain this steady perfusion pressure despite changes in mean arterial pressure (MAP) through autoregulation. When this autoregulation fails in the setting of sudden and severely elevated MAP, cerebral edema and microhemorrhages can occur. Edema occurs when the vascular endothelium is disrupted owing to elevated pressure causing leakage of plasma elements.[13] Symptoms can include headache, stupor, seizures, delirium, agitation, nausea/vomiting, and visual disturbances. Focal neurologic findings can occur, but are rare, and should raise the suspicion for ischemic stroke or cerebral hemorrhage.[14] Patients with long-standing hypertension have a better ability to tolerate increases in MAP without increasing cerebral perfusion. This ability is thought to be due to cerebral arteriolar hypertrophy, which reduces the transmission of the elevated pressure to the capillary bed. It is essential not to lower systemic BP too rapidly, as this can lead to a drop in cerebral perfusion pressure and cause ischemia. BP should be lowered within 2 to 6 hours of presentation to no more than 25% of the initial value.[15]

Myocardial Ischemia

Elevated systemic vascular resistance increases left ventricular (LV) myocardial wall tension and oxygen demand. In markedly elevated BP such as in hypertensive emergencies, myocardial perfusion may not be able to adequately maintain the increased myocardial oxygen demand, which can lead to myocardial ischemia and even infarction. Patients with long-standing hypertension may also have LV hypertrophy, which in itself increases myocardial oxygen demand. This increased LV mass can also cause some degree of coronary artery compression, leading to decreased luminal blood flow.[3] Preferred agents in treating patients with hypertensive emergencies with evidence of ischemia include nitrates that can lower LV preload and improve coronary blood flow as well as β-blockers that can reduce heart rate, decrease afterload, and improve diastolic coronary perfusion.[16] Hydralazine should be avoided, as it can induce a reflex tachycardia and increase cardiac work.

Acute Heart Failure

Acute heart failure presenting as acute pulmonary edema in a hypertensive crisis occurs with an incidence of 36%, making it the second most common sign of end-organ damage.[3] Heart failure can occur in a hypertensive crisis but it can also be a risk factor for the development of hypertensive crisis.[17]

It was initially thought that transient systolic dysfunction causes pulmonary edema in patients with hypertensive crisis, but this theory has been challenged. Gandhi and colleagues[18] used transthoracic echocardiography to evaluate LV ejection fraction during acute episodes of hypertensive pulmonary edema and found that the left ventricular ejection fraction was unchanged during the episodes as well as after treatment. However, they did observe segmental wall motion abnormalities after treatment. The investigators concluded that the cause of acute heart failure in patients with hypertensive crisis may be due to diastolic dysfunction secondary to ischemia.

Sodium nitroprusside is thought to be the best agent for acute pulmonary edema precipitated by a hypertensive crisis.[3] Sodium nitroprusside decreases both preload and afterload. It has a rapid onset of action and a short half-life. Cyanide toxicity is extremely rare. Thiocyanate toxicity is also uncommon and occurs only with high doses of nitroprusside in patients with renal insufficiency.[19] Angiotensin-converting enzyme (ACE) inhibitors such as enalapril can be used to reduce afterload and hence improve cardiac output.[20] A new third-generation dihydropyridine calcium-channel blocker, clevidipine, was shown in a small study to be effective in reducing BP without adverse events.[7] In this study, 89% of patients achieved target BP within 30 minutes of starting clevidipine. Clevidipine selectively inhibits extracellular calcium influx through L-type channels resulting in smooth muscle relaxation; thus it decreases peripheral vascular resistance. An advantage of clevidipine is that it undergoes metabolism by plasma esterases, thus it is independent of renal or hepatic function.[11] Loop diuretics such as furosemide are often used in combination with antihypertensive therapy to induce diuresis in hypertensive pulmonary edema. This common practice was recently challenged by a prospective, randomized, double-blinded placebo-controlled study in which the effectiveness of furosemide in lowering subjective perception of dyspnea was compared with placebo. The results showed no difference in the subjective perception of dyspnea between the 2 groups. Patients in the furosemide group required fewer antihypertensive medications, which led to a conclusion that furosemide may have some antihypertensive effect via direct venodilation. The results of the study challenge the practice of using loop diuretics to reduce the perception of dyspnea.[21]

Aortic Dissection

Aortic dissection is a rare but potentially deadly complication of a hypertensive crisis. Aortic dissection can be misdiagnosed as coronary ischemia, pleurisy, heart failure, stroke, musculoskeletal pain, or an acute abdomen. One must maintain a high index of suspicion, and cardiologists must be particularly aware that an aortic dissection can extend into the coronary arteries and present with both a history and ECG findings identical to those of an acute myocardial infarction. As far as a patient's initial presentation is concerned, one should remember the 3 Rs, namely rapid onset, ripping, and radiating pain in the chest, back, or both. Many diseases and conditions are associated with aortic dissection, but 75% of patients with acute aortic dissection have underlying hypertension[22,23] In the ED the diagnosis of aortic dissection is made using contrast-enhanced CT, magnetic resonance imaging, or transesophageal echocardiography (TEE), although in most settings CT is chosen because of the need for rapid diagnosis. A disadvantage of TEE is that it may not give sufficient visualization of the distal ascending aorta or the aortic arch.[22]

Once the diagnosis of aortic dissection is made, prompt treatment is essential because the death rate in acute aortic dissection may be as high as 1% per hour during the first 24 hours. A type-A dissection is a surgical emergency whereas a type-B dissection can often be managed medically. If the vascular surgery consultant determines that emergency surgery is not needed, prompt BP reduction to a target systolic BP of less than 120 mm Hg and reduction in heart rate to below 65 beats/min should be instituted. Intravenous β-blockade with esmolol or labetalol is usually started to reduce shear stress on the aorta. Other agents such as sodium nitroprusside are often added, and if the BP is refractory to multiple antihypertensive agents, reversible secondary causes of hypertension should be ruled out. Renal artery hypertension or acute pain from the dissection has to be considered as a possible cause of refractory hypertension. If the aortic dissection is complicated by organ ischemia, limb ischemia, or refractory pain, surgical or endovascular therapy may be necessary.[22,24]

Hypertensive Retinopathy

Arteriolar narrowing in patients with mild to moderate hypertension has been described since the late 1800s. Vessel narrowing and arteriolar wall thickening can be early signs of poorly controlled BP.[25] Retinopathy with bilateral flame-shaped hemorrhages and exudates (cotton-wool spots) usually indicates severe hypertension and is classified as grade III retinopathy. More advanced, grade IV retinopathy includes papilledema, which can be seen with hypertensive encephalopathy.[26] These fundoscopic findings of retinopathy in patients with hypertension have a low sensitivity. Also, there is a high rate of intraobserver and interobserver variability when it comes to identifying arteriolar narrowing through ophthalmoscopic examination. This variability decreases with grade III and IV retinopathy.[27] Some studies have shown an association between the degree of retinopathy and signs of end-organ damage such as LV hypertrophy, microalbuminuria, and coronary artery disease in women.[28,29] Ophthalmoscopy can be useful in recognizing acute end-organ damage in the form of papilledema in hypertensive encephalopathy, but the lack of arteriolar narrowing, retinal hemorrhages, exudates, or papilledema cannot be used to exclude a diagnosis.

Acute Renal Insufficiency

Renal insufficiency can be the cause or result of hypertensive crisis. There are changes in renal arteries in chronic hypertension, including endothelial dysfunction and impaired vasodilation. Thus renal autoregulation is altered, resulting in an increase of intraglomerular pressure with increasing systemic arterial pressure. This rise in pressure can cause ischemic injury and fibrosis.[3] Hypertensive emergency can occur in acute glomerulonephritis, hemolytic uremic syndrome, renal artery stenosis, patients on hemodialysis receiving erythropoietin with an accelerated rate of increase in hematocrit,[30] and in renal transplant patients, especially those on cyclosporin and corticosteroids.[10]

Clinical presentations that suggest renal involvement include proteinuria, elevated serum creatinine, hypokalemic metabolic alkalosis, and microangiopathic hemolytic anemia.[31] Uremia was historically the major cause of death until of hemodialysis and improved antihypertensive medications became available. The level of renal recovery relates to the degree of renal impairment at presentation and the underlying renal disorder. Minoxidil, a direct arteriolar vasodilator, is a potent, oral agent useful in malignant hypertension associated with renal failure. Minoxidil may cause reflex tachycardia and fluid retention.[31] ACE inhibitors such as captopril and enalapril are the drugs of choice for malignant hypertension in patients who present with scleroderma renal crises.[32] Fenoldopam, a selective dopamine-1 receptor agonist, which activates dopamine at the level of the kidney, is a recommended agent for patients with acute renal insufficiency because it increases renal perfusion. Calcium-channel blockers and β-blockers can also be used for lowering BP, although they have no effect on glomerular filtration.[3]

Hypertension in Pregnancy

Hypertension complicates 5% to 7% of all pregnancies, and unfortunately is still a leading cause of maternal and fetal morbidity and, rarely, mortality.[33–36] ED physicians and obstetricians often have to consider preterm delivery as the only viable option in the management of severe preeclampsia.

The hypertension of pregnancy is defined as a BP greater than 140 mm Hg systolic and/or greater than 90 mm Hg diastolic according to National High Blood Pressure Education Program.[37] Preeclampsia is a condition that needs to be distinguished from chronic hypertension, which usually is without complications and can be treated similarly to hypertension without pregnancy with treatment plans that are safe for the mother and fetus. Preeclampsia is primarily characterized by hypertension and proteinuria, but can also involve multiple organ systems. The proteinuria is defined by excretion of 300 mg per 24 hours, a urine protein/creatinine ratio of greater than 0.3, or a qualitative dipstick reading of 1+.[38] One potentially life-threatening complication of preeclampsia is the HELLP syndrome, characterized by some or all of the following signs: Hemolysis, abnormal Elevation of Liver enzyme levels (aspartate aminotransferase and lactate dehydrogenase), and Low Platelets (often <40,000/mL).[39]

There are multiple controversies related to both the pathophysiology and management of preeclampsia, but there is a general consensus that only delivery results in a true "cure".[34] De novo hypertension alone occurring after the 20th week of gestation in a nulliparous woman should, as a precaution, initially be treated as preeclampsia.[7] Preeclampsia has also been found to be a risk marker for future cardiovascular disease, so close postpartum risk-factor monitoring is strongly recommended.

Regarding treatment, there is a consensus that antihypertensive therapy should be given to lower the maternal risk of central nervous system complications in pregnant women with a sustained systolic BP greater than 160 mm Hg and/or diastolic BP greater than 110 mm Hg.[40] At lower BP levels between 140 and 159 mm Hg systolic and 90 and 105 mm Hg diastolic, there is no consensus on when and how to treat these levels of blood pressure. The antihypertensive drugs frequently used to treat severe hypertension in pregnancy include labetalol, hydralazine, nifedipine, and nitroprusside only as a last resort.[33,34] Methyldopa, a central adrenergic inhibitor, is the oral drug of choice.[34,36] Labetalol is an adrenergic blocking agent that has an oral and parental formulation with the extra advantage of being safe to use in breastfeeding women. Hydralazine was once considered the drug of choice in hypertensive emergencies, but a meta-analysis of multiple clinical trials found that compared with labetalol or nifedipine, hydralazine was associated with more cesarean sections, more placental abruption, more maternal oliguria, more adverse effects on fetal heart rate, and more maternal hypotension.[41] Nifedipine and magnesium sulfate have both been found to be effective in the treatment of hypertension associated with pregnancy, but it is important to remember that severe reductions in BP can occur when these agents are given together.

Postoperative Hypertension

Postoperative hypertension is defined as significantly elevated BP within the first 2 hours after surgery. The most common cause of postoperative hypertension is sympathetic activation and adrenergic surge. Reversible contributors to this sympathetic activation such as pain, hypoxemia, hypercarbia, hypothermia, volume overload, and anxiety should be treated first before administering antihypertensives unless end-organ damage is present.[42] Urinary retention after surgery is also thought to cause markedly elevated BP. Moreover, withdrawal from holding antihypertensives should be considered. In general, patients should not stop taking their home antihypertensive medications on the day of surgery, especially centrally acting agents such as clonidine and β-blockers. Patients with or without pre-existing hypertension can develop postoperative hypertension. Patients with poorly controlled hypertension are more likely to have postoperative hypertension.[43] Treatment should be focused on the cause of the hypertension and on whether the patient is able to take oral medications after the procedure. If possible, the patient's home medication can be given if there are no contraindications. β-Blockers should be avoided in certain instances such as profound bradycardia, heart block, severe chronic obstructive pulmonary disease, or acute heart failure.

Hyperadrenergic States

The hyperadrenergic states include pheochromocytoma; cocaine, amphetamine, and phencyclidine overdose; clonidine withdrawal; and monoamine oxidase (MAO) inhibitor–tyramine reaction. In these conditions there is a surge in catecholamine levels.[31] In a pheochromocytoma crisis and MAO inhibitor–tyramine reaction, phentolamine, phenoxybenzamine, or nitroprusside can be used to control BP. The use of β-blockers alone is not recommended for these conditions because it would result in an unopposed peripheral α-adrenergic vasoconstriction, which further

Table 3
Target blood pressure goals

Hypertensive Emergency	Target Blood Pressure
Hypertensive encephalopathy	MAP lowered by maximum 20% or to DBP 100–110 mm Hg within first hour then gradual reduction in BP to normal range over 48–72 h
Ischemic stroke	MAP lowered no more than 15%–20%, DBP not less than 100–110 mm Hg in first 24 h (thrombolytic protocols in stroke may allow slightly more aggressive management)
Ischemic stroke post-tPA	SBP <185 mm Hg or DBP <110 mm Hg
Intracerebral hemorrhage	MAP lowered by 20%–25%
Hypertensive retinopathy	MAP lowered by 20%–25%
Left ventricular failure	MAP to 60–100 mm Hg
Aortic dissection	SBP 100–120 mm Hg
Acute renal insufficiency	MAP lowered by 20%–25%
Pregnancy-induced hypertension	SBP 130–150 mm Hg and DBP 80–100 mm Hg
Postoperative hypertension	MAP lowered by 20%–25% (not based on published guidelines)
Myocardial ischemia/infarct	MAP to 60–100 mm Hg
Hyperadrenergic states	MAP lowered by 20%–25% (not based on published guidelines)

Abbreviations: DBP, diastolic blood pressure; MAP, mean arterial pressure; SBP, systolic blood pressure; tPA, tissue plasminogen activator.

increases BP.[19] Labetalol, which has both an α- and β-receptor antagonist effect, can also be used in a pheochromocytoma crisis; however, paradoxic hypertension may occur.[31] In the case of cocaine or amphetamine abuse, anxiolytics should be given first. Phentolamine can be added if hypertension persists after anxiolytics have been given.[44] Hypertension due to clonidine withdrawal should be treated by giving clonidine first.

SUMMARY

Management of hypertensive crisis in the ED will continue to challenge clinicians because of the lack of randomized clinical trials. Expert opinion and sound clinical judgment will continue to guide the management of hypertension crisis until such trials are completed. Hypertensive crisis persists largely because of medication nonadherence, poorly controlled chronic hypertension, substance abuse, and poor access to primary care. A few key principles should be noted: (1) verify BP readings before initiating treatment; (2) patients presenting with a hypertensive emergency should have their MAP reduced by 20% to 25% within the first hour, with the exception being ischemic stroke and aortic dissection as noted in **Table 3**; (3) hypertensive urgencies should be treated with oral, not parental, agents; (4) appropriate testing to differentiate hypertensive urgencies versus emergencies should be done; and (5) once BP is stabilized with parenteral therapy, the transition to oral therapy can begin within 6 to 12 hours.

REFERENCES

1. Deshmukh A, Kumar G, Kumar N, et al. Effect of joint national committee VII report on hospitalizations for hypertensive emergencies in the United States. Am J Cardiol 2011;108(9):1277–82.
2. Chobanian AV, Bakris GL, Black HR, et al. Seventh report of the Joint National Committee on prevention, detection, evaluation, and treatment of high blood pressure. Hypertension 2003;42:1206–52.
3. Aggarwal M, Khan I. Hypertensive crisis: hypertensive emergencies and urgencies. Cardiol Clin 2006;24:135–46.
4. Acelajado MC, Calhoun DA. Resistant hypertension, secondary hypertension, and hypertensive crises: diagnostic evaluation and treatment. Cardiol Clin 2010;28:639–54.
5. Elliott WJ. Clinical features and management of selected hypertensive emergencies. J Clin Hypertens 2004;6:587–92.
6. Keith NM, Waegner HP, Keronohan JW. The syndrome of malignancy hypertension. Arch Intern Med 1928;4:264–78.
7. Baumann BM, Cline DM, Pimenta E. Treatment of hypertension in the emergency department. J Am Soc Hypertens 2011;5:366–77.
8. Okada M, Matsumori A, Ono K, et al. Cyclic stretch up-regulates production of interleukin-8 and monocyte

chemotactic and activating factor/monocyte chemo-
attractant protein-1 in human endothelial cells. Arte-
rioscler Thromb Vasc Biol 1998;18:894–901.

9. Verhaar MC, Beutler JJ, Gaillard CA, et al. Progressive vascular damage in hypertension is associated
with increased levels of circulating P-selectin.
J Hypertens 1998;16:45–50.

10. Vaughan CJ, Delanty N. Hypertensive emergencies.
Lancet 2000;356:411–7.

11. Marik P, Rivera R. Hypertensive emergencies: an
update. Curr Opin Crit Care 2011;17:569–80.

12. Zampaglione B, Pascale C, Marchisio M, et al.
Hypertensive urgencies and emergencies: prevalence and clinical presentation. Hypertension 1996;
27:144–7.

13. Immink RV, van den Born BJ, van Montfrans GA,
et al. Impaired cerebral autoregulation in patients
with malignant hypertension. Circulation 2004;110:
2241–5.

14. Schwartz RB. Hyperperfusion encephalopathies:
hypertensive encephalopathy and related conditions. Neurologist 2002;8:22–34.

15. Gardner CJ, Lee K. Hyperperfusion syndromes:
insight into the pathophysiology and treatment of
hypertensive encephalopathy. CNS Spectr 2007;
12(1):35–42.

16. Frohlich ED. Target organ involvement in hypertension: a realistic promise of prevention and reversal.
Med Clin North Am 2004;88:1–9.

17. Tisdale JE, Huang MB, Borzak S. Risk factors for
hypertensive crisis: importance of out-patient blood
pressure control. Fam Pract 2004;21:420–4.

18. Gandhi SK, Powers JC, Nomeir A, et al. The
pathogenesis of acute pulmonary edema associated with hypertension. N Engl J Med 2001;344:
17–22.

19. Ram CV. Current concepts in the diagnosis and
management of hypertensive urgencies and emergencies. Keio J Med 1990;39:225–36.

20. Thomas L. Managing hypertensive emergencies in
the ED. Can Fam Physician 2011;57:1137–41.

21. Holzer-Richling N, Holzer M, Kerkner H, et al.
Randomized placebo controlled trial of furosemide
on subjective perception of dyspnoea in patients
with pulmonary oedema because of hypertensive
crisis. Eur J Clin Invest 2011;41:627–34.

22. Braverman AC. Aortic dissection: prompt diagnosis
and emergency treatment are critical. Cleve Clin J
Med 2011;78(10):685–96.

23. Hagan PG, Nienaber CA, Isselbacher EM, et al.
International Registry of Acute Aortic Dissection
(IRAD): new insights from an old disease. JAMA
2000;283:897–903.

24. Braverman AC, Thompson R, Sanchez L. Diseases
of the aorta. In: Bonow RO, Mann DL, Zipes DP,
et al, editors. Braunwald's heart disease. 9th edition.
Philadelphia: Elsevier; 2011.

25. Gunn RM. Ophthalmoscopic evidence of (1) arterial
changes associated with chronic renal diseases and
(2) of increased arterial tension. Trans Am Ophthalmol Soc 1892;12:124–5.

26. Wong TY, Mitchell P. Hypertensive retinopathy.
N Engl J Med 2004;351:2310–7.

27. Dimmitt SB, West JN, Eames SM, et al. Usefulness
of ophthalmoscopy in mild to moderate hypertension. Lancet 1989;20:1103–6.

28. Wong TY, Klein R, Klein BEK, et al. Retinal microvascular abnormalities, and their relation to hypertension, cardiovascular diseases and mortality. Surv
Ophthalmol 2001;46:59–80.

29. Shantha AU, Kumar AA, Bhaskar E, et al. Hypertensive retinal changes, a screening tool to predict
microalbuminuria in hypertensive patients: a cross-
sectional study. Nephrol Dial Transplant 2010;
25(6):1839.

30. Novak BL, Force RW, Mumford BT, et al. Erythropoi-
etin-induced hypertensive urgency in a patient with
chronic renal insufficiency: case report and review
of the literature. Pharmacotherapy 2003;23:265–9.

31. Kitiyakara C, Guzman NJ. Malignant hypertension
and hypertensive emergencies. J Am Soc Nephrol
1998;9:133–42.

32. Mouthon L, Bérezné A, Bussone G, et al. Scleroderma renal crisis: a rare but severe complication
of systemic sclerosis. Clin Rev Allergy Immunol
2011;40:84–91.

33. Lindheimer MD, Taler SJ, Cunningham FG. Hypertension in pregnancy. J Am Soc Hypertens 2010;
4(2):68–78.

34. Lindheimer MD, Taler SJ, Cunningham FG. Hypertension in pregnancy. J Am Soc Hypertens 2008;
2(6):484–94.

35. Villar J, Say L, Gulmezoglu AM, et al. Pre-eclampsia:
a health problem for 2000 years. In: Critchly H, MacLean A, Poston L, et al, editors. Pre-eclampsia.
London, England: RCOG Press; 2003. p. 189–207.

36. Ness RB, Roberts JM. Epidemiology of hypertension.
In: Lindheimer MD, Roberts JM, Cunningham FG,
editors. Chesley's hypertensive disorders in pregnancy. 2nd edition. Stamford (CT): Appleton & Lange;
1999. p. 43–65 (edition revision in press, May 2009,
Elsevier).

37. Report of the National High Blood Pressure Education Program Working Group on high blood pressure in pregnancy. Am J Obstet Gynecol 2000;
183:S1–22.

38. Shennan AH, Waugh J. The measurement of blood
pressure and proteinuria in pregnancy. In: Critchly H,
MacLean A, Poston L, et al, editors. Pre-eclampsia.
London, England: RCOG Press; 2003. p. 305–24.

39. Sibai BM. Diagnosis, controversies, and management of the syndrome of hemolysis, elevated liver
enzymes, and low platelet count. Obstet Gynecol
2004;103:981–91.

40. Magee LA, Abalos E, von Dadelszen P, et al. How to manage hypertension in pregnancy effectively. Br J Clin Pharmacol 2011;72(3):394–401.

41. Magee LA, Cham C, Waterman EJ, et al. Hydralazine for treatment of severe hypertension on pregnancy: meta-analysis. BMJ 2003;327:955–60.

42. Halpern NA. Today's strategies for treating postoperative hypertension. Immediate evaluation and targeted treatment are required. J Crit Illn 1995; 10(7):478–80, 483–90.

43. Haas CE, LeBlanc JM. Acute postoperative hypertension: a review of therapeutic options. Am J Health Syst Pharm 2004;61:1661–80.

44. Van den Born B, Beutler JJ, Gaillard C, et al. Dutch guideline for the management of hypertensive crisis—2010 revision. J Med 2011;69:248–55.

Blunt Cardiac Injury

Jeremy S. Bock, MD, R. Michael Benitez, MD*

KEYWORDS

- Blunt cardiac injury • Blunt aortic injury • Cardiac contusion • Commotio cordis

KEY POINTS

- Individuals with suspected blunt chest trauma who have only mild or no symptoms, a normal electrocardiogram (ECG), and are hemodynamically stable typically have a benign course and rarely require further diagnostic testing or long periods of close observation.
- Individuals with pain, ECG abnormalities, or hemodynamic instability represent a patient population in whom rapid evaluation of the heart (by echocardiography) and the great vessels (by advanced imaging) may be necessary.
- Although serious injuries are rare, many are associated with high mortality.

INTRODUCTION

Blunt chest trauma is associated with rapid deceleration, barotrauma, or compression injury of the heart. The spectrum of clinical outcomes related to such injury ranges from asymptomatic ectopic beats seen on electrocardiogram (ECG) to sudden death. A few of the most common patterns of blunt cardiac injury (BCI) are reviewed in this article.

ELECTRICAL DISTURBANCES

Individuals who experience chest pain or soreness following blunt chest trauma are frequently screened for BCI by ECG. Many support the notion that a normal screening ECG excludes the possibility of significant cardiac injury and predicts a benign cardiovascular course.[1–4] In a study of 333 individuals with blunt thoracic trauma, a normal screening ECG was associated with a negative predictive value of 98% for significant BCI.[1] These findings have been replicated by other groups.[5]

Although thought to be rare, the incidence of dysrhythmias and conduction disturbances following thoracic trauma is unknown because definitions vary by practice (ie, whether premature atrial or ventricular contractions are included).[6,7] Nevertheless, electrical disturbances requiring therapy are typically associated with a less favorable prognosis.[6] Such changes are not only a concern in their own right, but are often markers of more serious BCI.

Atrial Dysrhythmias

Sinus tachycardia is the most common ECG abnormality among trauma victims[8] and often reflects pain, catecholamine surge, and emotional disturbance. However, the possibility of major hemorrhage, myocardial rupture, pericardial tamponade, or tension pneumothorax must also be excluded, especially when hypotension is present. Sinus tachycardia is a normal or compensatory response in any of these clinical settings and the use of β-blockers should be avoided. Therapy appropriately directed at the underlying cause of the tachycardia, such as pain control, volume resuscitation, transfusion, or definitive correction of mechanical hemodynamic compromise, leads to gradual resolution of the sinus tachycardia.

Results from large case series suggest that ECG abnormalities other than sinus tachycardia are present in fewer 1% to 6% of patients with chest trauma.[7,9] Within this small fraction, atrial fibrillation (AF) is the most common. The author of one series reported AF on initial ECG in 9 of 240 patients with chest trauma (4%),[10] although prior history of persistent or paroxysmal AF was not

Division of Cardiology, University of Maryland School of Medicine, 110 South Paca Street, Seventh Floor, Baltimore, MD 21201, USA
* Corresponding author.
E-mail address: mbenitez@medicine.umaryland.edu

Cardiol Clin 30 (2012) 545–555
http://dx.doi.org/10.1016/j.ccl.2012.07.001
0733-8651/12/$ – see front matter © 2012 Elsevier Inc. All rights reserved.

excluded. This issue is important because of the high prevalence of AF in the general population, especially among older individuals.[11] Specific factors contributing to the development of new AF in patients with trauma may include catecholamine release, high prevalence of alcohol and drug use, electrolyte and acid-base derangements, anemia, and hypovolemia. These factors may be as important as the blunt impact in the initiation of AF. This possibility is supported by the finding that the incidence of AF in patients with thoracic trauma is similar to the incidence in those with head or abdominal trauma.[9]

In general, the treatment strategy of AF in patients with trauma should be similar to the strategy in the general population. Patients with rapid AF and hemodynamic compromise should be cardioverted according to advanced cardiac life support (ACLS) protocol. Asymptomatic hemodynamically stable patients may alternatively benefit from a more conservative rate-control strategy using β-blocker or calcium channel blocker drugs with consideration of delayed elective electrical cardioversion. In stable patients, cardioversion and anticoagulation for stroke prophylaxis should not be initiated in the emergency department, especially if the extent of injury and possibility of bleeding are not fully characterized.

Paroxysmal supraventricular tachycardia (PSVT) following BCI is rare but has been described in several series and case reports.[9] Initiation of these reentrant rhythms may reflect heightened adrenergic tone and an increased frequency of premature atrial ectopic beats in a patient with the intrinsic substrate (dual aortic valve [AV] nodal physiology) for this arrhythmia. It is appropriate to use vagal maneuvers or atrioventricular node (AVN) blocker medications such as adenosine to abruptly terminate PSVT. If the rhythm is recurrent, titration of oral β-blockers is recommended so long as this class is not contraindicated.

Conduction Disturbances

Atrioventricular and intraventricular conduction blocks related to BCI are not common but are well described.[12–14] Examples of transient, persistent, immediate, and delayed heart block following nonpenetrating trauma have all been reported. Immediate-term to short-term block may reflect direct trauma causing inflammation, edema, or stunning of specialized tissue. More extensive and permanent damage may occur secondary to localized necrosis and eventual fibrosis. Such possibilities have not been verified histopathologically because most patients with nonpenetrating chest trauma survive.

Right bundle branch block (RBBB) is the most frequently encountered conduction disturbance following trauma.[10,15] In the past, this has been attributed to the more anterior location of the right-sided cardiac structures.[16] However, RBBB, even when persistent, carries little if any long-term sequelae for patients unless other conduction disease is present.

Although first degree AVN block is the second most common conduction abnormality (after RBBB), complete AVN block is rare and usually transient.[15] In the absence of cardiac rupture or septal perforation, only a few cases of persistent complete heart block requiring a permanent pacemaker have been described in the setting of trauma.[12,14]

Generalized treatment paradigms cannot be based on the small number of available case reports of patients with heart block related to BCI. Patients who are hemodynamically stable with normal QRS duration and second-degree or third-degree block warrant close monitoring with the ability to escalate therapy if needed. Temporary transvenous demand pacing should be considered in patients with a widened QRS and advanced heart block, although there are no data to show that this alters outcomes. Patients with heart block who are hemodynamically unstable require immediate and thorough evaluation for definition of the root cause as well as consideration of transvenous pacing.

Commotio Cordis

Ventricular tachyarrhythmias (VT) and ventricular fibrillation (VF) are rare complications of BCI. Nevertheless, VT and VF are also the most lethal electrical events and have thus received the most scrutiny. Commotio cordis refers to sudden cardiac death (SCD) triggered by a brief, nonpenetrating, and low-energy blow to the precordium.[17,18] Such events are related to the induction of VF during a vulnerable period in the cardiac cycle and are not generally associated with structural injury to the heart.[19,20] Although the mechanism of commotio cordis remained mysterious for more than a century, a clear understanding of this entity has emerged in the last 15 years, largely because of the development of a contemporary experimental animal model[20,21] and commotio cordis registry.[22] Data from the Minneapolis Heart Institute Foundation registry suggest that commotio cordis is the second or third most common cause of SCD in young athletes.[22,23]

According to an analysis of 128 consecutive registry cases, approximately 78% of commotio cordis events occur in individuals younger than

18 years of age.[23] Sixty-two percent of these individuals were participating in a competitive sport at the time of their event. Those participating in baseball, softball, and ice hockey accounted for three-quarters of these deaths, with 81% occurring after an isolated blow to the precordium by the ball or puck. There was significant diversity in non–sports-related settings associated with commotio cordis including a toddler inadvertently hit in the chest by a plastic toy, a boy hit by a thrown snowball, and an adult man who died instantly after a low speed motor vehicle collision. It is not clear why 95% of individuals in the commotio cordis registry are male[23] but this is consistent with the observation that 89% of all reported SCDs in young athletes (including those attributed to hypertrophic obstructive cardiomyopathy and coronary anomalies) are also male.[22]

Some investigators have surmised that the predilection of commotio cordis for young people is related to a thin, underdeveloped, and compliant chest wall that readily transmits mechanical energy to the unprotected myocardium. This inadvertent precordial thump is translated to electrical energy that may incite a ventricular dysrhythmia during a vulnerable period of the cardiac cycle. Protective equipment for youth athletics using solid, high-velocity projectiles (ie, baseball, hockey, lacrosse) has been proposed as a means of prevention.[24,25] However, an analysis of 85 consecutive cases of commotio cordis found that 38% deaths occurred in athletes wearing standard chest protectors.[26] Further study of specific commercially available chest protectors showed that they offer protection against soft tissue injury but are inadequate in reducing the frequency of commotio cordis.[24]

Much of the improved understanding of the pathophysiology of commotio cordis is the result of an elegant animal model developed by Link and colleagues.[20] In this model, baseballs are propelled toward the precordium of anesthetized juvenile swine. Release of the projectile is timed by electrocardiogram (ECG) gating to impact the chest wall and cause a premature ventricular contraction (PVC) during a vulnerable portion of ventricular repolarization (10–30 milliseconds before the peak of the T-wave). Generation of VF by this mechanism is known as the R on T phenomenon. Investigators found that a little-league baseball propelled at 48 and 64 km/h (velocities typical for youth baseball) is able to trigger VF in 32% and 78% of correctly timed attempts, respectively.[25] Cardiac arrest seems to be instantaneous in this setting based on electrocardiographic and left ventricle (LV) catheter hemodynamic monitoring.[20,27] Based on these observations, it is reasonable to suspect commotio cordis in young male athletes who

suddenly collapse during competitive sports play, especially after being struck by a projectile.

Until recently, survival following a commotio cordis SCD was rare, even in those who received prompt bystander cardiopulmonary resuscitation (CPR) and defibrillation with an automatic electronic defibrillator (AED).[28] Investigators of an analysis of 128 consecutive cases to 2001 reported that 84% victims died and only 11% achieved complete neurologic and physical recovery after the event.[23] However, survival rates have improved substantially in the last several years, increasing to 35% of cases registered in the last decade. This finding probably reflects increased public awareness, bystander CPR training, public availability of AEDs, and implementation of community programs focused on minimizing delay to first defibrillator shock.[29–31] As is the experience with VF in other settings, the chance of successful defibrillation is inversely proportional to the duration of the arrhythmia.[23,32] Despite variability in successful resuscitation, prompt recognition of cardiac arrest with early external defibrillation remains the most important determinant of survival in commotio cordis.[23] The American Heart Association currently recommends the use of manual defibrillators, not AEDs, for infants and children less than 8 years of age with VF or pulseless VT.[33] This age range accounts for up to 15% to 20% commotio cordis cases. An initial energy dose of 2 to 4 J/kg is recommended for children and infants; however, doses greater than 4 J/kg may also be safe if lower energy shocks are ineffective.

Because VF is instantaneous following chest wall impact,[21] victims are typically either resuscitated successfully in the field or die before their arrival at an emergency center. Survivors with normal ECG and physical examination typically have a benign cardiovascular course and need only to be monitored for recurrent dysrhythmias. Because cardiac contusion and other structural injury is rare in these settings,[19,20,34] aggressive intervention and further diagnostic testing is generally not helpful in the emergency or trauma departments.

In summary, commotio cordis is a devastating, and frequently fatal, manifestation of blunt chest impact in young people. Early prehospital defibrillation is the single most important factor in minimizing mortality or survival with neurologic sequelae.

Other Ventricular Dysrhythmias

Sustained monomorphic or polymorphic VT following BCI should be treated according to standard ACLS protocols. These types of arrhythmias have rarely been reported in the absence of underlying structural heart disease, and full early evaluation, including echocardiography, is warranted to determine the need for urgent surgical or percutaneous intervention.

MYOCARDIAL CONTUSION
Subclinical Myocardial Contusion

Myocardial contusion (MC) is one of the most common, but ambiguous, cardiac diagnoses made following blunt chest trauma. The incidence of this complication is unknown because no consensus definition or uniform diagnostic criteria exist.[4] Some clinicians apply the label of MC to all patients experiencing chest soreness with mild increase of serum cardiac biomarkers following chest trauma. Others limit this diagnosis for those with frank cardiac dysfunction (ie, new segmental wall motion abnormalities or globally depressed cardiac contractility), life-threatening cardiac arrhythmias, or conduction disturbances. Conclusions about appropriate diagnostic tests, therapy, and outcomes are confounded by this lack of consensus.

Contusion or bruising of the heart may occur following a direct blow to the chest or rapid deceleration injury secondary to cardiac impact with the inner sternum. On histopathology, this is marked by intramyocardial hemorrhage, edema, and localized necrosis.[16] Many patients are screened for MC with serum cardiac biomarkers following chest trauma. Although this test is highly sensitive for detection of cardiomyocyte necrosis, many argue that an abnormal value in an otherwise stable patient offers no helpful diagnostic or prognostic information. Dowd and Krug[3] retrospectively reviewed 184 pediatric patients with traumatic injuries and discharge diagnoses of cardiac contusion over a 10-year period.[3] Among the 65 patients who were hemodynamically stable with normal screening ECG on arrival to the trauma center, not a single malignant arrhythmia or case of pump failure was observed. Further, investigators of a retrospective study of 71 adults admitted with the diagnosis of rule-out cardiac contusion reported no cardiac sequelae or mortality among hemodynamically stable patients with normal screening ECGs.[2] In contrast, the 13 patients who died, developed arrhythmias, or progressed to pump failure in this series each had abnormal ECGs on arrival.

In patients screened for subclinical MC with serum cardiac biomarkers, the clinical course and survival of those with abnormal results seems to be similar to those of patients with normal values if the patients are otherwise stable.[8,35] A retrospective review of 359 patients admitted for blunt chest trauma over a 4-year period found increased biomarkers in 30% of patients; however, only 5% of these patients developed subsequent arrhythmias or shock.[36] These 5% of patients could have been otherwise identified by their abnormal screening ECG or hemodynamic instability. One group found that only 7% of patients with chest trauma with cardiac troponin I (Tn I) levels greater than 1.5 ng/mL had clinically significant cardiac injuries manifested by cardiogenic shock, malignant arrhythmias, abnormal echocardiography, or depressed cardiac index less than 2.5 L/min/m^2.[1] Diagnosis of subclinical MC by echocardiography, gated cardiac radionuclide angiography (MUGA), or myocardial perfusion imaging similarly may not affect outcome in stable patients.[4,37,38] These and other studies suggest little if any clinical value of using serum biomarkers or functional testing to screen patients for subclinical MC if they are otherwise stable and have a normal ECG.

Clinically Significant MC

Severe BCI leading to frank myocardial dysfunction is often heralded by hypotension or other signs of cardiac failure such as new pulmonary congestion, end-organ hypoperfusion, malignant tachyrhythmias or bradyarrhythmias, or conduction disturbances. The mechanism of severe BCI is variable but often follows direct precordial impact, sudden deceleration, and cardiac bruising caused by impact with the internal sternum, or cardiac compression between the sternum and vertebral column. This condition most commonly occurs in the setting of motor vehicle accidents but may also occur in the setting of deceleration or crush injuries of the chest. When bruising, dysfunction, or arrhythmogenesis occur, the more anterior and thin-walled right heart chambers are more frequently involved compared with the left chambers and are also more prone to rupture (discussed later). Among patients who develop myocardial bruising and segmental wall motion abnormalities, arrhythmias and hypokinesia frequently resolve without intervention in 24 hours. Cardiac sequelae 1 year after a cardiac contusion in hemodynamically stable patients are rare.[8,39] Instances of permanent scar formation after severe cardiac contusions have been described but are also rare. In these cases, remodeling of the ventricle may result in formation of a ventricular aneurysm. Nevertheless, in the absence of hemodynamic or electrical instability, there seems to be little benefit to characterizing a cardiac contusion with markers of injury or segmental wall motion abnormalities on echocardiography.

In summary, cardiac contusion without chamber rupture is a nonspecific term often used to describe a spectrum of myocardial injuries that differ in mechanism and severity. The routine use of biomarkers or myocardial imaging in young and middle-aged hemodynamically stable adults with normal ECGs who are admitted for chest trauma seems to be of limited value. Although some groups advocate routine screening evaluation with serum biomarkers and use of echocardiography in cases of sternal and rib fractures,[6,40] it is not clear that this algorithm changes outcomes.

BCI WITH CHAMBER RUPTURE

A minority of patients affected by blunt thoracic injury develop rupture of the cardiac chambers. Survival is rare, with many individuals dying on the scene or during transport to the hospital.[41,42] Instant death is common in cases of rupture into an intact pericardium because of rapid hemopericardium and acute tamponade.[41] Those with contained ruptures who survive to first hospital encounter may have smaller tears in a cavity under lower pressure. Therefore hypotension in contained ruptures may be protective to some degree, which is supported by reports of patients who develop tamponade only after aggressive fluid resuscitation for hypotension. One literature review identified 23 case reports of 39 patients with rupture who survived to hospital admission.[43] On arrival, all 39 patients were severely hypotensive, 95% had evidence of increased central venous pressure, and 89% were tachycardic. The right ventricle (RV) was more commonly involved than the LV and the right atrium was more commonly involved than the left atrium.[43–45] These findings contrast with older reporting of an equal frequency of chamber rupture.[46] Mortality may reach more than 80% even among patients who survive transport to a level 1 trauma center.

Tamponade caused by contained rupture of the chambers is one of the most frequent causes of circulatory shock in patients with blunt chest trauma.[41] An estimated three-quarters of patients with rupture have other major associated injuries. However, many have hemodynamic instability out of proportion to the patient's apparent injuries or blood loss.[43,44] For this reason, all hypotensive patients with chest trauma should be rapidly evaluated by bedside echocardiogram. This technique allows differentiation of various cardiac causes of shock that may require different treatment pathways (ie, tamponade caused by hemopericardium vs primary ventricular failure). In cases of hemopericardium and impaired filling, even small-volume pericardiocentesis can rapidly, but temporarily, improve hemodynamics as a bridge to cardiac surgery.[43] Some experts think that left-sided thoracotomy or sternotomy is superior to pericardiocentesis if there is rapid deterioration in a patient's vital signs.

Uncontained chamber rupture caused by concomitant pericardial laceration has been reported in 6% to 10% of cases.[44,47] This variant is typically associated with even higher mortality than contained rupture because of rapid exsanguination into the thoracic cavity. In summary, rupture of the cardiac chambers is a rare event but carries a high mortality even among survivors to hospital admission. For this reason, immediate echocardiography or bedside ultrasonography is advised in all patients with chest trauma if they present with hypotension. In cases of early tamponade caused by a contained rupture, small-volume pericardiocentesis may sufficiently stabilize hemodynamics for definitive surgical repair. For rapidly deteriorating patients, thoracotomy or sternotomy provides better exposure, visualization, and access to the chest. A stepwise algorithm for identifying and evaluating BCI is shown in **Fig. 1**.

VALVULAR INJURY

Significant traumatic injury to the cardiac valves always results in valvular regurgitation. Although these events are thought to be rare,[45] the incidence is unknown because mild or moderate lesions can initially be subclinical. In asymptomatic individuals, mild functional regurgitation may represent a preexistent condition; regurgitation associated with structural damage, such as chordal rupture or leaflet avulsion, is more likely to be both more severe in nature and related to trauma. Acute severe disruption of the left-sided cardiac valves is often associated with rapid cardiovascular collapse.[48,49] Acute, severe aortic regurgitation (AR) or mitral regurgitation (MR) into a noncompliant, nonconditioned cardiac chamber results in pulmonary edema, respiratory failure, and hypotension.[48] Those with moderate left-sided valvular injuries may be initially stable, with development of heart failure symptoms over the course of weeks to years depending on the loss of structural integrity and regurgitant volume. Some sequelae may be insidious, as in the case of traumatic disruption of the tricuspid valve, which typically leads to symptomatic right ventricular dysfunction many years after injury.[50]

AV injury is thought to be the most common isolated valvular lesion following chest trauma. However, some investigators argue that this observation only reflects reporting bias caused by the high fatality rates of this particular lesion.[51]

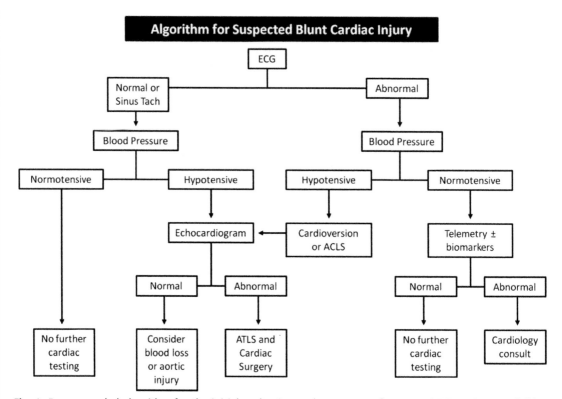

Fig. 1. Recommended algorithm for the initial evaluation and treatment of suspected BCI. Patients with blunt thoracic trauma who have a normal ECG and hemodynamics do well regardless of further laboratory or imaging studies. ATLS, advanced trauma life support.

Aortic cusp rupture or commissural avulsion probably occur secondary to a sudden and profound increase in intrathoracic pressure during a vulnerable period in early diastole when the transaortic gradient is highest and the AV is closed and therefore unsupported by the empty LV.[52] Patients with severe AV injury and AR typically manifest signs of cardiogenic shock. The typical decrescendo diastolic murmur may be short or absent because of rapid equalization of aortic and LV pressures and because the widened pulse pressure and physical findings associated with a large stroke volume are absent. Echocardiography, rather than physical examination, is the most rapid and reliable method for identification and quantification of acute aortic valvular injury. Urgent surgical consultation and often emergent repair are required because of shock or respiratory failure given the relative ineffectiveness of medical therapy and contraindication to percutaneous mechanical circulatory support (intra-aortic balloon counterpulsation).

Although isolated disruption of the mitral valve (MV) is especially rare, traumatic injury to the atrioventricular valves is more common than injury to the semilunar valves when concomitant chamber or septal rupture is present.[45] Isolated MV disruption

leading to acute, severe MR may occur secondary to a sudden increase in intraventricular pressure during systole when LV pressure is already high. Such profound LV pressure overwhelms the tensile strength of the papillary muscles or chordae, leading to mitral leaflet avulsion. Delayed mitral disruption may alternatively occur following papillary muscle contusion if there is progression to necrosis. Acute, severe MR generally leads to rapid pulmonary edema and circulatory shock. In contrast with severe AR, vasodilator medications and aortic balloon counterpulsation are critically important for stabilizing patients until emergency valve surgery can be performed.

CORONARY INJURY AND MYOCARDIAL INFARCTION

Traumatic injury to the coronary arteries, both in isolation and in association with other cardiac injuries, is uncommon but well described in the literature. Patterns of injury identified by angiography or autopsy include coronary occlusion, laceration, dissection, and aneurysm formation.[53–56] Clinical manifestations are variable but include immediate or delayed myocardial infarction, stable anginal symptoms, and sudden death. The electrocardiogram may show typical ST segment increase, and conscious patients may experience chest pain typical of myocardial ischemia or infarction. These signs and symptoms are not specific for coronary injury in the setting of blunt chest trauma, and, as previously discussed, can also be seen in the setting of MC. Echocardiography can help distinguish between the two, and the finding of a left ventricular regional wall motion abnormality, isolated to a coronary distribution (especially when congruent with electrocardiographic changes) should heighten concern for coronary injury. If traumatic coronary injury associated with symptoms or infarction is suspected, angiography and revascularization are possible and successful in certain settings. The benefits of surgical or percutaneous intervention must be balanced against the bleeding risks incurred with antiplatelet and antithrombotic therapy typically used in an interventional approach.

BLUNT AORTIC INJURY

High-energy chest trauma leading to rapid deceleration and traction is one of the principal causes of blunt aortic injury (BAI). This injury is commonly encountered in the setting of high-speed motor vehicle collisions, pedestrians struck, or falls from heights greater than 3 m. Horizontal deceleration creates shearing forces at the aortic isthmus, an anatomic transition zone between the almost immobile aortic arch and fixed descending thoracic aorta. Vertical deceleration displaces the heart caudally, placing traction on the ascending aorta. Other theories of forces leading to BAI are well described.[57]

Initial management of individuals with suspected BAI should follow the advanced trauma life support (ATLS) protocol. If patients exhibit circulatory or respiratory arrest or hemodynamic instability, ACLS management is recommended. Because chest radiographs are widely available, inexpensive, and can be performed quickly, it is often the initial test of choice for suspected BAI. One group found that widened or abnormal mediastinum may be present in up to 93% of individuals with BAI who survive to hospitalization.[58] Based on their data, sensitivity can be increased further toward 98% if other suggestive radiographic signs such as a left hemothorax, abnormal aortic knob, or left apical cap are considered. However, other investigators report false-negative chest radiographs in 44% and almost all studies report poor specificity of abnormal mediastinum for BAI.[59] In addition, tears limited to the intima and media, which may later progress, are most often missed

by plain radiographs. For these reasons, contrasted computed tomography (CT) remains the standard of care in most trauma centers.[60] Using intravascular ultrasound as the confirmatory diagnostic test, one group reported 100% sensitivity and 99% specificity of CT for detecting even minimal aortic injury (tears involving the intima and inner-most layer of the media).[59,61] Numerous reports indicate that CT is more reliable in establishing a diagnosis of BAI than aortography,[62] which is seldom used today. Diagnosis by transesophageal echocardiography can be considered for patients who are unstable and unsafe for transport to the CT scanner, although imaging of the transverse aortic arch is limited.[63] Three of the most common and fatal patterns of BAI and their recommended management are described later (**Fig. 2**).

Aortic Rupture and Contained Rupture

Aortic transection and free rupture caused by horizontal deceleration are associated with mortalities greater than 80% within the first 30 minutes of injury.[64–66] The remainder of victims typically have aortic tears contained by a thin layer of adventitia, fragile perivascular hematoma, or surrounding tissues. These individuals may survive to first hospital encounter but are at high risk for progression to free rupture if left untreated.[64,65] One report found that untreated, contained aortic rupture in patients reaching the hospital alive was associated with 30% death at 24 hours and 50% death at 7 days.[64]

Some have questioned whether the dismal survival rates reported in older series are inflated.[67] Individuals with aortic rupture found on autopsy frequently have other potentially fatal traumatic injuries. Regardless of this possibility, the threat of death is sufficiently high that surgical repair was traditionally delayed only for the purposes of stabilizing other emergency conditions. This long-assumed benefit of immediate repair was recently challenged by groups showing lower mortality among those who undergo delayed surgery (>24 hours after presentation) irrespective of aortic injury severity.[68] However, we think that the prospective studies used to support these conclusions are potentially limited by exclusion of patients too critical to randomize.[68] Retrospective studies showing better outcomes in patients undergoing delayed repair are also inherently biased because of the selection of patients with unstable aortic injuries for immediate repair.[69] Thus, mortality in the immediate repair group may be higher because of the severity of injury, having nothing to do with the timing of surgery. It

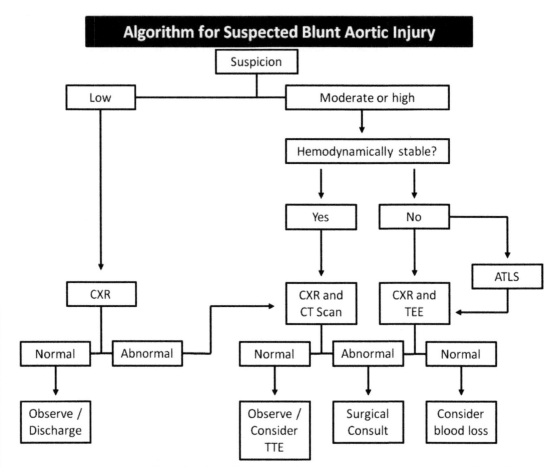

Fig. 2. Recommended algorithm for the initial evaluation and treatment of suspected BAI. CXR, chest radiograph; TEE, transesophageal echocardiography.

may be reasonable to delay repair in individuals with more stable aortic injuries for the purposes of resuscitation and treatment of more threatening conditions. Endovascular repair, rather than traditional open surgery, has been adopted by some centers as the preferred treatment of BAI in select patients. Results from a recent meta-analysis suggest that the endovascular approach is associated with lower mortality and reduced rates of paraplegia compared with open repair.[70] However, these findings were based on author-selected studies that were all retrospective and nonrandomized and thus prone to both selection and reporting bias. More recent comparisons of these 2 approaches show little difference in outcomes.[71]

In the emergency department, appropriate medical therapy to reduce shear stress on the aortic wall should be considered for all patients with aortic injury, especially those who are hypertensive. These include either β-blockers or combined α-blockers/β-blockers, which reduce

the slope of the arterial upstroke (ie, change in pressure [dP]/change in time [dt]) and lower heart rate. The use of a β-blocker that can be titrated, such as esmolol, is often preferred because these patients are at high risk of hemodynamic instability. Other antihypertensive agents that lead to reflex tachycardia, particularly vasodilators, are less appropriate but can be considered if refractory hypertension is present after initial β-blockade.

Aortic Dissection

Systemic hypertension remains the most important risk factor for thoracic aortic dissection.[72] Classic dissection associated with blunt chest trauma is rare compared with rupture.[64] Tears of the aortic intima frequently begin in the isthmus region. As blood enters beneath the intimal flap, there is separation from the media layer, and this false lumen may progress in a proximal or distal course. Although existing cystic medial necrosis is common, if not necessary, for the development of nontraumatic dissections, the presence of these changes is variable in individuals with dissection caused by trauma.

Any dissection, traumatic or otherwise, involving the ascending aorta or arch may be complicated by acute severe AR, coronary ischemia, free rupture into the pericardial space with tamponade, upper extremity ischemia, or occlusion of left carotid artery. Dissection flaps extending distally may compromise blood flow to the celiac, renal, or mesenteric branches. One large review found that chest pain was present in 73% of individuals with dissection.[72] Sharp chest pain is more common in individuals with proximal dissection; tearing back pain is associated with dissections distal to the origin of the left subclavian artery. Surgical outcomes are superior to outcomes of medical therapy in patients with proximal aortic dissection, whereas medical therapy remains the treatment of choice in uncomplicated dissections distal to the left subclavian artery. Endovascular therapy may be warranted in distal dissection complicated by threatened aortic rupture, progressive dissection despite medical therapy, or malperfusion syndromes. Whether dissections are managed medically or surgically, treatment with β-blockers followed by arterial vasodilators is appropriate in hemodynamically stable patients.

Aortic Pseudoaneurysm

Pseudoaneurysm refers to hematoma that forms outside of an arterial wall caused by vessel rupture contained only by surrounding tissues. The hematoma typically maintains communication with the arterial lumen through a narrow neck or point of rupture. The natural history of traumatic aortic pseudoaneurysms is usually one of progression, not stability. Although the time course is variable, pseudoaneurysms tend to expand and eventually rupture.[73] Saccular pseudoaneurysms may be suspected on plain film when large, but identification of small contained ruptures is best made by CT or magnetic resonance imaging. Depending on anatomy, these ruptures may be suitable for endovascular repair.

SUMMARY

Blunt chest trauma is associated with a spectrum of injuries to the heart and aorta that vary markedly in character and severity. The setting, signs, and symptoms of chest trauma (ie, motor vehicle collision, chest pain, hypotension) are often nonspecific for any particular injury. This variation represents a challenge to emergency providers who strive to resuscitate, diagnose, and seek appropriate expert consultation as quickly as possible.

Individuals with suspected blunt chest trauma who have only mild or no symptoms, a normal ECG, and are hemodynamically stable typically have a benign course. These individuals rarely require further diagnostic testing or long periods of close observation because these measures have not been shown to change outcomes. In contrast, individuals with pain, ECG abnormalities, or hemodynamic instability represent a different patient population in whom rapid evaluation of the heart by echocardiography and the great vessels by advanced imaging may be necessary. Although the serious injuries described earlier are rare, many are associated with high mortality.

REFERENCES

1. Velmahos GC, Karaiskakis M, Salim A, et al. Normal electrocardiography and serum troponin I levels preclude the presence of clinically significant blunt cardiac injury. J Trauma 2003;54:45–51.
2. Illig KA, Swierzewski MJ, Feliciano DV, et al. A rational screening and treatment strategy based on the electrocardiogram alone for suspected cardiac contusion. Am J Surg 1991;162:537–44.
3. Dowd MD, Krug S. Pediatric blunt cardiac injury: epidemiology, clinical features, and diagnosis. J Trauma 1996;40:61–7.
4. Fildes JJ, Betlej TM, Manglano R, et al. Limiting cardiac evaluation in patients with suspected myocardial contusion. Am Surg 1995;61:832–5.
5. Healy MA, Brown R, Fleiszer D. Blunt cardiac injury: is this diagnosis necessary? J Trauma 1990;30:137–46.
6. Maenza RL, Seaberg D, D'Amico F. A meta-analysis of blunt cardiac trauma: ending myocardial confusion. Am J Emerg Med 1996;14:237–41.
7. Ismailov RM, Ness RB, Redmond CK, et al. Trauma associated with dysrhythmias: results from a large matched case-control study. J Trauma 2007;62: 1186–91.
8. Lindstaedt M, Germing A, Lawo T, et al. Acute and long-term clinical significance of myocardial contusion following blunt thoracic trauma: results of a prospective study. J Trauma 2002;52:479–85.
9. Hadjizacharia P, O'Keefe T, Brown CV, et al. Incidence, risk factors, and outcomes for atrial arrhythmias in trauma patients. Am Surg 2011;77: 634–9.
10. Berk WA. ECG findings in nonpenetrating chest trauma: A review. J Emerg Med 1987;5:209–15.
11. Go AS, Hylek EM, Phillips KA, et al. Prevalence of diagnosed atrial fibrillation in adults: national implications for rhythm management and stroke prevention: the AnTicoagulation and Risk Factors in Atrial Fibrillation (ATRIA) Study. JAMA 2001;285:2370–5.

12. Benitez RM, Gold MR. Immediate and persistent complete heart block following a horse kick. Pacing Clin Electrophysiol 1999;22:816–8.

13. Pontillo D, Capezzuto A, Achilli A, et al. Bifasicular block complicating blunt cardiac injury. Angiology 1994;45:883–90.

14. Lazaros GA, Ralli DG, Moundaki VS, et al. Delayed development of complete heart block after blunt chest trauma. Injury 2004;35:1300–2.

15. Potkin RT, Werner JA, Trobaugh GB, et al. Evaluation of non-invasive tests of cardiac damage in suspected cardiac contusion. Circulation 1982;66:627–31.

16. Tenzer ML. The spectrum of myocardial contusion: a review. J Trauma 1985;25:620–7.

17. Maron BJ, Estes NA. Commotio cordis. N Engl J Med 2010;362:917–27.

18. Nesbitt AD, Cooper PJ, Kohl P. Rediscovering commotio cordis. Lancet 2001;357:1195–7.

19. Maron BJ, Poliac LC, Kaplan JA, et al. Blunt impact to the chest leading to sudden death from cardiac arrest during sports activities. N Engl J Med 1995; 333:337–42.

20. Link MS, Wang PJ, Pandian NG, et al. An experimental model of sudden death due to low-energy chest-wall impact (commotio cordis). N Engl J Med 1998;338:1805–11.

21. Link MS, Maron BJ, VanderBrink BA, et al. Impact directly over the cardiac silhouette is necessary to produce ventricular fibrillation in an experimental model of commotio cordis. J Am Coll Cardiol 2001; 37:649–54.

22. Maron BJ, Doerer JJ, Haas TS, et al. Sudden deaths in young competitive athletes: analysis of 1866 deaths in the United States, 1980-2006. Circulation 2009;119:1085–92.

23. Maron BJ, Gohman BA, Kyle SB, et al. Clinical profile and spectrum of commotio cordis. JAMA 2002;287:1142–6.

24. Weinstock J, Maron BJ, Song C, et al. Failure of commercially available chest wall protectors to prevent sudden cardiac death induced by chest wall blows in an experimental model of commotio cordis. Pediatrics 2006;117:e656–62.

25. Link MS, Maron BJ, Wang PJ, et al. Upper and lower limits of vulnerability to sudden arrhythmic death with chest-wall impact (commotio cordis). J Am Coll Cardiol 2003;41:99–104.

26. Doerer JJ, Haas TS, Estes NA, et al. Evaluation of chest barriers for protection against sudden death due to commotio cordis. Am J Cardiol 2007;99:857–9.

27. Link MS, Wang PJ, VanderBrink BA, et al. Selective activation of the K+ ATP channel is a mechanism by which sudden death is produced by low-energy chest-wall impact (commotio cordis). Circulation 1999;100:413–8.

28. Maron BJ, Wentzel DC, Zenovich AG, et al. Death in a young athlete due to commotio cordis despite prompt external defibrillation. Heart Rhythm 2005; 2:991–3.

29. Capucci A, Aschieri D, Piepoli MF, et al. Survival from sudden cardiac arrest via early defibrillation without traditional education in cardiopulmonary resuscitation. Circulation 2002;106:1065–70.

30. Myerburg RJ, Velez M, Rosenberg DG, et al. Automatic external defibrillators for prevention of out-of-hospital sudden death: effectiveness of the automatic external defibrillator. J Cardiovasc Electrophysiol 2003;14:S108–16.

31. Caffrey SL, Willoughby PJ, Pepe PE, et al. Public use of automated external defibrillators. N Engl J Med 2002;347:1242–6.

32. Winkle RA, Mead RH, Ruder MA, et al. Effect of duration of ventricular fibrillation on defibrillator efficacy in humans. Circulation 1990;81:1477–81.

33. Field JM, Hazinski MF, Sayre MR, et al. Executive summary: 2010 American Heart Association guidelines for cardiopulmonary resuscitation and emergency cardiovascular care. Circulation 2010; 122(Suppl):S640–56.

34. Deady B, Innes G. Sudden death of a young hockey player: case report of commotio cordis. J Emerg Med 1999;17:459–62.

35. Bertinchant JP, Polge A, Mohty D, et al. Evaluation of incidence, clinical significance, and prognostic value of circulating cardiac troponin I and T elevation in hemodynamically stable patients with suspected myocardial contusion after blunt chest trauma. J Trauma 2000;48:924–31.

36. Biffl WL, Moore FA, Moore EE, et al. Cardiac enzymes are irrelevant in the patient with suspected myocardial contusion. Am J Surg 1994;168:523–8.

37. Dubrow TJ, Mihalka J, Eisenhauer DM, et al. Myocardial contusion in the stable patient: what level of care is appropriate? Surgery 1989;106:267–73.

38. Gunnar WP, Martin M, Smith RF, et al. The utility of cardiac evaluation in the hemodynamically stable patient with suspected myocardial contusion. Am Surg 1991;57:373–7.

39. Sturaitis M, McCallum D, Sutherland G, et al. Lack of significant long-term sequelae following traumatic myocardial contusion. Arch Intern Med 1986;146: 1765–9.

40. Sybrandy KC, Cramer MJ, Burgersdijk C. Diagnosing cardiac contusion: old wisdom and new insights. Heart 2003;89:485–9.

41. Fulda G, Brathwaite CE, Rodriguez A, et al. Blunt traumatic rupture of the heart and pericardium: a ten-year experience (1979-1989). J Trauma 1991;31:167–72.

42. Perchinsky MJ, Long WB, Hill JG. Blunt cardiac rupture. The Emanuel Trauma Center experience. Arch Surg 1995;130:852–6.

43. Leavitt BJ, Meyer JA, Morton JR, et al. Survival following nonpenetrating traumatic rupture of cardiac chambers. Ann Thorac Surg 1987;44:532–5.

44. Brathwaite CE, Rodriguez A, Turney SZ, et al. Blunt traumatic cardiac rupture. A 5-year experience. Ann Surg 1990;212:701–4.

45. Parmley LF, Manion WC, Mattingly TW. Nonpenetrating traumatic injury of the heart. Circulation 1958;18: 371–96.

46. Bright EF, Beck CS. Non-penetrating wounds of the heart: a clinical and experimental study. Am Heart J 1935;10:293.

47. Liedtke AJ, DeMuth WE. Nonpenetrating cardiac injuries: a collective review. Am Heart J 1973;86: 687–97.

48. Schwaitzberg SD, Khalil KG. Isolated traumatic aortic valvular insufficiency with rapid pulmonary deterioration. Report of two cases. Arch Surg 1985;120:971–3.

49. McDonald ML, Orszulak TA, Bannon MP, et al. Mitral valve injury after blunt chest trauma. Ann Thorac Surg 1996;61:1024–9.

50. van Son JAM, Danielson GK, Schaff HV, et al. Traumatic tricuspid valve insufficiency: experience in thirteen patients. J Thorac Cardiovasc Surg 1994; 108:893–8.

51. Banning AP, Pillai R. Non-penetrating cardiac and aortic trauma. Heart 1997;78:226–9.

52. Prêtre R, Faidutti B. Surgical management of aortic valve injury after nonpenetrating trauma. Ann Thorac Surg 1993;6:1426–31.

53. Goel SS, Harvey JE, Penn M, et al. Images in cardiovascular medicine. Left anterior descending coronary artery occlusion secondary to blunt chest trauma. Circulation 2009;119:1975–6.

54. Suzuki I, Sato M, Hoshi N, et al. Coronary arterial laceration after blunt chest trauma. N Engl J Med 2000;343:742–3.

55. Ngaage DL, Singh SK, Bresnahan JF, et al. Chronic traumatic aneurysm of the left main coronary artery causing myocardial infarction. Ann Thorac Surg 2005;80:2383.

56. Carbone I, Francone M, Galea N, et al. Images in cardiology. Computed-tomography and magnetic resonance imaging assessment of traumatic left anterior descending coronary dissection causing acute myocardial infarction. J Am Coll Cardiol 2011;57:e3.

57. Neschis DG, Scalea TM, Flinn WR, et al. Blunt aortic injury. N Engl J Med 2008;359:1708–16.

58. Woodring JH. The normal mediastinum in blunt traumatic rupture of the thoracic aorta and brachiocephalic arteries. J Emerg Med 1990;8:467–76.

59. Demetriades D, Gomez H, Velmahos GC, et al. Routine helical computed tomographic evaluation

60. Melton SM, Kerby JD, McGiffin D, et al. The evolution of chest computed tomography for the definitive diagnosis of blunt aortic injury: a single-center experience. J Trauma 2004;56:243–50.

61. Malhotra AK, Fabian TC, Croce MA, et al. Minimal aortic injury: a lesion associated with advancing diagnostic techniques. J Trauma 2001;51:1042–8.

62. Fabian TC, Davis KA, Gavant ML, et al. Prospective study of blunt aortic injury: helical CT is diagnostic and antihypertensive therapy reduces rupture. Ann Surg 1998;227:666–76.

63. Smith MD, Cassidy JM, Souther S, et al. Transesophageal echocardiography in the diagnosis of traumatic rupture of the aorta. N Engl J Med 1995;332: 356–62.

64. Parmley LF, Mattingly TW, Manion WC, et al. Nonpenetrating traumatic injury to the aorta. Circulation 1958;17:1086–101.

65. Feczko JD, Lynch L, Pless JE, et al. An autopsy case review of 142 nonpenetrating (blunt) injuries of the aorta. J Trauma 1992;33:846–9.

66. Von Oppell UO, Dunne TT, De Groot MK, et al. Traumatic aortic rupture: twenty-year metaanalysis of mortality and risk of paraplegia. Ann Thorac Surg 1994;58:585–93.

67. Prêtre R, Chilcott M. Blunt trauma to the heart and great vessels. N Engl J Med 1997;336:626–32.

68. Demetriades D, Velmahos GC, Scalea TM, et al. Blunt traumatic thoracic aortic injuries: early or delayed repair: results of an American Association for the Surgery of Trauma prospective study. J Trauma 2009;66:967–73.

69. Pacini D, Angeli E, Fattori R, et al. Traumatic rupture of the thoracic aorta: ten years of delayed management. J Thorac Cardiovasc Surg 2005;129:880–4.

70. Xenos ES, Abedi NN, Davenport DL, et al. Meta-analysis of endovascular vs open repair for traumatic descending thoracic aorta rupture. J Vasc Surg 2008;48:1343–51.

71. Xenos ES, Bietz GJ, Davenport DL. Endoluminal versus open repair of descending thoracic aortic rupture: a review of the National Trauma Databank. Ther Adv Cardiovasc Dis 2011;5:221–5.

72. Hagan PG, Nienaber CA, Isselbacher EM, et al. The International Registry of Acute Aortic Dissection (IRAD): new insights into an old disease. JAMA 2000;283:897–903.

73. Prêtre R, LaHarpe R, Cheretakis A, et al. Blunt injury to the ascending aorta: three patterns of presentation. Surgery 1996;119:603–10.

I Passed Out: Now What?
General Approach to the Patient With Syncope

Ayman A. Hussein, MD, Anastasios Saliaris, MD*

KEYWORDS

- Syncope • Loss of consciousness

KEY POINTS

- When approaching a patient with reported transient loss of consciousness, it is essential to differentiate syncope from nonsyncopal causes. Clinicians should approach loss of consciousness with a wide differential diagnosis given different diagnostic and prognostic implications.
- It is important to identify patients with life-threatening conditions and those with red flags indicating an increased risk of sudden death.
- An initial approach to syncope consisting of a careful history, physical examination, and electrocardiograms is essential.

INTRODUCTION

Syncope is a transient loss of consciousness and postural tone characterized by a rapid-onset, short duration of symptoms with rapid and complete recovery. The term "syncope" is derived from the Greek words *syn* and *kopto* meaning "I cut" or "I interrupt," which in this case indicates interruption of the alert and conscious state. The underlying mechanism is transient global cerebral hypoperfusion.

When approaching a patient with reported transient loss of consciousness, it is essential to differentiate syncope from nonsyncopal causes. Many conditions can present with loss of consciousness but are not syncopal in nature. These include falls, metabolic disorders (hypoglycemia, hypoxia, hyperventilation with hypocapnia), intoxications, seizure disorders, cataplexy, drop attacks, transient ischemic attacks (vertebrobasilar or carotid origin), and psychogenic pseudo-syncope. Clinicians, therefore, should approach loss of consciousness with a wide differential diagnosis given different diagnostic and prognostic implications. This review will focus on causes of true syncope.

EPIDEMIOLOGY

Syncope is a common problem. More than 500,000 cases are diagnosed every year in the United States, accounting for up to 5% of emergency care visits and up to 3% of all hospital admissions.[1,2] In young populations, the prevalence in girls is twice that of boys.[3] In the general population, data from the Framingham Study[4] suggest that the incidence of syncope is 6.2 per 1000 person-years. This indicates that a person living 70 years has a 42% chance of experiencing a syncopal event during his or her lifetime. This estimate is based on the assumption that the incidence of syncope is constant over time. However, the incidence of syncope observed in the general population increases with age such that subjects older than 70 are at highest risk.[4] In patients older than 80, the incidence of syncope is 17 to 19 per 1000 person-years.[4] For elderly patients in long-term care facilities, the incidence may be as high as 6% per year, with the chance of a recurrent syncopal event being as high as 30%.[5] Overall, reports in the literature suggest that syncope is a common problem in the overall population but

Cardiac Arrhythmia and Electrophysiology, University of Maryland, 22 South Greene Street, Room N3W77, Baltimore, MD 21201, USA
* Corresponding author.
E-mail address: asaliari@medicine.umaryland.edu

Cardiol Clin 30 (2012) 557–566
http://dx.doi.org/10.1016/j.ccl.2012.07.014
0733-8651/12/$ – see front matter © 2012 Published by Elsevier Inc.

mainly in health care settings and long-term care facilities.

CAUSES OF SYNCOPE

Although syncope is benign and self-limited in most cases, it can imply imminent risk of sudden cardiac death, especially in patients with structural heart disease. Causes of syncope can be classified as follows:

- Syncope related to cardiac arrhythmia as primary cause
- Syncope related to structural cardiac or cardiopulmonary disease
- Syncope from cerebrovascular disease
- Neurally mediated or reflex syncope
- Syncope from orthostatic hypotension

The last 2 categories carry a good prognosis in general but the first 2 are associated with an increased risk of sudden death. The causes of syncope within each category are summarized in **Box 1**.

In a study evaluating 325 consecutive patients hospitalized for syncope, an underlying cause could not be identified in up to 25% of patients.[6] The most common identifiable causes included syncope of the vasovagal type (18%), followed by cardiac arrhythmias (18%), volume depletion (12%), acute coronary syndrome (7%), and structural heart disease (6%). Other causes, including drug overdose, pulmonary embolism, and cerebrovascular accidents, accounted for the remaining 13%. Other studies suggest that reflex or neutrally mediated syncope underlies up to 58% of all syncope cases and that cardiac disease underlies up to 23% of cases.[7] Unexplained syncope accounts for 18% to 41% of cases in some series.[7,8] The most common causes of syncope are reviewed in greater detail later.

Neurally Mediated Syncope

This is the most common type of syncope and usually carries an excellent prognosis.[4] In fact, patients with neurally mediated syncope in the absence of structural heart disease have similar morbidity and mortality as patients without syncope. The diagnosis of neurally mediated syncope includes vasovagal syncope, carotid sinus hypersensitivity, glossopharyngeal neuralgia, and situational syncope with loss of consciousness occurring in specific situations (eg, micturition, deglutition). Most patients with this type of syncope experience a prodrome of symptoms from increased vagal tone. These prodromal symptoms may include a feeling of warmth, lightheadedness,

---

Box 1
Causes of syncope

Neurally mediated

Vasovagal syncope

Carotid sinus syncope

Situational syncope

Acute hemorrhage

Cough, sneeze

Postexercise

Postprandial

Gastrointestinal stimulation (swallow, defecation, visceral pain)

Micturition, postmicturition

Others (weight lifting)

Glossopharyngeal neuralgia

Orthostatic hypotension

Primary autonomic failure (pure autonomic failure, multiple system atrophy, Parkinson disease)

Secondary autonomic failure (diabetic neuropathy, amyloid neuropathy)

Volume depletion (hemorrhage, diarrhea, Addison disease)

Postexercise

Postprandial

Drug-induced orthostatic syncope

Alcohol-induced orthostatic syncope

Primary cardiac arrhythmias

Sinus node dysfunction (including bradycardia/tachycardia syndrome)

Atrioventricular conduction system disease

Paroxysmal supraventricular and ventricular tachycardias

Inherited syndromes (long QT or short QT syndrome, Brugada syndrome)

Implanted device (pacemaker, implantable cardioverter-defibrillator) malfunction

Drug-induced arrhythmias

Structural cardiac or cardiopulmonary disease

Valvular disease

Acute myocardial infarction/ischemia

Obstructive cardiomyopathy

Atrial myxoma

Acute aortic dissection

Pericardial disease/tamponade

Pulmonary embolus/pulmonary hypertension

Vascular steal syndromes

pallor, diaphoresis, nausea, vomiting, or abdominal discomfort.

Reflex syncope can occur following numerous triggers but is most commonly seen with prolonged upright posture, warm environment, emotionally stressful events, and after eating, defecating, or urinating or immediately after exercise. In patients with neurally mediated syncope, a hypersensitive reflex often referred to as the Bezold-Jarish[9] reflex triggers a cascade of events that lead to syncope. In these patients, pressure receptors in underfilled atria, great veins, or left ventricle sense increased wall stress resulting in increased vagal afferent stimuli and a sudden withdrawal of sympathetic tone. This leads to bradycardia, decreased contractility, and vasodilation with a sudden drop in blood pressure and syncope.

For carotid sinus syncope, loss of consciousness results from direct mechanical stimulation of carotid baroreceptors and can be often reproduced by carotid massage. Common triggers include shaving, wearing a tight collar, and turning of the head.

A thorough history and physical examination are usually sufficient to recognize patients with reflex syncope. However, it is essential to keep in mind that neurally mediated syncope can have atypical presentations and more serious conditions should be considered, especially in patients with structural heart disease.

Orthostasis

This is a common cause of syncope and must be differentiated from vasovagal syncope. Orthostasis refers to a drop in blood pressure of greater than 20 mm Hg or a reflex tachycardia with greater than 25% increase in heart rate in response to position changes from sitting or lying down to upright. The resultant sudden drop in blood pressure may result in syncope. The autonomic nervous system typically responds to a change from sitting to upright posture by increasing sympathetic tone. In patients with autonomic dysfunction, either primary or secondary to various diseases, medication effect, or toxins, failure to increase sympathetic tone may lead to syncope. Hypovolemia, from dehydration or acute blood loss, is another important cause of orthostatic hypotension. In these patients, autonomic reflexes may be intact but low circulatory volumes are not sufficient to maintain appropriate blood pressure.

Cardiac Arrhythmias

Syncope can result from abnormal cardiac rhythms in association with altered hemodynamics and cerebral hypoperfusion. Both bradyarrhythmia and tachyarrhythmia can lead to syncope. Examples include sinus node dysfunction, abnormal atrioventricular conduction leading to heart block, and ventricular tachycardia. Supraventricular tachycardia can also occasionally result in syncope, although this is unlikely in patients with structurally normal hearts. When evaluating patients presenting with syncope, arrhythmia should be considered because syncope in these patients, even when transient, may be a premonitory sign of imminent risk of sudden cardiac death.

Syncope From Structural Cardiovascular Disease

In patients with structural heart disease, cardiac output may not be sufficient to meet circulatory demands and syncope may result. Examples include cardiac valvular disease, acute myocardial infarction or ischemia, obstructive cardiomyopathy, atrial myxoma, acute aortic dissection, pericardial disease including tamponade, pulmonary embolus, and pulmonary hypertension. In addition, patients with structural heart disease are at increased risk of developing arrhythmia and therefore may be at increased risk of sudden death.

Other Causes of Syncope

Other conditions may be associated with syncope and should be considered when approaching a patient with transient loss of consciousness.

- Neurologic syncope: This is a rare entity. In fact, most neurologic causes of loss of consciousness are associated with focal neurologic findings that exclude the diagnosis of syncope by definition. Examples include transient ischemic attacks with otherwise no focal findings, subclavian steal syndrome, subarachnoid bleeding, and complex migraine headaches. Nevertheless, one should keep in mind that syncope can present with convulsive activity but unlike seizure disorders, the loss of consciousness is usually brief without postictal state.
- Psychiatric syncope: This is typically observed in young patients without cardiac disease who present with recurrent episodes. Patients with true syncope, however, may seem confused or anxious as a result of transient cerebral hypoperfusion, rendering the differentiation of true syncope from psychogenic syncope difficult.
- Metabolic causes: These include hypoglycemia, hypoxia, alcohol toxicity, and alcohol-induced orthostasis.

- Rare causes: These include Takayasu arteritis, systemic mastocytosis, and carcinoid.

APPROACH TO THE PATIENT WITH SYNCOPE

A careful history and physical examination are often sufficient in the evaluation of young patients with vasovagal syncope. However, the evaluation may not be as easy in patients with atypical presentations. The general approach to the patient with syncope has been addressed in guidelines published from the European Society of Cardiology[10] and the American Heart Association/American College of Cardiology.[11] In general, the strategy emphasized the most is to identify high-risk patients (**Box 2**), especially when evaluating patients in emergency care settings. Conditions posing an immediate threat to life, such as pulmonary embolism, acute hemorrhage, or intracranial bleed, should be identified. It is also essential to identify patients with cardiac syncope who are at increased risk of sudden death.[4,12,13] This is especially true for patients with heart failure.[14]

INITIAL EVALUATION

The initial approach, consisting of a thorough history, physical examination, and ECG, may lead to the diagnosis in almost half of the patients.[15] In patients undergoing initial testing targeting a clinically suspected diagnosis, the initial approach can establish a diagnosis in 75% of the patients.[16] Extensive cardiovascular testing performed in patients without a clear diagnosis after the initial approach establishes a diagnosis in only 25%.[16]

Box 2
Syncope red flags

- Presence of structural heart disease
- Prior myocardial infarction
- Patients with pacemaker or defibrillator
- Syncope occurring during exercise
- Abnormal electrocardiogram (ECG)
- Family history of sudden death
- Syncope resulting in severe injury
- Frequent and recurrent episodes ($\geq$2 episodes in a 1-year period)
- Associated palpitations
- High-risk occupation, possible severe personal or collateral injury

---

History

When approaching a patient with syncope, it is essential to determine whether the event was true syncope or loss of consciousness from other causes, to identify patients with red flags (see **Box 2**) who are at increased risk of sudden death and to assess for any potential injury that happened as a consequence of the event.

- Patient's age: Syncope in young patients is often neurocardiogenic. Elements of the story suggesting more serious causes include loss of consciousness during exercise, family history of sudden cardiac death, history of congenital heart disease, or prolonged QT interval on ECG. In the elderly, syncope is usually associated with worse outcomes compared with younger patients.[17] These patients are more likely to have structural heart disease, more cardiovascular risk factors, dysautonomia, and orthostasis and are often on multiple medications, placing them at a higher risk of syncope. Adverse outcomes in this population may be related to the presence of heart disease instead of age itself.[18]
- Triggers and associated symptoms: The triggers and associated symptoms may suggest specific diagnoses. Dyspnea raises concern for pulmonary embolus or heart failure. Chest pain raises concerns for acute coronary syndrome or pulmonary embolus. Palpitations suggest that arrhythmia may be the underlying cause. Neurologic symptoms may suggest a neurologic cause, although, as noted, seizures may be seen with any disorder that leads to cerebral hypoperfusion. Certain triggers are associated with neurocardiogenic syncope, and the most typical of those are strong physical or emotional stress, micturition, defecation, coughing, swallowing, and prolonged standing in a warm environment. Specific triggers suggest situational syncope, whereas prodromal symptoms may suggest neurocardiogenic syncope, especially in younger patients. Patients with reflex syncope may experience feelings of warmth, nausea, vomiting, diaphoresis, or pallor, either before or shortly after the event. Factors suggesting seizures include aura symptoms, abrupt onset of symptoms with injury, tonic or tonic-clonic activity, head deviation, tongue biting, loss of bowel or bladder control, and postictal confusion.

- Position: The position in which the event occurs may help establish the diagnosis. Syncope after prolonged standing, especially in warm weather, suggests neurocardiogenic syncope. Syncope occurring in an upright position shortly after standing is usually related to orthostatic hypotension. The suspicion for arrhythmia should be high in patients with syncope in the sitting or supine position.[7]
- Onset: The presence of prodromal symptoms typically suggests neurocardiogenic syncope. The sudden onset of loss of consciousness without prodromal signs suggests arrhythmia.[17,19]
- Type of episode: Elements of the history help differentiate syncope from nonsyncopal causes of loss of consciousness. Syncope is usually associated with complete loss of consciousness, of sudden onset but short duration, with loss of postural tone and followed by immediate and complete recovery to baseline mental status. An episode with those characteristics is very likely to be syncope. When one of those elements is absent or in doubt, other causes of loss of consciousness should be considered.
- Syncope during exercise: Although neurocardiogenic syncope can rarely occur during exercise, this is exceedingly uncommon. Syncope during exercise is associated with an increased risk of sudden death[20,21] and therefore should raise the suspicion of arrhythmia or cardiac outflow obstruction (ie, hypertrophic obstructive cardiomyopathy, aortic stenosis). These patients should undergo a thorough evaluation for cardiac causes of syncope.
- Comorbid conditions: The presence of cardiac disease should raise the possibility of cardiac syncope. Preexisting neurologic conditions point toward neurologic causes such as seizures. In patients with a psychiatric history, syncope may be related to panic attacks or hyperventilation or secondary to medications or toxic substances, although cardiac causes should still be on the differential.
- Medications: Reviewing the patient's medications may help identify a culprit medication. Medications potentially associated with syncope include antihypertensives (calcium channel blockers, β-blockers, α-blockers, nitrates, and diuretics), antiarrhythmics, and medications affecting the QT interval (antipsychotics and antiemetics).
- Family history: Cardiac syncope must be considered in patients with a history of sudden death or early onset of cardiovascular disease in first-degree relatives.[22] Genetic disorders associated with syncope include long QT syndrome, Brugada syndrome, arrhythmogenic right ventricular cardiomyopathy, and idiopathic polymorphic ventricular tachycardia.

Physical Examination

A focused physical examination including vital signs and cardiovascular and neurologic examinations should be performed first. Further examination needs to focus on specific complaints and identify potential associated injuries. Certain findings on physical examination point toward specific causes.

- Abnormal vital signs: Orthostatic hypotension may be the cause of syncope in patients with orthostasis on physical examination. It is important to keep in mind, however, that vital signs are neither sensitive nor specific for the assessment of volume status or causes of syncope.[23,24] A blood pressure of 90 mm Hg or less in orthostatic patients is, however, highly suggestive of hypovolemia. Bradycardia or tachycardia suggests cardiac arrhythmia. Hyperventilation suggests panic attack or psychiatric causes but may also be related to a metabolic cause of syncope. Low oxygen saturations in patients with syncope suggest heart failure or pulmonary embolism as possible causes.
- Cardiac auscultation: Patients with abnormal auscultatory findings suggesting structural heart disease need more extensive workup to identify those at risk of sudden death. On auscultation, potential findings in association with syncope are murmurs (aortic stenosis, mitral stenosis, obstructive cardiomyopathy), presence of S3, S4, or gallop (heart failure), loud P2 (pulmonary hypertension), or plop (atrial myxoma).
- Lung examination: Crackles or wheezes on auscultation may be heard in patients with heart failure.
- Vascular examination: Palpation of pulses in the neck and all 4 extremities is important. Unequal pulses may be found in patients with aortic dissection. The presence of peripheral vascular disease may be a marker of systemic atherosclerosis including coronary disease. Carotid murmur

may be heard in carotid stenosis. Elevated jugular venous pressure suggests heart failure.

- Neurologic examination: Focal neurologic findings suggest neurologic causes of loss of consciousness. In patients with true syncope, patients return by definition to baseline neurologic function. It is important, however, to look for subtle neurologic abnormalities that may be related to a stroke or transient ischemic attack.
- Other associations of physical examination findings: When approaching a patient with possible syncope, it also important to consider the following:
  ○ Look for injuries; some of those may be serious, especially if head trauma is involved.
  ○ Lateral tongue laceration may suggest seizure.
  ○ Incontinence suggests seizure.
  ○ Rectal examination is performed to rule out gastrointestinal bleed.
  ○ A focused examination to address the patient's complaints or history is important.

Electrocardiography

Although it is not a component of the physical examination, the importance of obtaining a 12-lead ECG for patients with syncope cannot be overstressed. This should be part of the initial evaluation of every patient with syncope. Despite its low diagnostic yield, it is inexpensive and easy to obtain and will help to identify patients with a potential arrhythmic cause of their syncope. Electrocardiographic findings suggestive of arrhythmia include[10]:

- Bifascicular block (defined as left bundle branch block or right bundle branch block combined with left anterior or left posterior fascicular block)
- Other intraventricular conduction abnormalities (QRS duration ≥ 0.12 second)
- Mobitz I second-degree atrioventricular block
- Asymptomatic sinus bradycardia (<50 beats per minute), sinoatrial block, or sinus pause (>3 seconds) in the absence of negative chronotropic medications[10]
- Preexcited QRS complexes, suggesting Wolff-Parkinson-White syndrome
- Long or short QT intervals
- Right bundle branch block pattern with ST-segment elevation in leads V_1 to V_3 (Brugada syndrome)

- Negative T waves in right precordial leads, epsilon waves, and ventricular late potentials suggestive of arrhythmogenic right ventricular cardiomyopathy
- Q waves suggesting myocardial infarction

Some electrocardiographic findings are diagnostic for arrhythmia-related syncope.[10] These include:

- Persistent sinus bradycardia less than 40 beats per minute
- Repetitive sinoatrial blocks or sinus pauses greater than 3 seconds[10]
- Mobitz II second- or third-degree atrioventricular block
- Alternating left and right bundle branch block
- Ventricular tachycardia or rapid paroxysmal supraventricular tachycardia
- Pacemaker or implantable cardioverter-defibrillator malfunction with cardiac pauses

In acute or in-hospital settings, telemonitoring may help identifying arrhythmias or ECG features in association with arrhythmia-related syncope.[25]

OTHER TESTING

Numerous tests can be used for the evaluation of patients with possible syncope. However, the diagnostic yield is the highest when testing strategies are guided by the clinical presentation and initial evaluation. Routine laboratory tests obtained in patients with acute syncope include complete blood counts, glucose levels, basic metabolic panel, and electrolytes; others should be considered depending on the clinical scenario. The following testing strategy is recommended as the initial approach by the 2009 guidelines from the European Society of Cardiology[10]:

- Carotid sinus massage in patients older than 40 years
- Echocardiogram when there is previous known heart disease or data suggestive of structural heart disease or syncope secondary to cardiovascular cause
- Immediate ECG monitoring when there is a suspicion of arrhythmic syncope
- Orthostatic challenge (lying to standing orthostatic test or head-up tilt testing) when syncope is related to the standing position or there is suspicion of a reflex mechanism
- Other less-specific tests such as neurologic evaluation or blood tests indicated only when there is suspicion of nonsyncopal transient loss of consciousness

Carotid Sinus Massage

This may help identifying patients with carotid hypersensitivity. A positive response with long pauses (>3 seconds) or with a drop in blood pressure of greater than 50 mm Hg is diagnostic and is highly predictive of the occurrence of spontaneous asystolic episodes. This maneuver should be avoided in patients with recent stroke or transient ischemic attack and those with carotid murmurs, unless a Doppler study is done and confirms no carotid stenosis.

Orthostatic Challenge

This can be performed with active standing and serial measurements of blood pressure or with tilt table testing, a modality that is more widely used in clinical practice. One should keep in mind that orthostatic challenge testing, including tilt table testing, has limited specificity, sensitivity, and reproducibility. It should be reserved for patients suspected to have neurocardiogenic syncope but in whom the initial evaluation failed to confirm the diagnosis. In this subset of patients, it performs fairly well in identifying patients susceptible to reflex syncope. In patients without structural heart disease, reproducing syncope is diagnostic. However, in patients with structural heart disease, other cardiovascular causes of syncope should still be ruled out even with a positive tilt test. Another application of this test modality in patients with syncope is the identification of patients with orthostatic syndromes.[10]

Echocardiography

This modality should be considered for patients suspected to have structural heart disease on the initial evaluation. Our practice typically maintains a low threshold for requesting echocardiograms on patients presenting with syncope. It can identify patients with left ventricular dysfunction, segmental wall motion abnormalities, valvular disease, hypertrophic cardiomyopathy, and pericardial or aortic disease.[26] It may also suggest pulmonary embolism in patients with right ventricular dysfunction or elevated pulmonary pressures. The presence of severe aortic stenosis, obstructive tumor or thrombus, cardiac tamponade, or aortic dissection is considered diagnostic as a cause for syncope. The presence of other structural heart disease is only suggestive but not diagnostic of cardiac syncope, and further testing is often required. In emergency settings, bedside echocardiography is increasingly used in clinical practice, but its role is not well established in patients with syncope.

Cardiac Monitoring

This is usually indicated for patients suspected of having arrhythmia-related syncope. In-hospital telemetry, 24- to 48-hour Holter monitors, or longer-term event recorder monitors may provide useful information regarding arrhythmia in patients with syncope. Their diagnostic value is, however, limited because they provide little to no information if syncope does not occur during the monitoring period.[8,27] An asymptomatic arrhythmia does not prove arrhythmia-related syncope, but the absence of arrhythmia during an event essentially rules out arrhythmia as the cause of syncope.[27] Electrocardiographic monitoring is diagnostic when tachyarrhythmia or bradyarrhythmia is documented during the event.

Holter Monitoring

Short-term cardiac monitors (24- to 48-hour Holter monitoring) may be useful, but their diagnostic yield is very limited because of the intermittent nature of syncope. They help in diagnosing fewer than 3% of patients, but they may be helpful in selecting patients for electrophysiologic invasive studies.[28] Short-term monitors are generally useful only in patients experiencing syncope on a daily basis.

External Event Recorders

External event recorders allow longer periods of monitoring and have better diagnostic yields than short-term monitors.[27] They can usually be ordered in up to 30-day intervals. These recorders temporarily store several minutes of electrophysiologic data. The patient is provided with a trigger button that allows them to activate the device after the event and thereby permanently store a tracing from the time of the event.[29] To provide the highest diagnostic yield, the patient should be instructed to activate the monitor during any syncopal prodrome or immediately after experiencing a syncopal event. Although most of these recorders are capable of autorecording bradycardic or tachycardic events that meet certain preprogrammed criteria, their diagnostic yield remains limited by the dependence on patient activation.

Implantable Loop Recorders

In patients with infrequent syncope occurring at less than 1- or 2-month intervals in whom noninvasive testing fails to establish a diagnosis, implantable loop recorders may be helpful. These are typically implanted in left parasternal or precordial regions and have a battery life of up to 36 months. These devices can be activated either by the patient or according to programmed algorithms for tachycardia and bradycardia detection thresholds. The most commonly observed rhythms in association with syncope with these devices are transient bradyarrhythmias. Symptoms in association with normal sinus rhythm are also common.[30,31]

For patients with neurocardiogenic syncope, loop recorders can establish the diagnosis better than provocative testing. However, sinus node and atrioventricular node dysfunction are hard to differentiate from neurocardiogenic syncope on loop recorders. In patients with structural heart disease, especially those with previous myocardial infarction, early provocative testing may be preferred to loop recorders because they allow early treatment planning. However, in patients without structural heart disease, loop recorders may be the preferred strategy.[30–32] Loop recorders seem to be safe and cost effective.[32]

The current guidelines recommend loop recorders for early-phase evaluation of patients with recurrent syncope of uncertain origin who have no high-risk criteria and a high likelihood of recurrence within the battery life of the device and of those with high-risk features in whom extensive workup failed to lead to a diagnosis or specific treatment, as well as for the assessment of whether bradycardia is a culprit in patients with suspected reflex syncope with frequent or traumatic episodes before considering pacemaker insertion.

Exercise Testing

Exercise testing may be indicated in patients with a high likelihood of coronary disease and ischemia and those with syncope during exercise. It is imperative, however, to rule out aortic stenosis or hypertrophic cardiomyopathy before exercise testing. The diagnostic yield of exercise testing is low but it may be helpful in the following settings[10]:

- It is considered diagnostic when syncope is reproduced during or immediately after exercise in the presence of ECG abnormalities or severe hypotension.
- It is also considered diagnostic when Mobitz II second- or third-degree atrioventricular block develops during exercise even without syncope.
- In patients younger than 40 years, hypotension during exercise may indicate left main coronary artery disease or hypertrophic cardiomyopathy, as potential underlying structural heart disease in association with syncope.

- In patients with prolonged QT interval, failure of the QT to shorten suggests a congenital QT syndrome.

Patients with suspected ischemia on exercise testing may benefit from cardiac catheterization. In patients with exertional syncope who are suspected to have anomalous coronary artery origin as the cause of their events, coronary angiography is often not required to establish the diagnosis. In those patients, cardiac magnetic resonance imaging or computed tomography may be sufficient for the diagnosis. Cardiac magnetic resonance imaging or computed tomography may also be helpful in patients suspected to have arrhythmogenic right ventricular dysplasia, cardiac sarcoidosis, or other infiltrative disease process as an underlying cause of syncope.

Invasive Electrophysiologic Studies

These are very useful with the highest diagnostic yield being in patients with structural heart disease who have otherwise no indications for implantable cardioverter-defibrillators. In such patient populations, electrophysiologic studies (EPS) may be positive in up to 50% of patients.[33] EPS are recommended for patients with ischemic heart disease when arrhythmia-related syncope is suspected and in patients with bundle branch block when other testing fails to establish the diagnosis. It is important to keep in mind that an ischemia workup is often required in patients with ischemic heart disease before performing EPS.[11] Although EPS is often useful in the evaluation of syncope caused by malignant tachycardias, such as ventricular tachycardia, its use in diagnosing bradycardia-mediated syncope is somewhat limited.

Useful Tips for the Clinician: Risk Stratification

The overall approach to the patient with syncope based on what we discussed may be complex and very costly. A simple approach to identify patients who need testing consists of the following:

- History, physical examination, and ECG are very important in the initial evaluation.
- The clinical features and associated symptoms are very helpful and may suggest specific diagnoses.
- Identify the red flags in association with risk for sudden death (see **Box 2**).
- Syncope during exertion needs serious investigation.
- High-risk features require early and intensive workup on an inpatient basis.
- Single or rare episodes in patients with low-risk features do not usually necessitate

invasive diagnostic workup. The diagnosis in most of these patients is reflex syncope.

- Workup is indicated in low-risk patients with recurrent episodes or serious injury even if the history suggests reflex syncope.

REFERENCES

1. Day SC, Cook EF, Funkenstein H, et al. Evaluation and outcome of emergency room patients with transient loss of consciousness. Am J Med 1982;73:15–23.
2. Silverstein MD, Singer DE, Mulley AG, et al. Patients with syncope admitted to medical intensive care units. JAMA 1982;248:1185–9.
3. Ganzeboom KS, Colman N, Reitsma JB, et al. Prevalence and triggers of syncope in medical students. Am J Cardiol 2003;91:1006–8. A8.
4. Soteriades ES, Evans JC, Larson MG, et al. Incidence and prognosis of syncope. N Engl J Med 2002;347:878–85.
5. Lipsitz LA, Wei JY, Rowe JW. Syncope in an elderly, institutionalised population: prevalence, incidence, and associated risk. Q J Med 1985;55:45–54.
6. Sule S, Palaniswamy C, Aronow WS, et al. Etiology of syncope in patients hospitalized with syncope and predictors of mortality and rehospitalization for syncope at 27-month follow-up. Clin Cardiol 2011; 34:35–8.
7. Alboni P, Brignole M, Menozzi C, et al. Diagnostic value of history in patients with syncope with or without heart disease. J Am Coll Cardiol 2001;37: 1921–8.
8. Kapoor WN. Evaluation and outcome of patients with syncope. Medicine (Baltimore) 1990;69:160–75.
9. Chang-Sing P, Peter CT. Syncope: evaluation and management. A review of current approaches to this multifaceted and complex clinical problem. Cardiol Clin 1991;9:641–51.
10. Task Force for the Diagnosis and Management of Syncope, European Society of Cardiology (ESC), European Heart Rhythm Association (EHRA), et al. Guidelines for the diagnosis and management of syncope (version 2009). Eur Heart J 2009;30: 2631–71.
11. Strickberger SA, Benson DW, Biaggioni I, et al. AHA/ACCF scientific statement on the evaluation of syncope: from the American Heart Association Councils on Clinical Cardiology, Cardiovascular Nursing, Cardiovascular Disease in the Young, and Stroke, and the Quality of Care and Outcomes Research Interdisciplinary Working Group; and the American College of Cardiology Foundation in collaboration with the Heart Rhythm Society. J Am Coll Cardiol 2006;47:473–84.
12. Kapoor WN, Karpf M, Wieand S, et al. A prospective evaluation and follow-up of patients with syncope. N Engl J Med 1983;309:197–204.
13. Quinn JV, Stiell IG, McDermott DA, et al. Derivation of the San Francisco syncope rule to predict patients with short-term serious outcomes. Ann Emerg Med 2004;43:224–32.
14. Middlekauff HR, Stevenson WG, Stevenson LW, et al. Syncope in advanced heart failure: high risk of sudden death regardless of origin of syncope. J Am Coll Cardiol 1993;21:110–6.
15. Linzer M, Yang EH, Estes NA 3rd, et al. Diagnosing syncope. Part 1: value of history, physical examination, and electrocardiography. Clinical Efficacy Assessment Project of the American College of Physicians. Ann Intern Med 1997;126:989–96.
16. Sarasin FP, Louis-Simonet M, Carballo D, et al. Prospective evaluation of patients with syncope: a population-based study. Am J Med 2001;111: 177–84.
17. Calkins H, Shyr Y, Frumin H, et al. The value of the clinical history in the differentiation of syncope due to ventricular tachycardia, atrioventricular block, and neurocardiogenic syncope. Am J Med 1995; 98:365–73.
18. Kapoor WN, Hanusa BH. Is syncope a risk factor for poor outcomes? comparison of patients with and without syncope. Am J Med 1996;100:646–55.
19. Krahn AD, Klein GJ, Yee R, et al. Predictive value of presyncope in patients monitored for assessment of syncope. Am Heart J 2001;141:817–21.
20. Sakaguchi S, Shultz JJ, Remole SC, et al. Syncope associated with exercise, a manifestation of neurally mediated syncope. Am J Cardiol 1995;75:476–81.
21. Colivicchi F, Ammirati F, Biffi A, et al. Exercise-related syncope in young competitive athletes without evidence of structural heart disease. Clinical presentation and long-term outcome. Eur Heart J 2002;23:1125–30.
22. Driscoll DJ, Jacobsen SJ, Porter CJ, et al. Syncope in children and adolescents. J Am Coll Cardiol 1997; 29:1039–45.
23. Sarasin FP, Louis-Simonet M, Carballo D, et al. Prevalence of orthostatic hypotension among patients presenting with syncope in the ED. Am J Emerg Med 2002;20:497–501.
24. Baraff LJ, Schriger DL. Orthostatic vital signs: variation with age, specificity, and sensitivity in detecting a 450-mL blood loss. Am J Emerg Med 1992;10: 99–103.
25. Bass EB, Curtiss EI, Arena VC, et al. The duration of Holter monitoring in patients with syncope. is 24 hours enough? Arch Intern Med 1990;150:1073–8.
26. Sarasin FP, Junod AF, Carballo D, et al. Role of echocardiography in the evaluation of syncope: a prospective study. Heart 2002;88:363–7.
27. Sivakumaran S, Krahn AD, Klein GJ, et al. A prospective randomized comparison of loop recorders versus Holter monitors in patients with syncope or presyncope. Am J Med 2003;115:1–5.

28. Bachinsky WB, Linzer M, Weld L, et al. Usefulness of clinical characteristics in predicting the outcome of electrophysiologic studies in unexplained syncope. Am J Cardiol 1992;69:1044–9.

29. Linzer M, Pritchett EL, Pontinen M, et al. Incremental diagnostic yield of loop electrocardiographic recorders in unexplained syncope. Am J Cardiol 1990;66:214–9.

30. Krahn AD, Klein GJ, Yee R, et al. Randomized assessment of syncope trial: conventional diagnostic testing versus a prolonged monitoring strategy. Circulation 2001;104:46–51.

31. Farwell DJ, Freemantle N, Sulke AN. Use of implantable loop recorders in the diagnosis and management of syncope. Eur Heart J 2004;25: 1257–63.

32. Krahn AD, Klein GJ, Yee R, et al. The high cost of syncope: cost implications of a new insertable loop recorder in the investigation of recurrent syncope. Am Heart J 1999;137:870–7.

33. Linzer M, Yang EH, Estes NA 3rd, et al. Diagnosing syncope. Part 2: unexplained syncope. Clinical Efficacy Assessment Project of the American College of Physicians. Ann Intern Med 1997;127:76–86.

Acute Management of Atrial Fibrillation
From Emergency Department to Cardiac Care Unit

Hiroko Beck, MD, Vincent Y. See, MD*

KEYWORDS

- Atrial fibrillation • Cardioversion • Rate control • Rhythm control • Stroke • Thromboembolism
- Arrhythmia • Anticoagulation

KEY POINTS

- Atrial fibrillation is a complex disorder resulting from various causes that include reversible causes and progressive arrhythmic substrates that underlie initiation, recurrence, persistence, and progression of atrial fibrillation.
- Primary management goals include (1) accurate diagnosis, (2) clinical stabilization, (3) recognition and treatment of reversible causes and risk factors, (4) symptom management with rate and/or rhythm control, and (5) prevention of cardioembolic events.
- Atrial fibrillation may present with heterogeneous symptoms and severity that affect quality of life to varying degrees and may cloud initial evaluation.
- Restoration and maintenance of sinus rhythm have the primary goal of symptom control. This may not be required in all patients in the absence of mortality benefit but may improve quality of life.
- Multiple tools are available to stratify thromboembolic and hemorrhagic risks to guide optimal and safe methods of stroke prevention, which must be determined acutely and reassessed chronically.

INTRODUCTION

Atrial fibrillation (AF) has challenged physicians for more than 800 years since it was initially described by Maimonides in 1187.[1] Despite improved understanding of mechanism and therapy, optimal strategies to manage AF remain unclear.[2] Acute management goals include diagnosis, clinical stabilization, symptom control of rate and/or rhythm, thromboembolic stroke prevention, and treatment of reversible causes. Optimized and individualized therapy based on these goals allows smooth transition from acute to long-term AF care and risk modification.

Definition

AF is a supraventricular tachyarrhythmia characterized by rapid, chaotic atrial activity with fibrillatory or absent P waves on electrocardiography (ECG) that vary in amplitude and morphology, and with atrial rates that frequently exceed 300 beats per minute (bpm) (**Fig. 1**). In the presence of intact atrioventricular (AV) conduction, the

Disclosures: None.
Cardiac Electrophysiology Section, Division of Cardiology, Department of Medicine, University of Maryland School of Medicine, University of Maryland Medical Center, N3W77, 22 South Greene Street, Baltimore, MD 21201, USA
* Corresponding author.
E-mail address: vsee@medicine.umaryland.edu

Cardiol Clin 30 (2012) 567–589
http://dx.doi.org/10.1016/j.ccl.2012.07.007

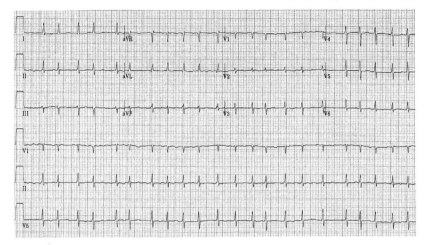

Fig. 1. AF with rapid ventricular response.

ventricular response rate is typically irregularly irregular with chaotic, rapid, and varying RR intervals. Abnormal AV conduction may blunt ventricular response rates. Atrial flutter (AFL) has been classified in multiple ways but is typically characterized by rapid, organized atrial activity at 250 to 350 bpm with negative sawtooth waves in the inferior ECG leads II, III, aVF and positive or biphasic waves in lead V1 (**Fig. 2**). Despite the organized nature of AFL, long-term complications and stroke

risk are similar to those of AF.[3,4] Recommendations made in this article include AFL unless otherwise specified.

Epidemiology

AF is the most common arrhythmia, with estimated incidence of more than 75,000 and prevalence of more than 2.2 to 2.3 million in the United States and more than 6 million in the European Union

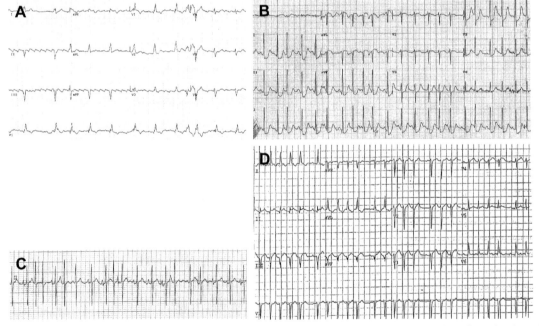

Fig. 2. Rhythms that may imitate AF. (*A*) Atrial flutter: typical negative sawtooth P waves in the inferior leads and positive P waves in V1 with variable atrioventricular block. (*B*) Sinus tachycardia with frequent atrial premature beats. (*C*) Multifocal atrial tachycardia: more than 3 discrete P wave morphologies are highlighted. (*D*) Atrial tachycardia with Mobitz I, second degree AV block (Wenckebach). (*Courtesy of* Stephen W. Smith, MD, Hennepin County Medical Center and University of Minnesota [*B*].)

(EU).[5–7] In the Medicare population, AF prevalence increased 5% per year between 1993 and 2007.[8] AF accounts for one-third of US hospitalizations with more than 529,000 annual discharges.[5,6] AF hospital admissions have increased 66% in the past 20 years.[9] Growth of the aging population and prevalent cardiopulmonary disorders, including hypertension, coronary artery disease (CAD), heart failure (HF), and valvular disease, contribute to increasing AF incidence (**Table 1**).[5,7] Systemic disorders including obesity, diabetes, and bronchopulmonary disease contribute to increasing AF prevalence, morbidity, and mortality, including HF and stroke.[10–14]

Approximately 15% to 20% of ischemic stroke is attributed to AF.[5,15,16] The ischemic stroke rate among patients with nonvalvular AF averages 5% per year, increases with age, and is 2 to 7 times the rate in patients without AF.[5,15,16]

AF is associated with increased overall and cardiovascular mortality.[17] Whether this is caused by AF or associated comorbid risks is unclear. However, interventions to maintain sinus rhythm (SR) once AF has occurred have not shown mortality benefit and highlight the importance of cardiovascular risk prevention.[18,19]

Causes and Pathophysiology

The pathophysiology of AF is multilayered and complex. Some reversible causes of AF include thyroid dysfunction, pain, and infection, and post-surgical states are associated with high rates of spontaneous conversion on correction of these conditions (see **Table 1**).[7,15] Approximately 50% of all AF in the emergency department (ED) spontaneously reverts to SR within 48 hours.[20] Whether this represents resolution of acute triggers or early events in AF natural history may be difficult to discriminate.

AF risk factors such as cardiopulmonary disease and aging initiate structural and electrophysiologic remodeling that underlie the recurrence, persistence, and progression of AF. AF begets further AF with progressive alterations in cardiomyocytes, cardiac fibroblasts, interstitial and microvascular architecture, systemic inflammatory state, cell coupling, left atrial (LA) dilatation, and

---

Table 1
Causes, risk factors, and associated conditions for AF

Reversible Conditions Associated with AF	Conditions Associated with Left Atrial Arrhythmic Substrate and AF
Alcohol intake (holiday heart syndrome)	Aging
Postoperative stress	Cardiovascular disease
Postcardiothoracic surgery (early)	• Hypertension
Pain	• Valvular disease
Infection	○ Mitral, aortic
Sepsis/systemic inflammatory response syndrome	• CAD
Myocardial infarction	• Heart failure
Pericarditis	○ Systolic, diastolic
Myocarditis	• Left ventricular hypertrophy
Pulmonary embolism	• Cardiomyopathy
Pneumonia	○ Hypertrophic
Asthma/chronic obstructive pulmonary disease exacerbation	○ Idiopathic/dilated
	○ Primary electrical
Hyperthyroidism	• Congenital heart disease
Electrolyte abnormality	○ Atrial septal defect
Autonomic tone	○ Other congenital defects
Sympathetic	• Infiltrative disorders
Parasympathetic (or vagal)	○ Amyloidosis
Associated underlying arrhythmia:	• Inflammatory sarcoidosis
• Atrial flutter	Familial/genetic
• Wolff-Parkinson-White syndrome	Pulmonary
• Atrioventricular node reentry tachycardia	• Chronic obstructive pulmonary disease
	• Obstructive sleep apnea
	Chronic kidney disease
	Systemic
	• Obesity
	• Diabetes mellitus

ion channels.[2,21] Atrial refractory properties, downregulation of L-type inward Ca^{2+} current, and upregulation of inward rectifier potassium (K^+) currents are altered within hours of AF onset.[7]

Classification

AF classifications presented in the 2006 American College of Cardiology (ACC)/American Heart Association (AHA)/European Society of Cardiology (ESC) and 2010 ESC Guidelines for AF are most commonly used because of their simplicity and clinical relevance (**Box 1**).[7,15] Asymptomatic AF episodes occur in patients with symptomatic AF.[22] Whether termination with antiarrhythmic therapy (AAT) or cardioversion alters paroxysmal or persistent AF designations varies with the 2006 or 2010 guidelines.[7,15] Long-standing persistent AF includes episodes of more than 1 year that frequently progress to permanent AF. Permanent

AF has been unsuccessfully cardioverted or accepted within a long-term rate-control strategy.

The natural history of AF typically includes clusters of initially brief, rare paroxysms that evolve to longer and more frequent episodes. Among patients without conditions that promote AF, the long-term risk of continued AF is 2% to 3%.[23] Over 25 years, ~31% of patients with paroxysmal or persistent AF progress to permanent AF.[23]

Socioeconomic Ramifications

AF is one of the most substantial economic burdens on the US health care system. Symptoms, sequelae, and psychological stress contribute to health care use, impaired quality of life, and likely loss of occupational productivity.[24,25] AF accounted for 276,000 ED and hospital outpatient visits in 2001.[26] Between 1996 and 2001, hospital discharges with a primary diagnosis of AF increased 34%.[5] In 2004, the estimated annual cost per patient was $3600.[27] Medicare expenditures related to AF have been estimated at $16 billion annually.[28]

Acute Evaluation in the ED

Successful transition of AF care depends on initial risk stratification and acute management. Initial AF assessment occurs in various inpatient or outpatient settings but often starts in the ED. Recommendations in this article are relevant to any site of initial AF management.

MANAGEMENT GOALS

Acute management of AF begins with accurate diagnosis, treatment of underlying causes and risks, acute stabilization, symptom control with rate and/or rhythm control, thromboembolic stroke risk stratification and modification, and transition to chronic management to prevent recurrence and complications of AF (**Fig. 3**).

Diagnosis

Focused but thorough history, including medical and procedural history, social and medication history, family history, physical examination, laboratory testing, and cardiac imaging, may elucidate AF patterns and causes.[7,15] Medication history identifies prior AF therapy and potential drug interactions. Family history increases AF risk 2-fold if any family member (and 4.7-fold if any family member aged <60 years) is affected by AF.[29] Physical examination frequently reveals an irregular pulse rate by palpation or auscultation. Essential examination features include signs of underlying causes, end-organ hypoperfusion, and HF.

Box 1
Classification of AF

First detected: no previously detected AF; duration and onset may be unknown.

Paroxysmal: recurrent episodes that self-terminate in less than 7 days.

Persistent: recurrent episodes that last more than 7 days

Long-standing persistent: persistent AF of more than 1 year's duration.

Permanent: ongoing long-term episodes accepted as part of a rate-control strategy or refractory to rhythm control.

Lone: AF in age less than 60 years in absence of clinical or echocardiographic findings of cardiopulmonary disease including hypertension. Prognosis in relation to mortality and thromboembolism is favorable.

Nonvalvular: episodes occur in absence of rheumatic mitral valve disease, a prosthetic heart valve, or mitral valve repair.

Secondary: episodes occur as a result of reversible causes such as acute myocardial ischemia, cardiac surgery, pericarditis, myocarditis, hyperthyroidism, or acute pulmonary disease.

Silent: asymptomatic episodes. Appreciation of subtle symptoms may develop. May also be paroxysmal, persistent, or permanent.

These terms typically apply to episodes of AF of more than 30 seconds in duration without reversible cause.

Classifications of AF are not mutually exclusive.

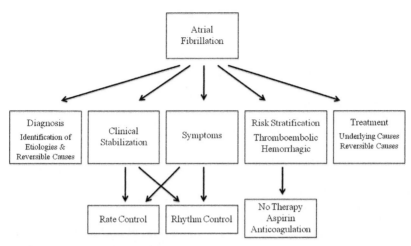

Fig. 3. Summary of acute management goals in AF.

AF presentations may vary with profound, subtle, or no symptoms. Initial manifestations may include hemodynamic instability, palpitations, cardiomyopathy, and stroke. More often, symptoms are subtle and nonspecific, including altered exercise tolerance, exertional dyspnea, and fatigue. AF may resolve before evaluation, and ambulatory cardiac rhythm monitoring may identify paroxysmal arrhythmias.

Diagnosis of AF requires high-quality ECG interpretation. AF frequently presents with rapid ventricular response (RVR) defined by ventricular rate more than 100 bpm (see **Fig. 1**). Other supraventricular tachyarrhythmias may mimic AF (see **Fig. 2**). Discriminating characteristics of these rhythms are reviewed in **Table 2**.

AF may present as wide complex tachycardia that may be challenging to differentiate from

Table 2
Discriminating characteristics of rhythms that imitate AF

	P Waves	Rhythm	Rate (bpm)
AF	Lack of organized or discernible P waves Coarse fibrillatory waves may mimic atrial flutter	Irregularly irregular QRS	Atrial: 300–600 Ventricular: normal, tachycardia, bradycardia
Multifocal atrial tachycardia	≥3 different P wave morphologies	Irregular Irregularly irregular	Atrial: >100–250 Ventricular: variable but often RVR rate
Sinus tachycardia with premature atrial complexes	Preservation of sinus P waves with intermittent PACs that may differ in P wave morphology	May seem irregular	Sinus P wave morphology and normal P wave axis >100 PACs with different coupling interval and morphology vs sinus
Atrial flutter	Counterclockwise or typical: (−) sawtooth pattern in inferior leads and (+) or biphasic in V1 Clockwise: opposite P wave findings Atypical: none of the waves listed earlier, usually with abnormal atrial substrate such as prior atrial ablation or cardiac surgery	P waves: regular QRS: regular or irregular	Atrial rate ~300 2:1 AV block frequently → ventricular rate ~150 (or multiples of atrial rate) Atrial rate and AV conduction may slow with AAT

Abbreviation: PAC, premature atrial contraction.

ventricular tachycardia. Preexisting bundle branch block (BBB), rate-related BBB, or aberrant conduction may manifest with wide complex tachycardia (**Fig. 4**). AAT or digoxin (Lanoxin) may regularize AF and require altered ECG sweep speed or duration for diagnosis.

On diagnosing AF, ECGs should be further reviewed for signs of predisposing factors, structural heart disease (SHD), or critical conditions that alter acute management. Some conditions apparent on ECG that predispose to AF risk include atrial enlargement, left ventricle (LV) hypertrophy, myocardial ischemia or myocardial infarction (MI), pulmonary conditions, pericardial disease, drug toxicity, hypothermia, and metabolic derangements (**Fig. 5**; see **Table 1**).

Assessment and Therapeutic Plan

Initial assessment includes determination of cardiopulmonary stability, symptom onset and severity, and thromboembolic versus hemorrhagic risk (see **Fig. 3**). Understanding AF causes, patterns, and stability stratifies patient risk and disposition. Detection of reversible or exacerbating causes allows rapid treatment and risk reduction (see **Table 1**). Evaluation for CAD is frequently initiated, but myocardial ischemia may contribute to, or result from, AF. Coronary evaluation should be tailored to CAD pretest probability based on signs and symptoms.

Echocardiography is an essential part of overall AF evaluation to determine cardiac structure and function. However, acute use of echocardiography is not recommended for AF alone and should be tailored to clinical suspicion of critical causes based on appropriateness guidelines.[30]

Acute Management of Patients with Symptoms or Hemodynamic Instability

Initial triage is determined by hemodynamic stability and symptoms. Myocardial ischemia, hypotension, angina, or HF prompts urgent therapy. Urgent electrical direct current cardioversion (DCC) is recommended in unstable scenarios while diagnostic assessment continues. If AF onset is within 48 hours, DCC may be performed without transesophageal echo (TEE) or systemic anticoagulation with stroke prevention directed by individualized risk stratification (**Fig. 6**; **Table 3**A–F). If onset is unknown or longer than 48 hours, TEE is recommended to evaluate for atrial thrombi. In the absence of anticoagulation, atrial thrombi are observed in 13% of patients, with 90% of thrombi found in the LA appendage.[31] If urgency of DCC precludes TEE, concurrent low-molecular-weight heparin (LMWH) or bolus intravenous (IV) heparin with infusion to achieve therapeutic activated partial thromboplastin time levels 2 times the upper limits of the reference range is recommended. Following cardioversion, atrial stunning, despite electrical systole, results in impaired atrial contraction in proportion to AF duration.[32] Atrial contractility usually improves within several days but may take 3 to 4 weeks.[15,32] Most thromboembolic events occur within 10 days, with 80% within 3 days.[33] Anticoagulation with vitamin K antagonism (VKA) to target International Normalized Ratio (INR) 2.0 to 3.0, direct thrombin inhibition, or factor Xa inhibition is recommended for at least 4 weeks during the highest thromboembolic risk period.[7,15]

Multiple methods of thromboembolic and hemorrhagic risk stratification have been described

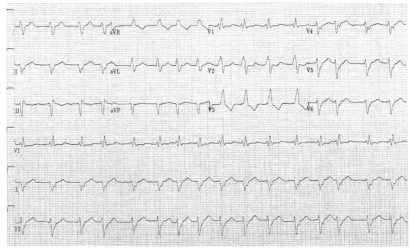

Fig. 4. AF with aberrancy presenting with wide complex rhythm.

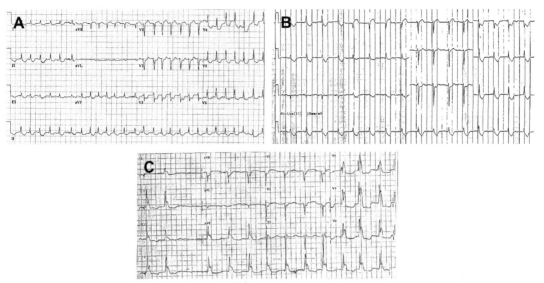

Fig. 5. Electrocardiographic clues to critical conditions coinciding with acute AF presentations. (*A*) Myocardial ischemia. (*B*) Digitalis toxicity: atrial tachycardia with AV block and repolarization abnormalities. (*C*) Hypothermia: AF, bradycardic ventricular response, and J or Osborne wave repolarization abnormalities. (*Courtesy of* Philip Podrid, MD, Boston University School of Medicine and West Roxbury Veteran's Affairs Medical Center [*B*, *C*].)

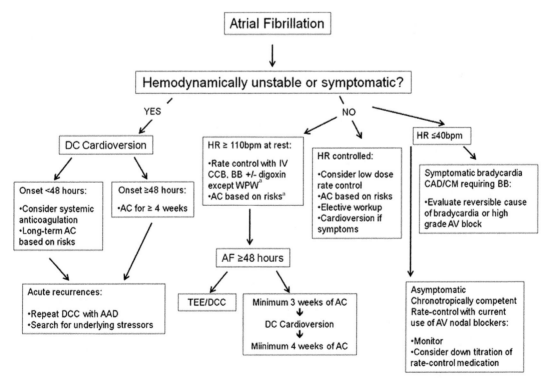

Fig. 6. Proposed approach to acute management of AF. Anticoagulation refers to vitamin K antagonists, direct thrombin inhibitors, or factor Xa inhibitors described in **Table 6**. Assumes identification and treatment of reversible causes and/or exacerbating risk factors highlighted in **Table 1** and **Fig. 3**. [a] Specific management goals in Wolff-Parkinson-White (WPW). AAD, antiarrhythmic drugs; AC, anticoagulation; BB, β-blocker; CCB, calcium channel blocker; CM, cardiomyopathy; HR, heart rate.

Table 3 Indices to stratify thromboembolic and hemorrhagic risks and associated thromboprophylaxis recommendations
(A) CHADS2 point system
(B) CHADS2 stroke risk
(C) CHADS-VASC point system
(D) CHADS-VASC stroke risk
(E) HAS-BLED score
(F) HAS-BLED hemorrhage risk

and validated. Among them, the CHADS2 (congestive heart failure, hypertension, age 75 years or older, diabetes mellitus, stroke or TIA or thromboembolism) and CHADS-VASC (vascular disease, age 65–74 years, sex category) scores (see **Table 3**A–F) are commonly used because of their simplicity and predictive value.[34,35] Thromboembolic and hemorrhagic risks must be balanced. HAS-BLED (hypertension, abnormal renal/liver function, stroke, bleeding history or predisposition, labile INR, elderly [>65 years], and concomitant drugs/alcohol) is a simple means of hemorrhagic risk stratification (see **Table 3**A–F).[36]

AF in the Stable Patient

Approximately 50% of all patients evaluated in the ED spontaneously convert from AF within 48 hours.[20] Among patients with spontaneous termination, 40% remained AF free for more than 5 years,[37] whereas others have described a 10% recurrence rate in the first year and 5% per year thereafter.[7] These findings may represent the resolution of reversible AF causes and/or early time points in AF natural history. In such settings, it is reasonable to monitor and rate-control patients while evaluation is initiated (see **Fig. 6**). Initial rate-control agents include β-blockers or nondihydropyridine calcium channel blockers (CCB). If

Table 3A CHADS2 score		
	CHADS2 Risk Factor	**Score**
C	Congestive HF	1
H	Hypertension	1
A	Age >75 y	1
D	Diabetes mellitus	1
S	Prior stroke or TIA[a]	2

[a] Systemic but noncerebrovascular thromboembolism included as stroke/TIA equivalent.
Abbreviation: TIA, transient ischemic attack.

these agents are contraindicated or inadequate, digoxin or amiodarone (Cordarone, Nexterone, Pacerone) may be considered in the absence of manifest preexcitation.[15] If rate control is refractory to multiple medications with continued symptoms or hemodynamic compromise, cardioversion is appropriate with concurrent cardioembolic risk modification.

In the presence of cardiovascular disease or persistent AF, AF recurrence rates are high after cardioversion. In the absence of mortality benefit from SR maintenance, initial rate control is appropriate unless patients are hemodynamically unstable or symptomatic. Patients refractory to or intolerant of AAT may benefit from electrophysiology consultation.

Management of AF in Specific Scenarios

CAD and acute coronary syndrome
Dual antiplatelet therapy is recommended following acute coronary syndrome (ACS) and percutaneous coronary intervention (PCI). The prevalence of major bleeding with concurrent warfarin (Coumadin, Jantoven), aspirin, and clopidogrel (Plavix) is 2.6% to 4.6% at 30 days and 7.4% to 10.3% at 1 year.[7] Recent guidelines have recommended bare metal rather than drug eluting stents to allow short-term triple therapy if chronic anticoagulation is anticipated. Because warfarin and aspirin are similarly effective for secondary prevention of coronary events,[38,39] recent guidelines have recommended either anticoagulation alone for stable CAD or anticoagulation plus antiplatelet monotherapy following ACS and adequate time following PCI.[7] Development of AF during MI is associated with adverse short-term and long-term prognoses.[40]

AF and bradycardia
AF is typically associated with RVR, but AV conduction disease or AV nodal antagonists may result in slow ventricular rates. Distinguishing slow ventricular response from high-grade AV block may be challenging (**Fig. 7**). Regularized bradycardia with underlying AF and absence of AV nodal antagonists should prompt evaluation for high-grade AV block and potential pacing indications.

Tachy-brady syndrome describes sudden oscillations between paroxysmal AF and frequently associated sinus node dysfunction (SND). Tachy-brady syndrome may limit AF medication titration or result in symptomatic bradycardia, sinus pauses, or syncope (see **Fig. 7**).

Cardiac implantable electronic devices
Patients with implantable cardiac rhythm devices such as pacemakers or implantable cardioverter-defibrillators (ICD) may present with AF. Fibrillatory

Table 3B
Thromboembolic risk and treatment recommendations by CHADS2 score

CHADS2 Score	Adjusted Stroke Rate Per Year (%)	Thromboembolism Prevention AHA/ACC/ESC 2006	Thromboembolism Prevention ESC 2010
0	1.9	Aspirin 81–325 mg Consider no therapy	Aspirin or no therapy
1	2.8	Anticoagulation or aspirin: based on major risk factors Anticoagulation favored: (1) Female age >75 y; LVEF <35%	Age >75 y: Anticoagulation Age <75 y: Anticoagulation or aspirin
2	4.0	Anticoagulation	Anticoagulation
3	5.9	Anticoagulation	Anticoagulation
4+	8.5	Anticoagulation	Anticoagulation

Major risk factors: prior thromboembolic event; age >75 years in 2010 guidelines versus female age >75 years in 2006 guidelines.

2010 ESC guidelines have transitioned to a risk factor rather than risk score approach to thromboembolism prophylaxis.
Abbreviation: LVEF, left ventricular ejection fraction.

waves may be observed between ventricular paced complexes or with temporary pacing inhibition. Patients with ICDs may present with AF/RVR and inappropriate ICD therapy.[41] ICD shocks that effectively cardiovert or defibrillate ventricular arrhythmias may not cardiovert AF.

Ventricular preexcitation and Wolfe-Parkinson-White syndrome

Immediate DCC is recommended for preexcited AF with rapid tachycardia or hemodynamic instability (see **Fig. 6**; **Fig. 8**). RR intervals less than 250 milliseconds between consecutive preexcited QRS complexes suggest increased risk of preexcited AF degenerating to ventricular fibrillation and SCD.[42] because preexcitation reflects antegrade electrical fusion between decremental AV nodal and nondecremental accessory pathway conduction, AV nodal blockers including β-blockers, nondihydropyridine CCB, digoxin, and adenosine are contraindicated for preexcited AF.[15] If DCC is not immediately available, AATs that slow both accessory pathway and AV nodal conduction (including amiodarone, ibutilide, or procainamide) are reasonable.[15]

Pregnancy

AF is rare in pregnancy, but AF recurrence is common if previously diagnosed. Rate-control options include β-blockers, nondihydropyridine CCB, and digoxin, although first-trimester β-blocker use may be associated with growth retardation. Flecainide has been used for both pregnant and fetal arrhythmias. Amiodarone may have

Table 3C
CHADS-VASC score

	CHADS-VASC Risk Factor	Points	Thromboprophylaxis
C	Congestive heart failure/LV dysfunction	1	Risk Score
H	Hypertension	1	Risk Score
A	Age >75 y	2 (Major)	Anticoagulation
D	Diabetes mellitus	1	Risk Score
S	Stroke/TIA/TE	2 (Major)	Anticoagulation
V	Vascular disease (prior myocardial infarction, peripheral artery disease, or aortic plaque)	1	Risk score
A	Age 65–74 y	1	Risk score
S C	Sex category (ie, female gender)	1	Risk score

Age >75 years and prior thromboembolic events are weighted major clinical risk factors for recurrent thromboembolism with recommendations for oral anticoagulation for thromboprophylaxis. Risk score refers to risk factor–based determination of thromboprophylaxis medication.
Abbreviation: TE, thromboembolism.

Table 3D
Thromboembolic risk and treatment recommendations by CHADS-VASC score

CHADS-VASC Score	Adjusted Stroke Rate (%/y)	Thromboprophylaxis Recommendations
0	0	Aspirin or no therapy
1	1.3	Anticoagulation preferred rather than aspirin Anticoagulation if >1 major risk factor[a]
2	2.2	Anticoagulation
3	3.2	Anticoagulation
4	4.0	Anticoagulation
5	6.7	Anticoagulation
6	9.8	Anticoagulation
7	9.6	Anticoagulation
8	6.7	Anticoagulation
9	15.2	Anticoagulation

[a] Major risk factors are: (1) age >75 years and (2) prior thromboembolic event.

negative fetal effects. DCC is recommended in unstable patients. Thromboembolism prophylaxis should be tailored to pregnancy stage and teratogenic and stroke risks.[7,15]

Rate-Control Targets

A randomized trial comparing lenient (<110 bpm) and strict (previously recommended <80 bpm at rest and <110 bpm with moderate exercise) heart rate control revealed noninferiority of lenient rate control in a primary outcome of cardiovascular death, HF and stroke hospitalization, systemic embolism, major bleeding, arrhythmic events, life-threatening adverse effects of rate-control drugs, and pacemaker or defibrillator implant.[43] Lenient rate control was easier to achieve.[43]

Consultation and Admission

Varying presentations, stability, and symptoms preclude unified recommendations for admission.

First AF with stable hemodynamics and rate control absent symptoms or reversible causes may not require admission. Refractory tachycardia and hemodynamic instability may benefit from critical care evaluation. Critical coexisting issues or AF sequelae including MI pulmonary embolism, CVA, or sepsis may require critical care and cardiovascular specialty management.

Communication with primary care physicians and cardiologists is essential in overall AF management. Cardiac electrophysiologists provide subspecialty insight with particular attention to AAT or interventional therapy. Surgical or medical issues influence decisions regarding thromboembolic versus hemorrhagic risks. Drug interactions may result in significant morbidity, mortality, and rehospitalization (**Boxes 2** and **3**, **Table 4**).

Table 3E
HAS-BLED risk score

	HAS-BLED Risk Factor	Points
H	Hypertension	1
A	Abnormal liver and renal function (1 point each)	1 or 2
S	Stroke	1
B	Bleeding	1
L	Labile INRs	1
E	Elderly (eg, >65 y)	1
D	Drugs or alcohol (1 point each)	1 or 2

Abbreviation: INR, international normalization ratio.

Table 3F
HAS-BLED score and hemorrhagic risk

HAS-BLED Score	Bleeds Per 100 Patient-Years
0	1.13
1	1.02
2	1.88
3	3.74
4	8.70
5	12.50
6	0.0
7	…
8	…
9	…
Any score	1.56

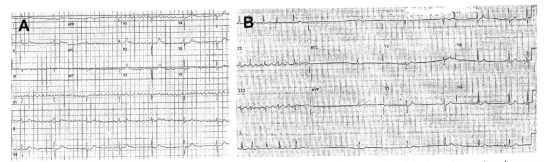

Fig. 7. AF associated with bradycardia. (*A*) AF with high-grade atrioventricular block and junctional escape rhythm. (*B*) Tachy-brady syndrome with paroxysmal AF termination and conversion pause before onset of sinus bradycardia. (*Courtesy of* P. Podrid, MD).

Atrial arrhythmias occur in 30% to 50% patients following cardiothoracic surgery. AF occurring late after cardiothoracic surgery suggests altered electroanatomic substrate that may benefit from arrhythmia consultation.[44] AF or AFL following cardiac transplant may represent rejection and should prompt evaluation by a transplant cardiologist.[45]

PHARMACOLOGIC STRATEGIES
Rate Control

Acute rate control may be achieved by IV or oral agents depending on desired time to onset, degree of tachycardia, symptoms, and hemodynamic stability. The optimal time over which to achieve rate control is unknown. β-Blockers, nondihydropyridine CCB, and digoxin are the mainstay of rate control (**Table 5**). Negative inotropy and chronotropy associated with β-blockers and CCB may precipitate HF, bradycardia, and AV block. Concurrent β-blocker and CCB administration is either not recommended or should be used cautiously.

β-Blockers

β-Blockers are first-line rate-control agents. In the AFFIRM (Atrial Fibrillation Follow-up Investigation of Rhythm Management) study, β-blockers were superior to CCB in achieving rate targets.[22] β-Blockers differ in adrenergic receptor and receptor subtype selectivity. Patients with obstructive lung disease may tolerate β-blockade, but cautious monitoring is recommended regardless of selectivity. β-Blockers with concurrent α-blockade may precipitate vasodilation and hypotension. Esmolol is an IV β-blocker with rapid onset and offset that may be associated with large infusion volumes. Renal versus hepatic drug elimination may direct β-blocker selection. β-Blockers may aid treatment of AF in hyperadrenergic states.

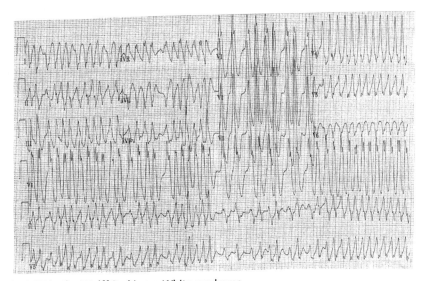

Fig. 8. Preexcited AF in the Wolff-Parkinson-White syndrome.

Calcium Channel Antagonists: Nondihydropyridine

Nondihydropyridine CCBs are effective for AF rate control. CCB may be preferred in patients with bronchospastic or obstructive pulmonary disease. CCB should be used with caution or avoided in HF

with LV systolic dysfunction because of negative inotropic effects. Short-acting IV CCBs require continuous infusion that may influence disposition.

Cardiac Glycosides

Digoxin is a purified cardiac glycoside that both inhibits the Na^+/K^+ ATPase and potentiates vagal tone, which slows AV node conduction. Positive inotropy without vasodilation makes digoxin useful in HF and hypotension. Benefits have been observed with concurrent β-blockers or CCB but not for digoxin monotherapy.

Narrow therapeutic window, renal clearance, and drug interactions (see **Boxes 2** and **3**, **Table 4**) via the cytochrome P450 system require cautious initiation and monitoring of digoxin. Digitalis toxic rhythms include delayed afterdepolarization-triggered ventricular arrhythmias and atrial tachycardia with complete AV block (see **Fig. 5**).[46] DCC is contraindicated in digitalis toxicity, because this may induce ventricular fibrillation that is particularly defibrillation resistant.[15]

Antiarrhythmic Medications in Rate Control

Amiodarone has multiple effects including antagonism of β-receptors and calcium, sodium, and potassium channels. Amiodarone may not effectively cardiovert AF but does augment rate control.

Pharmacologic Cardioversion

Pharmacologic cardioversion of AF is successful in ~30% to 50% of cases, in contrast with ~90% with DCC.[47] Pharmacologic cardioversion requires telemetry observation but no anesthesia. Oral or IV AAT available for cardioversion vary between the United States and EU (see **Table 5**). Prevention of thromboembolism, regardless of method, is reviewed later and in **Table 3A–F**.

Rhythm Control

The goal of maintaining SR is amelioration of AF symptoms. Rhythm control strategies have not shown reduction of mortality or complications.[18,19,22] Despite a history of multiple AAT used for AF rhythm control, currently recommended drugs are flecainide (Tambocor), propafenone (Rhythmol), dofetilide (Tikosyn), sotalol (Betapace, Sorine), amiodarone, and dronedarone (Multaq) (see **Table 5**).

Amiodarone
Amiodarone exerts multiple effects including sodium (I_{Na}), potassium (I_{Kr}, I_{Kur}, I_{to}, I_{KAch}), calcium (I_{CaL}), funny current (I_f), and β-receptor blockade that vary between acute and chronic administration. Amiodarone is the most commonly

Table 4
Drug-drug interactions frequently encountered in AF management

Drugs	Drug Metabolism	Increased Effect	Decreased Effect
Antiarrhythmic Medications			
Amiodarone	CYP2C9 CYP2D6 CYP3A4[a] P-glycoprotein[b]	Digoxin Warfarin Dofetilide Flecainide Lidocaine (no effect if added) β-blockers Calcium channel blockers Fluoroquinolones Cyclosporine Protease inhibitors Theophylline Grapefruit juice	Bile acid sequestrant
Dofetilide	Renal cation transport system	QT prolonging drugs Megestrol Trimethoprim Verapamil Cisapride Cimetidine	—
Flecainide	CYP2D6	Amiodarone	—
Ibutilide	Hepatic Renal	Amiodarone Cisapride Class IA and III AAD QT prolonging drugs	—
Lidocaine	CYP1A2 CYP2B6 CYP3A4[a]	Nonselective β-blockers HIV protease inhibitors Amiodarone if added	CYP450 inducers (eg, rifampicin)
Propafenone	CYP1A2 CYP2D6 CYP3A4[a]	Digoxin (>80% patients) Warfarin	Rifampicin
Sotalol	Renal	Class IA and III AAD Digoxin QT prolonging drugs	Magnesium hydroxide Aluminum oxide
Rate-Control Agents			
Adenosine	Adenosine deaminase: Blood, tissue	AV nodal blockers Dipyridamole Carbamazepine	Caffeine products Theophylline
β-Blocker	Liver Renal	Other AV nodal blockers	β-Agonists
Calcium channel blocker	Verapamil: CYP3A4[a], P-glycoprotein Diltiazem: CYP3A4[a]	Other AV nodal blockers	β-Agonists
Digoxin	P-glycoprotein[b]	Amiodarone	—
Anticoagulants			
Warfarin	CYP2C9 VKORC1 CYP3A4[a]	Digoxin Amiodarone Propafenone Verapamil	Vitamin K Diet and drugs Genetic variation ↓ or ↑

Grapefruit juice should be avoided in medications that involve the [a] CYP3A4 and [b] P-glycoprotein systems
Abbreviations: HIV, human immunodeficiency virus; VKORC1, vitamin K epoxide reductase complex.

Table 5
Pharmacologic therapy used in acute management of AF. Class definitions and Level of evidence (LOE) are based on those conventionally used in ACC/AHA/ESC guidelines

(A) Medical Therapy for Rate Control of AF

Drug Indication Class LOE	Loading Dose	Onset	Maintenance Dose	Major Side Effects
Esmolol Class I, LOE C	500 µg/kg IV more than 1 min	5 min	60–200 µg/kg/min IV	↓BP, HB, ↓HR, asthma, HF
Metoprolol Class I, LOE C	2.5–5 mg IV bolus over 2 min; up to 3 doses	5 min	NA	↓BP, HB, ↓HR, asthma, HF
Diltiazem Class I, LOE B	0.25 mg/kg IV over 2 min	2–7 min	5–15 mg/h IV	↓BP, HB, HF
Verapamil Class I, LOE B	0.075–0.15 mg/kg IV over 2 min	3–5 min	NA	↓BP, HB, HF
Amiodarone Class IIa, LOE C	150 mg over 10 min Oral loads may vary	Days	0.5–1 mg/min IV 200 mg daily (may vary)	↓BP, HB, pulmonary toxicity, skin discoloration, hypothyroidism, hyperthyroidism, corneal deposits, optic neuropathy, warfarin interaction, sinus bradycardia, conduction defects, phlebitis, drug-drug interactions (see **Table 4**)
Digoxin Class I, LOE B	0.25 mg IV each 2 h, up to 1.5 mg	60 min or more	0.125–0.375 mg daily IV or oral	Digitalis toxicity, HB, ↓HR Not recommended as monotherapy

(B) Medical Therapy for Cardioversion of AF and/or Maintenance of SR

Drugs Indication Class Level of Evidence	Dosing	Major Adverse Effects
Amiodarone Class IIA, LOE A	Intravenous or oral Refer to Table 5A for details	Drug-drug interactions CYP450 P-glycoprotein Higher risk of ventricular proarrhythmia with: Prolonged QT SHD Depressed LV function Bradycardia

Drug (Class, LOE)	Dosing	Risk Factors / Comments
Ibutilide, Class I (IIA for persistent), LOE A	IV 1 mg over 10 min; If AF/AFL persists after 10 min, an additional 1 mg infusion may be considered	Electrolytes: hypokalemia, hypomagnesemia; Addition of diuretics, QT prolonging drugs; Renal dysfunction; Rapid dose increase; Female gender; Excessive QT increase after initiation of drug; Previous proarrhythmia; Torsades de pointes (not dose dependent); Stop infusion if arrhythmia terminates, ventricular arrhythmias, or significant ↑ QTc; No concurrent class III AAT for at least 4 h after or within 5 half-lives
Sotalol (for SR maintenance, not cardioversion)	Oral 80, 120, 160 mg	Torsades de pointes; Monitor with renal failure; May be used but with caution in heart failure
Dofetilide, Class I, LOE A	Registered prescribers; CrCl-based dosing; 500, 250, 125 µg oral BID	Torsades des pointes; No HR slowing or bradycardia effects
Flecainide, Propafenone, Class I, LOE A	Oral (United States); Oral or IV (United States or EU)	Higher risk of ventricular proarrhythmia with: QRS >120 ms; Structural heart disease; Depressed LV function; Concomitant VT; Rapid ventricular rate; Rapid dose increase; Addition of negative inotropes; Excessive QRS widening >150%

Abbreviations: BID, twice daily; CrCl, creatinine clearance; HB, heart block; HR, heart rate; HF, heart failure.

prescribed AAT for AF despite not being approved by the US Food and Drug Administration for AF. Data are conflicting regarding rates of cardioversion (IV ~52%; oral ~28%) at 24 hours.[7,15] Time to cardioversion is delayed versus class IC agents.

Amiodarone effectively maintains SR (>60% over 16 months).[7,15,24] It is tolerated in the presence of SHD.

Adverse effects and intolerance are common (15%–20%) with amiodarone.[48] QT prolongation is frequent, but torsades de pointes (TDP) is uncommon.[49] SB and AV conduction abnormalities are common. Metabolism via the CYP3A4, CYP2C9, and P-glycoprotein pathways results in multiple drug interactions with verapamil (Calan, Covera, Isoptin, Verelan), digoxin, statins, and warfarin (see **Boxes 2** and **3**, **Table 4**).[46] Long-term adverse effects depend on dose and duration and include corneal deposits; photosensitivity; and pulmonary, thyroid, and liver toxicity. Phlebitis and hypotension are common with IV administration. Amiodarone-AAT interactions increase proarrhythmia risk; cessation of class I or III AAT for at least 3 to 5 half-lives is recommended. Amiodarone cessation for at least 3 months is recommended before initiation of dofetilide.

Class III antiarrhythmic therapy

Ibutilide Ibutilide is a class III AAT with predominant I_{Kr} antagonism approved for acute IV administration to convert AF or AFL with estimated rates of 44% over 90 minutes.[50] Minimal changes in sinus rate, PR interval, or QRS duration are observed. TDP occurs in 3% to 5% of cases independent of dose.[51] Telemetry observation is recommended for at least 4 hours.[46,52] Class IA and III AAT are contraindicated within 4 hours of ibutilide infusion.

Dofetilide Dofetilide is effective for the conversion to and maintenance of SR in populations with and without HF. Estimated conversion rates are ~87% within 30 hours with 58% to 79% suppression of AF at 1 year. Dose-dependent QTc prolongation and TDP risks require inpatient loading by certified prescribers in the United States. Renal impairment and prolonged QTc limit dofetilide use.

Sotalol Sotalol is effective at maintaining SR with rates of ~37% at 1 year, but is ineffective for cardioversion.[7,15] QTc prolongation and TDP are significant adverse effects that require ECG monitoring at initiation. Renal insufficiency, bronchospasm, QT prolongation, and HF require cautious initiation.

Dronedarone Dronedarone is a deiodinated designed molecule resembling amiodarone. Dronedarone is less effective than amiodarone for SR maintenance but reduces AF hospitalizations and recurrence. It is contraindicated in decompensated or recent decompensated HF and permanent AF because of increased mortality. Adverse effects include bradycardia and gastrointestinal intolerance. Concerns regarding liver toxicity and cardiovascular events in ischemic heart disease have surfaced, but so far without specific recommendations.

Class IC antiarrhythmic medications

Oral flecainide and propafenone have estimated net conversion rates of 38%.[7,15] Both maintain SR at ~30% to 35% over 1 year with reduced AF recurrence and duration. These drugs are contraindicated in the context of MI, CAD, and SHD based on increased sudden death in the Cardiac Arrhythmia Suppression Trial (CAST).[53] Both are sodium channel blockers that exhibit use dependence with QRS prolongation at increased heart rates. Propafenone and flecainide may slow and organize AF to AFL leading to 1:1 AFL that is often poorly tolerated (**Fig. 9**). Concurrent AV nodal blockade is recommended; propafenone has mild β-blocker activity.[46] Both are ineffective for termination of persistent AF or AFL. Adverse effects include neurologic effects, hypotension, and bradycardia.

Flecainide A single oral dose of flecainide 300 mg has cardioversion rates of 75% to 91% at 8 hours. In Europe, IV flecainide cardioversion rates are 67% to 92%. QRS widening more than 25% may portend increased proarrhythmia risk; some advocate exercise testing for QRS duration.[54]

Propafenone Propafenone conversion rates are ~56% at 2 to 6 hours with a single 600-mg oral dose. IV propafenone is available in Europe with termination rates of 40% to 90%.

Quinidine

Quinidine was one of the earliest AAT to show efficacy in maintaining SR. Its use is limited by increased mortality attributed to proarrhythmia based on meta-analysis.

Vernakalent

Vernakalent is a multichannel blocker with predominant blockade of atrial potassium (I_{to}, I_{KACh}, I_{Kur}) and late sodium (I_{NaL}) currents. IV vernakalent is approved in the EU but pending in the United States for acute AF conversion. Oral vernakalent is initiating phase II testing. No proarrhythmia has been described thus far.

Thromboembolic Risk Reduction

Current oral anticoagulation options are vitamin K antagonists (warfarin), direct thrombin inhibitors

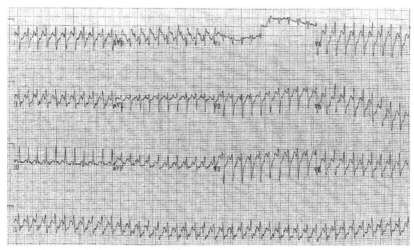

Fig. 9. Atrial flutter with 1:1 atrioventricular conduction.

(dabigatran; Pradaxa) or factor Xa inhibitors (rivaroxaban; Xarelto) (**Table 6**). Two factor Xa inhibitors are pending US Food and drug Administration (FDA) approval (apixaban) or further phase III data (edoxaban). Antiplatelet therapy is less effective than anticoagulation but may be considered in low-risk patients without SHD. CHADS2 or CHADS-VASC risk scores help determine thromboembolic risk and appropriate prophylaxis (see **Table 3**A–F). Anticoagulation risk with VKA may be acceptable and underused in elder adults.[55]

Suboptimal real-world time in therapeutic range (TTR) and inconvenience of monitoring limit the usefulness of VKA. In contrast, disadvantages of newer agents include costs, lack of antidote, lack of assay, and limited long-term data regarding adverse effects. Enthusiasm surrounded the direct thrombin inhibitor, ximeligatran, until escalating short-term liver toxicity forced its market withdrawal. Whether VKA or newer oral anticoagulants should be used as first line remains controversial.[56,57]

Table 6
Approved antithrombotic medical therapy for prevention of thromboembolic events

Anticoagulant	Mechanism	Dosing	Pros	Cons
Warfarin (Coumadin)	Vitamin K antagonist	Dosing by INR 2.0–3.0	Cost Experience Long-term data Monitoring: INR Reversibility	INR monitoring and costs Variable dose response Drug interactions Food interactions
Dabigatran (Pradaxa)	Direct thrombin inhibitor	150 mg orally BID CrCl 15–30 mL: 75 mg BID CrCl <15 mL: not recommended	Monitoring: none Diet: no restrictions	Caution with renal dysfunction, elderly No monitoring or antidote
Rivaroxaban (Xarelto)	Factor Xa inhibitor	20 mg orally daily CrCl 30–50 mL: caution CrCl <30 mL: not recommended Child-Pugh class B or C liver failure: avoid	Once-daily dosing Monitoring: none Diet: no restrictions	Caution with renal/hepatic dysfunction, elderly Bridging: ↑ thromboembolic events on drug cessation

Abbreviation: BID, twice daily; CrCl, creatinine clearance.

Vitamin K antagonists

VKA have established relative risk reduction (RRR) of stroke (~64%) and mortality (~26%) versus control and ~39% RRR of stroke versus aspirin.[7,15,58] Hemorrhagic risks are a major concern but may be reduced to less than 1% per year with appropriate monitoring targeting INR of 2 to 3.[7] Drug interactions, diet and lifestyle, genetic variation, and adherence influence dose response and TTR. Recent randomized trials of anticoagulants have described a ~60% rate of TTR.[59–61]

Direct thrombin/factor II inhibitors

Dabigatran is an oral, direct thrombin inhibitor approved by the FDA in 2010 for thromboembolism prophylaxis in nonvalvular AF. Dabigatran is not recommended in patients with valvular disease, prosthetic valves, severe renal insufficiency (glomerular filtration rate [GFR] <15 mL/min), advanced liver disease with impaired clotting function, and advanced age.[59,62]

Factor Xa inhibitors

Novel oral factor Xa inhibitors (rivaroxaban, apixaban) have emerged as noninferior alternatives to warfarin in nonvalvular AF. Rivaroxaban is FDA approved for prevention of thromboembolic events in nonvalvular AF with once-daily dosing. However, anticoagulant bridging is recommended because of increased thromboembolism rates on rivaroxaban withdrawal.[61,63] Rivaroxaban is not recommended in patients with valvular disease or impaired renal or hepatic function.

FDA review of apixaban for prevention of AF embolic events is pending.

Antiplatelet therapy

Anticoagulant therapy with VKA is superior to dual antiplatelet therapy with aspirin plus clopidogrel for thromboprophylaxis.[64] Although aspirin plus clopidogrel reduced stroke in patients with AF not amenable to anticoagulation, a significantly increased risk of bleeding was observed compared with aspirin alone.[65] Anticoagulation has been prominently recommended rather than antiplatelet therapy between the 2006 ACC/AHA/ESC and 2010 ESC guidelines.[7,15]

AF Prevention

Upstream therapies including antagonism of the renin-angiotensin-aldosterone axis, statins, and polyunsaturated fatty acids may delay development or progression of AF but have no benefit in acute AF.

NONPHARMACOLOGIC STRATEGIES
Cardioversion

Electrical cardioversion is a widely available and highly successful method of restoring SR in up to 90% of patients.[47] The benefit of rhythm control for death, stroke, and HF remain absent,[50] but cardioversion may be necessary for symptomatic and unstable AF.

Electrical cardioversion uses direct current energy. Biphasic waveforms use less energy and reduce tissue injury. Synchronization to the QRS complex is critical to avoid inadvertent T wave shock and ventricular fibrillation induction.

Review of the procedure, anticoagulation plan, and informed consent are required. Adequate skin preparation improves electrode contact. Anterolateral or anteroposterior (AP) positions maximize energy vectors through the LA. Dedicated airway, hemodynamic, and rhythm monitoring is required. Applied pressure with electrically inert material may improve electrode contact. Advanced cardiac life support recommendations for first shock are 120 to 360 J.

Unsuccessful DCC may occur for various reasons at any interface between the defibrillator and the patient (**Table 7**). Immediate or early recurrence of AF may be confused with unsuccessful DCC. Patch or paddle position, contact, and connections must be confirmed. Increased energy output may be used; many practitioners initially cardiovert at higher energy. AP patch repositioning may improve shock vectors. Addition of AAT can be considered. Although acute success of cardioversion is high, recurrence rates relate to arrhythmic substrate including LA size, AF duration, and valvular dysfunction.

Ablation of AF for Rhythm Control

AF ablation may be performed using various catheter-based or surgical techniques to electrically isolate AF triggers or modify atrial substrate to maintain SR for symptomatic relief. This typically involves electrical pulmonary vein isolation (PVI), because the most common electrophysiologic AF triggers emanate from sites of automaticity in the LA–pulmonary vein junctions.[66] Although definitions of recurrence, follow-up, and methods vary, studies indicate freedom from recurrent atrial arrhythmia in the range of 39% to 79.4% after 3-year to 6-year follow-up.[67–72] AF ablation is recommended to candidates with symptomatic, recurrent AF refractory to, or intolerant of, at least 1 AAT; AF ablation may be considered before AAT for paroxysmal AF.[71]

Although ablation is performed electively for long-term AF management, acute recurrence and complications (**Table 8**) may require expedited acute evaluation. Death and atrioesophageal fistula occur in less than 1%. Cerebrovascular events (1%–2%), cardiac tamponade (1%–6%), major or

Table 7
DCC: troubleshooting and complications

Issues	Management
Cardioversion: unsuccessful	Unsuccessful vs immediate/early recurrence of AF?
	Patch position
	Patch contact
	Apply pressure during shock with electrically inert material
	Check connections
	Antiarrhythmic medication
	Repeat shock
	Repeat shock with higher energy
Ventricular fibrillation	Avoidance: synchronize shock to QRS
	Defibrillation: switch shock to asynchronous
Bradycardia	Transcutaneous pacing
Asystole	Confirm ventricular capture
Pulseless electrical activity	Advanced cardiac life support
Immediate or early recurrence of AF	Frequent cause of failed cardioversion
	Repeat cardioversion
	Antiarrhythmic medication

minor hemorrhage (∼5%), and pulmonary vein stenosis (0%–10%) estimates vary.[69,70,73,74] Iatrogenic atypical atrial flutter may occur in 2% to 14%.[74]

Recurrent arrhythmias including AF, atrial tachycardia, and atypical AFL are common within the first 3 months of ablation and may not predict success. Many electrophysiologists recommend rhythm control in this period, although this practice is of unclear benefit.[75] Patients having AF ablation are typically anticoagulated for at least several months.

Ablation of Atrial Flutter for Rhythm Control

AFL typically involves a macroreentrant circuit between the tricuspid annulus, inferior vena cava, and crista terminalis. Rate control of AFL may be more challenging. The cavotricuspid flutter isthmus is frequently amenable to ablation with favorable acute and long-term success at low complication rates; AFL ablation may be considered as first-line therapy.

Ablation for Rate Control of AF

AV junction ablation may be considered for patients intolerant of, or unable to achieve, adequate AF rate control and are not optimal AF ablation candidates. AV junction ablation is ∼90% effective for symptom relief but requires acceptance of heart block and pacemaker implant.[76] Because AF remains present, thromboembolic risks remain unmodified after this procedure. Heightened TDP risk observed immediately following AV junction ablation is ameliorated by short-term increased pacing rates.[76]

Left Atrial Appendage Occlusion for Prevention of Thromboembolism

LA appendage occlusion devices have emerged and may be considered for nonacute thromboembolism risk reduction when anticoagulation is contraindicated.

Self-management Strategies

Education, understanding of signs and symptoms, and adherence to medication, lifestyle modification, and follow-up may reduce ED visits for AF. Risk modification including trigger avoidance, weight reduction, and treatment of underlying conditions must be reinforced.

Pill-in-pocket antiarrhythmic therapy
Some patients are appropriate candidates for ambulatory cardioversion using oral flecainide or propafenone as discussed earlier (see **Table 5**).[77] This strategy should be initiated in a monitored setting.[15]

Anticoagulation monitoring
Some patients with appropriate compliance and stable warfarin dosing may perform point-of-care home INR monitoring.

Evaluation and Reassessment

Regardless of treatment strategy, reevaluation of symptoms, hemodynamics, comorbidities, and

Table 8
AF ablation: complications, evaluation, and management

Complications	Presentation	Management
Cerebrovascular event TIA vs stroke	Altered mental status and focal deficits; diagnosis may be delayed until recovery	Neurologic consultation Head CT, MRI, and MRA of the brain Anticoagulation, thrombolysis, or intervention May be embolism caused by thrombus or air

Vascular complications
  Arteriovenous fistula
  Pseudoaneurysm
  Hematoma
	Within 1 d to 1 wk
	May be asymptomatic
	Groin swelling, pain, thrills, pop
	Retroperitoneal bleed: back pain
		Serial examinations, blood counts. Transfusion if appropriate
		Femoral ultrasound. CT scan for retroperitoneal bleed
		Anticoagulation management varies with severity
		Interventional vascular/vascular surgery consultation

Pericardial effusion Cardiac tamponade	During procedure or within days: dyspnea, hypotension, shock	Hemodynamic monitoring; cardiac silhouette on fluoroscopy Echocardiography (intracardiac, transthoracic, transesophageal) Reversal of anticoagulation Pericardiocentesis: may require surgical repair
Pulmonary vein stenosis	Rapid or insidious: weeks -months Variable symptoms including dyspnea, hemoptysis, bronchitis	CT angiography to evaluate pulmonary veins Possible balloon dilation/stent placement
Atrial-esophageal fistula Esophageal injury	Insidious: 1–5 wk after ablation Fever, malaise, neurologic symptoms, gastrointestinal bleed, hemoptysis, hematemesis Requires high index of suspicion	CT scan or MRI Surgery for fistula Endoscopy: may exacerbate fistula Esophageal temperature probe Esophageal barium swallow Proton pump inhibitors
Phrenic nerve palsy	Usually periprocedural Dyspnea, cough, hiccup, effort intolerance, diaphragmatic increase	Favorable prognosis: frequently recovers without intervention
Atrial arrhythmias AF Atypical atrial flutter Atrial tachycardia	AF: may be common in first 3 mo without impact on long-term outcome AT/atypical AFL: may be challenging to control with AAT or rate control	Rhythm monitor: transtelephonic, Holter, implantable Contact electrophysiology Cardioversion Antiarrhythmic drug Electrophysiology study/ablation

Abbreviations: CT, computed tomography; MRA, magnetic resonance angiography; MRI, magnetic resonance imaging.

stroke risk is essential both acutely and chronically. Communication among primary care physicians, cardiologists, and electrophysiologists facilitates successful long-term care. Reassessment of underlying conditions and adequate rate control aids treatment of symptoms.

SUMMARY

Key goals of acute AF management include accurate diagnosis, clinical stabilization, modification of underlying causes and risks, amelioration of symptoms by rate or rhythm control, and stratification and prevention of thromboembolic stroke. Because clinical manifestations of AF vary greatly, management must be individualized. Evolving methods of risk assessment and therapy may augment therapeutic options to prevent and reduce AF and associated sequelae. Appropriate selection of AF management tools and strategies benefits from collaboration among emergency, primary, cardiovascular, and cardiac rhythm physicians.

REFERENCES

1. Rosner F. Maimonides' medical writing. Translated and annotated by Fred Rosner, MD. Haifa (Israel): The Maimonides Research Institute; 1989.
2. Prystowsky EN. The history of atrial fibrillation: the last 100 years. J Cardiovasc Electrophysiol 2008; 19(6):575–82.
3. Seidl K, Hauer B, Schwick PA, et al. Risk of thromboembolic events in patients with atrial flutter. Am J Cardiol 1998;82:580–3.
4. LeLorier P, Humphries KH, Krahn A, et al. Prognostic differences between atrial fibrillation and atrial flutter. Am J Cardiol 2004;93(5):647–9.
5. Roger VL, Go AS, Lloyd-Jones DM, et al. Heart disease and stroke statistics-2011 update: a report from the American Heart Association. Circulation 2011;123(4):e18–209.
6. Go AS, Hylek EM, Phillips KA, et al. Prevalence of diagnosed atrial fibrillation in adults: national implications for rhythm management and stroke prevention: the Anticoagulation and Risk Factors in Atrial Fibrillation (ATRIA) study. JAMA 2001;285:2370–5.
7. Camm AJ, Kirchhof P, Lip GY, et al. Guidelines for the management of atrial fibrillation: the task force for the management of atrial fibrillation of the European Society of Cardiology (ESC). Eur Heart J 2010;31(19):2369–429.
8. Piccini JP, Hammill BG, Sinner MF, et al. Incidence and prevalence of atrial fibrillation and associated mortality among Medicare beneficiaries, 1993-2007. Circ Cardiovasc Qual Outcomes 2012;5:85–93.
9. Friberg J, Buch P, Scharling H, et al. Rising rates of hospital admissions for atrial fibrillation. Epidemiology 2003;14:666–72.
10. Levy S, Maarek M, Coumel P, et al. Characterization of different subsets of atrial fibrillation in general practice in France: the ALFA study. Circulation 1999;99:3028–35.
11. Gami AS, Pressman G, Caples SM, et al. Association of atrial fibrillation and obstructive sleep apnea. Circulation 2004;110:364–7.
12. Wanahita N, Messerli FH, Bangalore S, et al. Atrial fibrillation and obesity-results of a meta-analysis. Am Heart J 2008;155(2):310–5.
13. Krahn AD, Manfreda J, Tate RB, et al. The natural history of atrial fibrillation: incidence, risk factors, and prognosis in the Manitoba Follow-Up Study. Am J Med 1995;98:476–84.
14. Maggioni AP, Latini R, Carson PE, et al. Valsartan reduces the incidence of atrial fibrillation in patients with heart failure: results from the Valsartan Heart Failure Trial. Am Heart J 2005;149:548–57.
15. Fuster V, Rydén LE, Cannom DS, et al. ACC/AHA/ESC 2006 guidelines for the management of patients with atrial fibrillation: a report of the American College of Cardiology/American Heart Association Task Force on Practice Guidelines and the European Society of Cardiology Committee for Practice Guidelines (Writing Committee to Revise the 2001 Guidelines for the Management of Patients with Atrial Fibrillation). Circulation 2006;114:e257–354.
16. Wolf PA, Abbott RD, Kannel WB. Atrial fibrillation as an independent risk factor for stroke: the Framingham Study. Stroke 1991;22:983–8.
17. Benjamin EJ, Wolf PA, D'Agostino RB, et al. Impact of atrial fibrillation on the risk of death: the Framingham Heart Study. Circulation 1998;98(10):946–52.
18. Van Gelder IC, Hagens VE, Bosker HA, et al. A comparison of rate control and rhythm control in patients with recurrent persistent atrial fibrillation. N Engl J Med 2002;347:1834–40.
19. Roy D, Talajic M, Nattel S, et al. Rhythm control versus rate control for atrial fibrillation and heart failure. N Engl J Med 2008;358:2667–77.
20. Dell'Orfano JT, Patel H, Wobrette DL, et al. Acute treatment of atrial fibrillation: spontaneous conversion rate and cost of care. Am J Cardiol 1999;83:788–90.
21. Davies MJ, Pomerance A. Pathology of atrial fibrillation in man. Br Heart J 1972;34:520–5.
22. Wyse DG, Waldo AL, DiMarco JP, et al, Atrial Fibrillation Follow-up Investigation of Rhythm Management (AFFIRM) investigators. A comparison of rate control and rhythm control in patients with atrial fibrillation. N Engl J Med 2002;347:1825–33.
23. Jahangir A, Lee V, Friedman PA, et al. Long-term progression and outcomes with aging in patients with lone atrial fibrillation: a 30-year follow-up study. Circulation 2007;115(24):3050–6.

24. Singh BN, Singh SN, Reda DJ, et al. Amiodarone versus sotalol for atrial fibrillation. N Engl J Med 2005;352:1861–72.

25. Rohrbacker NJ, Kleinman NL, White SA, et al. The burden of atrial fibrillation and other cardiac arrhythmias in an employed population: associated costs, absences, and objective productivity loss. J Occup Environ Med 2010;52(4):383–91.

26. Coyne KS, Paramore C, Grandy SG, et al. Assessing the direct costs of treating nonvalvular atrial fibrillation in the United States. Value Health 2005;9(5):348–56.

27. Le Heuzey JY, Paziaud O, Piot O, et al. Cost of care distribution in atrial fibrillation patients: the COCAF study. Am Heart J 2004;147:121–6.

28. Lee WC, Lamas GA, Balu S, et al. Direct treatment cost of atrial fibrillation in the elderly American population: a Medicare perspective. J Med Econ 2008; 11:281–98.

29. Fox CS, Parise H, D'Agostino RB Sr, et al. Parental atrial fibrillation as a risk factor for atrial fibrillation in offspring. JAMA 2004;291(23):2851–5.

30. Douglas PS, Garcia MJ, Haines DE, et al. ACCF/ASE/ AHA/ASNC/HFSA/HRS/SCAI/SCCM/SCCT/SCMR 2011 appropriate use criteria for echocardiography: a report of the American College of Cardiology Foundation Appropriate Use Criteria Task Force, American Society of Echocardiography, American Heart Association, American Society of Nuclear Cardiology, Heart Failure Society of America, Heart Rhythm Society, Society for Cardiovascular Angiography and Interventions, Society of Critical Care Medicine, Society of Cardiovascular Computed Tomography, and Society for Cardiovascular Magnetic Resonance. J Am Coll Cardiol 2010. http://dx.doi.org/10.1016/ j.jacc.2010.11.002. published online before print November 19, 2010.

31. Manning WJ, Silverman DI, Katz SE, et al. Impaired left atrial mechanical function after cardioversion: relation to the duration of atrial fibrillation. J Am Coll Cardiol 1994;23(7):1535–40.

32. Khan IA. Atrial stunning: determinants and cellular mechanisms. Am Heart J 2003;145:787–94.

33. Berger M, Schweitzer P. Timing of thromboembolic events after electrical cardioversion of atrial fibrillation or flutter: a retrospective analysis. Am J Cardiol 1998;82:1545–7.

34. Gage BF, Waterman AD, Shannon W, et al. Validation of clinical classification schemes for predicting stroke: results from the National Registry of Atrial Fibrillation. JAMA 2001;285(22):2864–70.

35. Lip GY, Nieuwlaat R, Pisters R, et al. Refining clinical risk stratification for predicting stroke and thromboembolism in atrial fibrillation using a novel risk factor-based approach: the Euro Heart Survey on Atrial Fibrillation. Chest 2010;137(2):263–72.

36. Pisters R, Lane DA, Nieuwlaat R, et al. A novel user-friendly score (HAS-BLED) to assess 1-year risk of major bleeding in patients with atrial fibrillation: the Euro Heart Survey. Chest 2010;138(5):1093–100.

37. Kerr R, Humphries KH, Talajic M, et al. Progression to chronic atrial fibrillation after initial diagnosis of paroxysmal atrial fibrillation: results from the Canadian Registry of Atrial Fibrillation. Am Heart J 2005; 149:489–96.

38. Smith P, Arnesen H, Holme I. The effect of warfarin on mortality and reinfarction after myocardial infarction. N Engl J Med 1990;323(3):147–52.

39. Hurlen M, Abdelnoor M, Smith P, et al. Warfarin, aspirin, or both after myocardial infarction. N Engl J Med 2002;347:969–74.

40. Lopes RD, Pieper KS, Horton JR, et al. Short- and long-term outcomes following atrial fibrillation in patients with acute coronary syndromes with or without ST-segment elevation. Heart 2008;94(7): 867–73.

41. Van Rees JB, Borleffs CJ, de Bie MK, et al. Inappropriate implantable cardioverter-defibrillator shocks: incidence, predictors, and impact on mortality. J Am Coll Cardiol 2011;57(5):556–62.

42. Klein GJ, Bashore TM, Sellers TD. Ventricular fibrillation in the Wolff-Parkinson-White syndrome. N Engl J Med 1979;301:1080–5.

43. Van Gelder IC, Groenveld HF, Crijns HJ, et al. Lenient versus strict rate control in patients with atrial fibrillation. N Engl J Med 2010;362(15):1363–73.

44. See VY, Roberts-Thompson KC, Stevenson WG, et al. Atrial arrhythmias after lung transplantation: epidemiology, mechanisms at electrophysiology study, and outcomes. Circ Arrhythm Electrophysiol 2009;2(5):737–41.

45. Dasari TW, Pavlovic-Surjance B, Patel N, et al. Incidence, risk factors, and clinical outcomes of atrial fibrillation and atrial flutter after heart transplantation. Am J Cardiol 2010;106(5):737–41.

46. Zipes DP, Jalife J. Cardiac electrophysiology. Philadelphia: Saunders; 2009.

47. Kirchhof P, Monnig G, Wasmer K, et al. A trial of self-adhesive patch electrodes and hand-held paddle electrodes for external cardioversion of atrial fibrillation. Eur Heart J 2005;26:1292–7.

48. Goldschlager N, Epstein AE, Naccarelli GV, et al. A practical guide for clinicians who treat patients with amiodarone: 2007. Heart Rhythm 2007;4(9):1250–9.

49. Hohnloser SH, Klingenheben T, Singh BN. Amiodarone-associated proarrhythmic effects. A review with special reference to torsade de pointes tachycardia. Ann Intern Med 1994;121(7):529.

50. Wyse DG. Cardioversion of atrial fibrillation for maintenance of sinus rhythm: a road to nowhere. Circulation 2009;120:1444–52.

51. Li H, Easley A, Barrington W, et al. Evaluation and management of atrial fibrillation in the emergency department. Emerg Med Clin North Am 1998;16: 389–403.

52. Pfizer. Ibutilide (Corvert) [package insert]. [Online]; 2006. Available at: http://www.pfizer.com/files/products/uspi_corvert.pdf. Accessed March 29, 2012.

53. Echt DS, Liebson PR, Mitchell LB, et al. Mortality and morbidity in patients receiving encainide, flecainide, or placebo - the Cardiac Arrhythmia Suppression Trial. N Engl J Med 1991;324:781–8.

54. Zimetbaum P. Antiarrhythmic drug therapy for atrial fibrillation. Circulation 2012;125:381–9.

55. Hylek EM, Evans-Molina C, Shea C, et al. Major hemorrhage and tolerability of warfarin in the first year of therapy among elderly patients with atrial fibrillation. Circulation 2007;115(21):2689–96.

56. Ansell J. New oral anticoagulants should not be used as first-line agents to prevent thromboembolism in patients with atrial fibrillation. Circulation 2012;125:165–70.

57. Granger CB, Armaganijan LV. New oral anticoagulants should be used as first-line agents to prevent thromboembolism in patients with atrial fibrillation. Circulation 2012;125:159–64.

58. Hart RG, Pearce LA, Aguilar MI, et al. Meta-analysis: antithrombotic therapy to prevent stroke in patients who have nonvalvular atrial fibrillation. Ann Intern Med 2007;146:857–67.

59. Connolly SJ, Ezekowitz MD, Yusuf S, et al. Dabigatran versus warfarin in patients with atrial fibrillation. N Engl J Med 2009;361:1139–51.

60. Granger CB, Alexander JH, McMurray JJ, et al. Apixaban versus warfarin in patients with atrial fibrillation. N Engl J Med 2011;365(11):981–92.

61. Patel MR, Mahaffey KW, Garg J, et al. Rivaroxban versus warfarin in nonvalvular atrial fibrillation. N Engl J Med 2011;365(10):883–91.

62. Wann LS, Curtis AB, Ellenbogen KA, et al. 2011 ACCF/AHA/HRS Focused update on the management of patients with atrial fibrillation (update on dabigatran). J Am Coll Cardiol 2011;57:1330–7.

63. Jannsen Pharmaceuticals. Rivaroxaban (Xarelto) [package insert]. [Online] 12/2011. Available at: http://www.xareltohcp.com/sites/default/files/pdf/xarelto_0.pdf#zoom=100. Accessed March 29, 2012.

64. Connolly S, Pogue J, Hart R, et al. Clopidogrel plus aspirin versus oral anticoagulation for atrial fibrillation in the Atrial fibrillation Clopidogrel Trial with Irbesartan for prevention of Vascular Events (ACTIVE W): a randomised controlled trial. Lancet 2006;367(9526):1903–12.

65. Connolly SJ, Pogue J, Hart RG, et al. Effect of clopidogrel added to aspirin in patients with atrial fibrillation. N Engl J Med 2009;360:2066–78.

66. Haïssaguerre M, Jaïs P, Dipen C, et al. Spontaneous initiation of atrial fibrillation by ectopic beats originating in the pulmonary veins. N Engl J Med 1998;339:659–66.

67. Weerasooriy R, Khairy P, Litalien J, et al. Catheter ablation for atrial fibrillation: are results maintained at 5 years of follow-up? J Am Coll Cardiol 2011;57:160–6.

68. Gaita F, Caponi D, Scaglione M, et al. Long-term clinical results of 2 different ablation strategies in patients with paroxysmal and persistent atrial fibrillation. Circ Arrhythm Electrophysiol 2008;1:269–75.

69. Hussein AA, Saliba WI, Martin DO, et al. Natural history and long-term outcomes of ablated atrial fibrillation. Circ Arrhythm Electrophysiol 2011;4:271–8.

70. Sorgente A, Tung P, Wylie J, et al. Six year follow-up after catheter ablation of atrial fibrillation: a palliation more than a true cure. Am J Cardiol 2012;109:1179–86.

71. Calkins H, Brugada J, Packer DL, et al. HRS/EHRA/ECAS expert consensus statement on catheter and surgical ablation of atrial fibrillation: recommendations for personnel, policy, procedures and follow up. Europace 2007;9:335–79.

72. Calkins H, Brugada J, Cappato R, et al. 2012 HRS/EHRA/ECAS expert consensus statement on catheter and surgical ablation of atrial fibrillation: recommendations for patient selection, procedural techniques, patient management and follow-up, definitions, endpoints, and research trial design: a report of the Heart Rhythm Society (HRS) task force on catheter and surgical ablation of atrial fibrillation. Europace 2012;9:632–96.

73. Holmes DR, Monahan KH, Packer D, et al. Pulmonary vein stenosis complicating ablation for atrial fibrillation. JACC Cardiovasc Interv 2009;2:267–76.

74. Wazni O, Wilkoff B, Saliba W. Catheter ablation for atrial fibrillation. N Engl J Med 2011;365:2296–304.

75. Leong-Sit P, Roux JF, Zado E, et al. Antiarrhythmics after ablation of atrial fibrillation (5A study): six-month follow-up study. Circ Arrhythm Electrophysiol 2011;4(1):11–4.

76. Betts TR. Atrioventricular junction ablation and pacemaker implant for atrial fibrillation: still a valid treatment in appropriately selected patients. Europace 2008;10:425–32.

77. Alboni P, Botto GL, Baldi N, et al. Outpatient treatment of recent-onset atrial fibrillation with the "pill-in-the-pocket" approach. N Engl J Med 2004;351:2384–91.

Novel Patterns of Ischemia and STEMI Equivalents

Benjamin J. Lawner, DO, EMT-P[a,b,*],
Jose V. Nable, MD, NREMT-P[a], Amal Mattu, MD[a]

KEYWORDS

- Myocardial infarction • STEMI • Wellens' syndrome • Posterior myocardial infarction
- Left bundle branch block • STEMI-equivalents

KEY POINTS

- Although STEMI criteria are well established, interest is emerging in other cardiac conditions that also benefit from timely intervention, specifically "STEMI equivalents," which warrant similarly aggressive and definitive intervention.
- Electrocardiographic changes consistent with cardiac ischemia include (1) the de Winter ST/T complex, (2) ST elevation in lead aVR, (3) pathologic ST changes in the presence of left bundle branch block, and (4) Wellens' phenomenon.
- Increased awareness about the STEMI equivalents facilitates communication between emergency physicians and cardiologists.
- Ultimately, agreement about the need for percutaneous cardiac intervention improves core measure metrics, such as the door-to-balloon time, and likewise improves patient outcomes.

INTRODUCTION

Diagnosis of ST-segment elevation myocardial infarction (STEMI) is time sensitive. After characteristic electrocardiogram (ECG) changes are noted, clinicians must take the necessary steps to activate a cardiac catheterization laboratory and attempt reperfusion. The axiom of "time is muscle" affects nearly every medical professional involved in emergency cardiac care. Emergency physicians must strive to obtain an ECG within 10 minutes of someone presenting with chest pain or an anginal equivalent. Often acting solely on the basis of the initial ECG interpretation, cardiologists mobilize entire teams to avert ischemic consequences. The imperative of diagnostic accuracy further contributes to the challenges associated with catheterization laboratory activation. Although STEMI criteria are well established, there is emerging interest in other cardiac conditions that also benefit from timely intervention. Specifically, "STEMI equivalents" warrant similarly aggressive and definitive intervention. This article focuses on ECG changes consistent with cardiac ischemia including (1) the de Winter ST/T complex, (2) ST elevation in lead aVR, (3) pathologic ST elevation in the presence of bundle branch block, and (4) Wellens' syndrome. This article also reviews the ECG presentation of posterior wall MI (PWMI). Many of the STEMI equivalents represent proposed additions to future American College of Cardiology/American Heart Association guidelines

The authors have nothing to disclose.
[a] Department of Emergency Medicine, University of Maryland School of Medicine, 110 South Paca Street, 6th Floor, Suite 200, Baltimore, MD 21201, USA; [b] Baltimore City Fire Department, 301 E. Fayette Street, Baltimore, MD 21202, USA
* Corresponding author. Department of Emergency Medicine, University of Maryland School of Medicine, 110 South Paca Street, 6th Floor, Suite 200, Baltimore, MD 21201.
E-mail address: blawn001@umaryland.edu

with respect to use of the catheterization laboratory.[1] Increased awareness about these conditions facilitates communication between emergency physicians and cardiologists. Ultimately, agreement about the need for percutaneous cardiac intervention improves core measure metrics, such as the door-to-balloon time, and likewise improves patient outcomes.

LEFT MAIN CORONARY ARTERY OCCLUSION: FACILITATING RECOGNITION AND THE IMPORTANCE OF LEAD aVR

Acute left main coronary artery occlusion is a dangerous condition that requires prompt recognition. Indeed, the left main coronary artery perfuses a large segment of the heart's anterior wall. Consequences related to a delay in reperfusion include lethal dysrhythmia and cardiogenic shock. Fortunately, acute left main occlusion is a rare event. Because the clinical presentation of acute left main coronary artery occlusion is potentially catastrophic, a timely and accurate ECG diagnosis is vital to good patient outcomes. The existence of collateral coronary circulation may contribute to the relative infrequency of this condition. Prediction of an acute occlusion is of prime importance, and the ECG provides valuable clues to the diagnosis. Yamaji and colleagues[2] prospectively studied the ECGs of 16 patients with angiographically confirmed left main coronary artery obstruction. The ECGs were compared with patients with confirmed occlusion of the left anterior descending (LAD) artery and right coronary artery. Fourteen (88%) of 16 patients with acute left main obstruction displayed ST-segment elevation in lead aVR. Furthermore, the elevation in aVR was of greater amplitude than the elevation observed in lead V_1. The authors additionally report that the ratio of ST-segment elevation (aVR/V_1) helps distinguish between a left main and a LAD lesion. With approximately 80% sensitivity and specificity, patients with acute left main obstruction displayed greater amplitude of ST-segment elevation in lead aVR. **Fig. 1** showcases pathologic ST elevation in lead aVR.

In 2007, Rostoff and colleagues[1] analyzed data from several clinical trials that examined ST-segment changes in lead aVR. The authors

acknowledge the challenges inherent in using aVR to predict occlusion of the left main coronary artery. The lack of prospective studies coupled with different criteria for ST-segment elevation (using a cutoff of 0.05 mV as opposed to 0.1 mV) contributes to a degree of diagnostic uncertainty. However, the data pooled from three studies validate the examination of lead aVR. ST-segment elevation in aVR predicted left main coronary artery occlusion with a sensitivity of 77.6% and a specificity of 82.6%. Rostoff and colleagues[1] confirm ST-segment elevation in aVR as a "reliable predictor of acute occlusion of the LMCA." More recently, a 2011 analysis of the Manitoba cardiogenic shock registry affirmed the close link between ECG findings and cardiac anatomy.[3] One hundred ninety-one patients with MI met the study's inclusion criteria, and 53 (28%) of cases demonstrated ST-segment elevation in aVR. Of those patients, 111 (58%) survived to hospital discharge. Sixteen of 53 (30%) had left main coronary artery stenosis of ($\geq$50%) and 24 (45%) of 53 exhibited significant proximal LAD coronary artery disease. This study is significant in that it examines the use of lead aVR within a notably sicker cohort, namely those patients with cardiogenic shock. The authors conclude that ST-segment elevation in aVR is an adequate predictor of coronary anatomy and reliably predicts the presence of significant stenosis and triple-artery disease. Ducas and colleagues[3] highlight ST-segment elevation in aVR as a "particular parameter to identify an easy predictor of life threatening coronary disease." Not surprisingly, 30-day mortality rates were lower in patients who experienced resolution of aVR ST-segment elevation after reperfusion therapy.[3]

The prognostic value of lead aVR underscores its clinical importance. In addition to its association with left main disease, aVR abnormalities are linked with increased mortality. In the study by Yamaji and coworkers,[2] death occurred more frequently in those patients who had a higher magnitude of ST-segment elevation in lead aVR. Using a cut off value of 0.15 mV, ST elevation predicted death with 75% specificity and sensitivity. In a study by Kosuge and colleagues,[4] more than 300 patients with ST-segment deviation of greater than or equal to 0.5 mm were included. At 90 days, only ST-segment elevation in aVR and positive

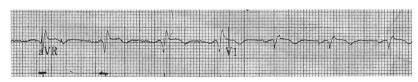

Fig. 1. Pathologic ST-segment elevation in lead aVR.

troponin values emerged as independent predictors of death or MI. Not surprisingly, patients with positive troponins and aVR findings had the highest incidence of left main coronary artery or three-vessel disease.[4] The study by Kosuge and colleagues[4] excluded patients with ST-segment elevations in leads other than aVR. Accordingly, the study corroborates the assertion that ST-segment elevation in lead aVR has important prognostic and therapeutic considerations.

Barrabes and colleagues[5] corroborated the association between ST-segment elevation in aVR and poor short-term prognosis. Seven hundred seventy-five patients were included in a study that examined admissions to the hospital's coronary care unit. One hundred thirty-four of these patients (17.3%) had greater than or equal to 0.1 mV of ST-segment elevation. Lead aVR elevation was associated with increased age, vital sign abnormalities, and the presence of previous angina. ST-segment elevation in aVR was the only initial electrocardiographic variable that persisted as an independent predictor of death. Even after the authors excluded ECGs that demonstrated ST-segment elevation in lead V_1 or met the criteria for LVH, lead aVR retained its predictive ability. In-hospital morbidity was similarly linked to ST-segment elevation in aVR. Patients with greater than or equal to 0.1 mV of ST-segment elevation in aVR more frequently required coronary artery bypass grafting.[5]

COMING OUT OF ISOLATION: THE PWMI

Despite mandatory and widespread scrutiny of emergent ECGs, a significant percentage of MI is missed on the initial ECG. More effective use of the ECG may contribute to increased accuracy and precision when searching for evidence of ischemia. The PWMI may evade detection because it may occur in conjunction with inferior wall changes. Furthermore, PWMI may also present in isolation. Unless posterior leads are obtained with regularity, ST-segment changes that reflect the changes of PWMI can be overlooked.[6]

Acute PWMI reportedly occurs in 15% to 20% of acute MIs.[6,7] The right coronary artery, by way of its posterior descending branches, perfuses the heart's posterior wall. The left circumflex artery also supplies blood to the posterior wall.[8] PWMI often occurs in conjunction with injury to the inferior or lateral wall of the left ventricle. Although less common, posterior wall infarction can also occur in relative isolation. The incidence of isolated PWMI is estimated at anywhere from 5% to 10%.[6,9]

Recognition of the isolated PWMI presentation begins with a search for a prominent R wave in lead V_1. Although high-amplitude precordial R waves result from other conditions, the presence of a tall R wave in lead V_1 is an abnormal finding.[9,10] Indeed, the initial R wave observed in V_1 is usually small in amplitude because septal depolarization occurs in a left-to-right direction. Tall R waves, defined as an R/S ratio of equal to or greater than one, coupled with ST-segment depression in leads V_1 through V_2 indicate ischemia of the heart's posterior wall. Upright T waves are observed in leads V_1 through V_3. **Fig. 2** displays the ECG changes typical of posterior wall infarction. The anterior precordial leads appear as an inverted reflection of the heart's posterior wall. Simplistically, the ST-depression would actually appear as ST-segment elevation in a true posterior ECG lead.

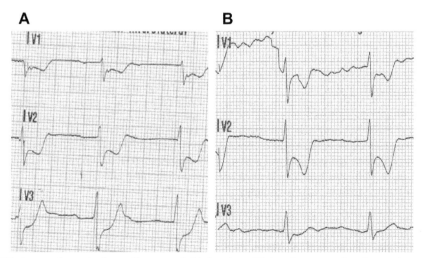

Fig. 2. (*A*) ECG changes in posterior wall myocardial infarction. (*B*) Another example of posterior wall ischemia.

Timely recognition of posterior wall injury is important. ECG changes associated with PWMI indicate a worse prognosis when appearing in conjunction with more widespread ST-segment elevation.[6] The tall R waves, ST-segment depression, and upright T waves that herald posterior wall injury reflect extension of a more massive infarction when seen alongside ST-segment elevation in inferior or anterior leads. It is well established that the risks of cardiogenic shock and lethal dysrhythmia increase in proportion to the magnitude of the MI. Emergency clinicians must avoid diagnosing ST depression in the early precordial leads as a non–ST-segment MI. PWMI is a condition benefiting from acute reperfusion therapy.[6,7] Physicians and others charged with the review of initial ECGs should remain vigilant for R wave and ST segment pathology in leads V_1 through V_3.

TO INCREASE DETECTION, LOOK TO THE POSTERIOR

Fortunately, relatively simple and inexpensive strategies exist to increase detection of the PWMI. The standard electrode placement does not directly reflect injury current traveling toward the patient's posterior surface. Indeed, the endocardial surface of the posterior wall faces traditionally placed anterior chest leads.[11] It logically follows that the use of additional or posterior electrodes may increase the sensitivity of the ECG in the detection of PWMI injury currents. Somers and colleagues[11] reviewed the application and usage of posterior leads (V_7 through V_9). The authors maintain that use of a 15-lead ECG increases the sensitivity for posterior wall ischemia to approximately 90%. Zalenski and colleagues[12] studied 149 admitted patients with suspected acute coronary syndromes. A standard 12-lead was obtained and was immediately followed by tracings from leads V_4R, V_8, and V_9. In 43 (28.9%) of 149 of patients, additional "major abnormalities," such as ST-segment deviation, Q waves, and T-wave inversion, were detected. The authors concluded that there was "an eightfold increase in the odds of detecting ST elevation." Importantly, ECG criteria for thrombolytic therapy were "uniquely" present on additional ECG leads.[12] In a subsequent trial, Zalenski and colleagues[13] enrolled 603 adults with suspected acute coronary syndrome and compared the accuracy of a standard 12-lead ECG with one that included right ventricular and posterior leads. Approximately 2% of patients without ST-segment elevation on the initial 12-lead displayed unique elevation of greater than 1 mm on leads V_7 through V_9. In this subgroup of patients, unique ST-segment elevation also increased the positive predictive value for acute

MI. The authors acknowledge several important limitations. First, they cautioned that ST-segment elevation in "non standard" leads cannot be used with the same confidence. Incorporating additional leads resulted in an overall 7% decrease in specificity for acute MI. Furthermore, a single cardiologist masked to patient outcome interpreted all study ECGs. This scenario is therefore not representative of actual clinical practice when an ECG finding is usually linked to a clinical presentation concerning for acute coronary syndrome. Simply stated, the routine use of posterior wall electrodes may heighten the provider's suspicion for isolated PWMI and subsequently increase detection.

Wung and Drew[14] attempted to validate the ECG criteria for PWMI in patients undergoing angiography. The authors studied 53 subjects who received elective left circumflex coronary angioplasty. Continuous 15-lead ECGs were recorded during balloon occlusion to capture the ECG changes accompanying a model of posterior wall ischemia. Patients who had suffered a previous MI, displayed significant collateral flow during angiography, or who experienced a balloon deflation duration of less than 60 seconds were excluded. A total of 49% of patients displayed ST-segment elevation of greater than 1 mm in the posterior ECG leads. Another 45% of patients had posterior ST-segment elevation of 0.5 to 1 mm. The authors' conclusions affirm the value of additional leads and suggest that a lowering of the diagnostic criteria from 1 to 0.5 mm would significantly improve the sensitivity of the posterior leads.[13]

PROXIMAL LAD OCCLUSION AND THE DE WINTER ST/T WAVE COMPLEX

de Winter and colleagues[15] describe a pattern consistent with a proximal LAD occlusion in which there is a 1- to 3-mm ST-segment depression in the precordial leads with an upsloping morphology. The ST segments then join tall and symmetric T waves. They found this pattern evident in 30 of 1532 patients who were diagnosed with an anterior MI. The tall and symmetric T waves that de Winter and colleagues[16] describe in this pattern are persistent. This is in contrast to hyperacute T waves, not uncommonly associated as an early but transient finding with STEMI.

Another study by Verounden and colleagues[17] found that this same pattern was associated with anterior MI. Of 1890 patients who underwent percutaneous coronary intervention (PCI) for an anterior MI, 35 had this ECG pattern. Of these 35 patients, 23 had a proximal LAD artery occlusion. The remaining had occlusions of the distal LAD. The authors hypothesize that the lack of ST-segment elevation could be because the very large transmural area of injury from a proximal LAD occlusion generates no injury currents. In this study, the authors conclude that approximately 2% of patients with anterior MI may present with the described ECG pattern.

This ECG pattern consisting of ST-segment depression, upsloping ST segment, followed by persistently tall and symmetric T waves, must be recognized as a potential finding in patients with anterior MI caused by a proximal LAD lesion (**Fig. 3**). Given the subtlety of this pattern, which has no ST-segment elevation, it certainly is possible for the described finding to be attributed incorrectly to ischemia as opposed to infarction. Patients with this ECG pattern and presenting with chest pain or other symptoms of ischemia should be considered candidates for immediate reperfusion therapy.

WELLENS' SYNDROME

In 1982, Wellens' group described an ECG pattern associated with patients with a critical stenosis of the proximal LAD artery.[18] Leads V_2 and V_3 (and sometimes V_4) demonstrate either biphasic or inverted T waves. It should be noted, however, that unlike the de Winter ST/T wave complex, Wellens' syndrome is not an acute process. The pattern may manifest persistently over a period of weeks. Physicians may often find the characteristic ECG pattern in a pain-free patient.[19] In their original study, Wellens group found this ECG pattern was not uncommon, with 18% of patients admitted for unstable angina demonstrating the described pattern.[18]

Although approximately one-quarter of patients with Wellens' syndrome present with biphasic T waves in the mid-precordial leads (**Fig. 4**A), most patients have inverted T waves[20] (see **Fig. 4**B). These ECG patterns are highly specific for disease of the LAD artery. In a follow-up study by de Zwaan and colleagues[21] of 188 patients who presented to a hospital with angina and Wellens' syndrome ECG criteria, all patients were found by angiogram to have greater than 50% stenosis of the proximal LAD artery.

Although Wellens' syndrome may progress to an anterior MI, asymptomatic patients may be evaluated by nonemergent angiography.[7] It should be noted, however, that these patients are certainly at risk for left ventricular dysfunction.[19] Given the associated proximal LAD critical stenosis, stress testing is potentially inappropriate in these patients because they are at significant risk for infarction.[22] Of note, half the patients in the original Wellens study demonstrated the pattern at the time of admission, whereas the remainder of the patients demonstrated the abnormality later during the first 24 hours of admission.[18] This further highlights the importance of obtaining serial ECGs in patients presenting to the hospital with symptoms concerning for acute MI.

LEFT BUNDLE BRANCH BLOCK AND ACUTE MI

Left bundle branch block (LBBB) has long been considered to be a predictor of increased mortality and morbidity in patients with acute MI.[23] It has been hypothesized that large infarctions of sufficient size were needed to affect the bundle branch conduction system, because of the poor prognostic indictor of LBBB in patients with acute MI.[24] LBBB has been shown to be associated with decreased ejection fraction, possibly one reason why this ECG pattern is associated with increased mortality and morbidity.[25] As such, patients presenting with LBBB in the setting of chest pain or other ischemic equivalent have for years been treated as aggressively as patients with STEMI. Current recommendations by the American College of Cardiology/American Heart Association stipulate that patients with new or presumably new LBBB should undergo immediate reperfusion therapy.[26]

Despite these recommendations, patients with new or presumably new LBBB often do not receive immediate reperfusion therapy. The Acute Coronary Treatment and Intervention Outcomes Network Registry—Get With the Guidelines enrolled more than 46,000 patients with either STEMI or new LBBB.[27] In this study, 94% of patients with STEMI received acute reperfusion (PCI or fibrinolytics), compared with only 48% of patients with new or presumably new LBBB. Only 64% of patients with LBBB received revascularization (PCI or bypass grafting), compared with 92% of patients presenting with STEMI. Clearly, clinicians often opt not to follow American Heart Association recommendations regarding immediate reperfusion therapy.

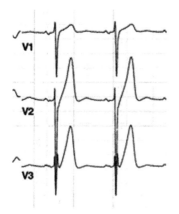

Fig. 3. de Winter ST/T wave complex.

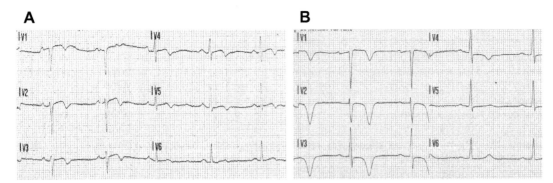

Fig. 4. Wellens' syndrome. (*A*) One manifestation of Wellens' syndrome is the presence of biphasic T waves in the anterior precordial leads. (*B*) Wellens' syndrome commonly presents with deep T-wave inversions in the anterior precordial leads.

Recent literature has called into question the necessity of immediate reperfusion for patients presenting with LBBB. Only a minority of patients with a new or presumed new LBBB are diagnosed with MI.[28] In an observational cohort study by Chang and colleagues,[29] 7937 patients presenting to an emergency department with chest pain were followed. Of the 55 patients who had a new or presumed new LBBB, four were ultimately diagnosed with an acute MI. The rate of acute MI in patients with new or presumed new LBBB was no different than patients with no LBBB or the group of patients with an old LBBB.

Sgarbossa and colleagues[30] describe three ECG criteria they found to be predictive of acute MI in patients with LBBB: (1) ST-segment elevation concordant with the QRS complex (**Fig. 5**A); (2) ST-segment depression in leads V_1, V_2, or V_3 (see **Fig. 5**B); and (3) ST-segment elevation of greater than 5 mm discordant from the QRS complex (see **Fig. 5**C).

In the original study, the Sgarbossa criteria were found to be very specific, but not sensitive, for

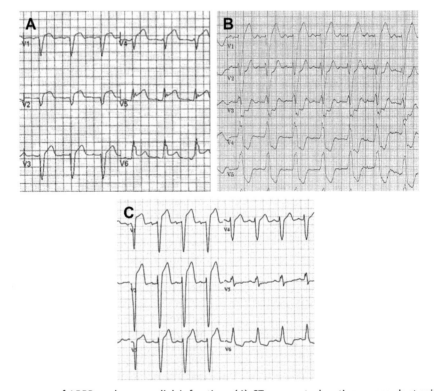

Fig. 5. The presence of LBBB and myocardial infarction. (*A*) ST-segment elevation concordant with the QRS complex. (*B*) ST-segment depression in leads V_1, V_2, or V_3. (*C*) ST-segment elevation of greater than 5 mm discordant from the QRS complex.

determining which patients with an LBBB were having an MI. A recent study found that MI was diagnosed in 86% of patients with concordant ST-segment changes (criteria 1 or 2), compared with 28% of patients without concordant changes.[28] Criterion 3 was noted to be less specific for acute MI. Another study by Al-Faleh and coworkers[31] also validated the use of the Sgarbossa criteria. Forty-nine percent of patients with LBBB who met the Sgarbossa criteria had elevated cardiac biomarkers.

The Sgarbossa criteria can be applied as a scoring system to improve specificity (**Table 1**). Concordant ST-segment elevation is given a score of 5, ST-segment depression in the anterior leads is scored 3, whereas ST-segment elevation of greater than 5 mm is given a score of 2.[30] A study at the Mayo Clinic enrolled 892 patients included in a suspected STEMI protocol.[32] Thirty-six of these patients had a new or presumably new LBBB. A total score of 5 or greater was 100% specific for acute MI, but only 14% sensitive. The study's authors conclude that this low sensitivity limits the usefulness of the Sgarbossa criteria in diagnosing acute MI routinely. However, the greatest use of the Sgarbossa criteria lies in the very high specificity.

It has been estimated that the false-positive rate for catheterization laboratory activation is approximately 10%.[33] The presence of an LBBB alone is a not uncommon factor associated with false-positive activations. However, the very high specificity of the Sgarbossa criteria in the presence of an LBBB, especially the presence of criteria 1 or 2, means that the catheterization laboratory should certainly be activated if the criteria are present. However, the low sensitivity of the criteria means that clinicians should not rely on their absence to rule out acute MI. Given the accumulating evidence of the lower prevalence of acute MI than previously believed in patients with LBBB, it has been suggested that a new or presumed new LBBB by itself may not warrant activation of the catheterization laboratory. Rather, patients with an LBBB should be evaluated emergently in the catheterization laboratory if they have Sgarbossa criteria 1 or 2, if they seem unstable, or if cardiac biomarkers are elevated.[7]

PACEMAKERS COMPLICATE INTERPRETATION OF ISCHEMIA

The presence of a pacemaker may potentially confound the evaluation of an ECG in a patient presenting with a potential acute MI. With most pacemakers having an initiating impulse in the right ventricle, depolarization progresses from the right to left ventricle.[34] Furthermore, the ST segments are expected to be discordant from the terminal portion of the QRS complex.

In a study by Sgarbossa and colleagues,[35] the "rule of appropriate discordance" is found to be helpful in evaluating the ECG of a patient with a pacemaker. The authors studied the approximately 41,000 patients in the GUSTO trial, of which 32 had a ventricular pacemaker.[23] The finding of discordant ST-segment elevation was found to be 53% sensitive and 88% specific for acute MI.[35] Concordant ST-segment elevation of greater than 1 mm was found to be 18% sensitive and 94% specific.[35] Similarly, ST-segment depression of greater than 1 mm in leads V_1, V_2, or V_3 was 29% sensitive and 82% specific for acute MI.[35] Therefore, similar to the Sgarbossa criteria developed for LBBB, this similar set of criteria for evaluating ECGs of patients with a pacemaker is highly specific, but not very sensitive in identifying patients with acute MI. **Fig. 6** showcases concordant ST-segment elevation and discordant ST-segment elevation measuring greater than 5 mm.

Given that the Sgarbossa criteria developed for patients with pacemakers are again highly specific, but not sensitive, for acute MI, these patients present challenging cases to the clinician. The risk of false-positive activations of the catheterization laboratory is high if the clinician does not take into account other indications that the patient may be experiencing an acute MI, such as patient instability, comparison of old ECGs, and elevated cardiac biomarkers.

Table 1
Sgarbossa's criteria (when the ischemia is suspected in the presence of a left bundle branch block or paced rhythm)

ST-Segment Change	Measurement	Score
Concordant ST-segment elevation	>1 mm	5
Concordant ST-segment depression in V_1 through V_3	>1 mm	3
Inappropriately discordant ST-segment elevation	>5 mm	2

The Sgarbossa criteria can be applied as a scoring system to improve specificity. The low sensitivity of the criteria, however, limits their usefulness in the diagnosis of acute myocardial infarction.

Data from Sgarbossa EB, Pinski SL, Barbagelata A, et al. Electrocardiographic diagnosis of evolving acute myocardial infarction in the presence of left bundle-branch block. GUSTO-1 (Global Utilization of Streptokinase and Tissue Plasminogen Activator for Occluded Coronary Arteries) Investigators. N Engl J Med 1996;334(8):481–7.

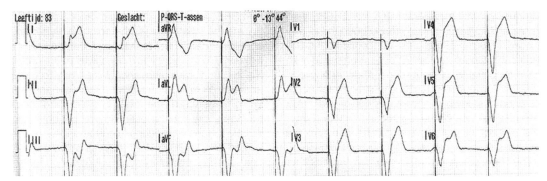

Fig. 6. Paced rhythm and myocardial infarction. (*Courtesy of* M.M. Meuwissen, Amphia Breda, The Netherlands; and *From* http://ECGpedia.org/. Accessed March 18, 2012; with permission.)

ACTIVATION OF THE CARDIAC CATHETERIZATION LABORATORY: FUTURE DIRECTIONS

The decision to send a patient for immediate reperfusion is predicated on more than the interpretation of a single, diagnostic ECG. STEMI guidelines are clear with respect to contiguous ST-segment elevation and the presence of reciprocal change. However, the emergent ECG provides the clinician with information far in excess of classic STEMI criteria. As the collective knowledge base expands, emergency physicians and cardiologists alike must widen their focus to include conditions that are linked to the need for aggressive reperfusion therapy. A collaborative discussion that integrates evidence-based guidelines ideally facilitates definitive care for at-risk patients. Tools to increase the ECGs sensitivity for PWMI are readily available. A closer inspection of the traditional 12-lead, or more routine use of posterior leads, will help identify the PWMI that occurs in isolation. Accordingly, the ability to recognize novel patterns of ischemia, such as the de Winter ST/T wave complex and ST-segment elevation in lead aVR, may facilitate accurate and timely reperfusion. Close scrutiny and increased awareness of "STEMI equivalents" helps identify ECG findings more clearly associated with the need for urgent reperfusion.

REFERENCES

1. Rostoff P, Piwowarska W, Gackowski A. Electrocardiographic prediction of acute left main coronary artery occlusion. Am J Emerg Med 2007;25(7):852–5.
2. Yamaji H, Iwasaki K, Kusachi S. Prediction of acute left main coronary artery obstruction by 12-lead electrocardiography. J Am Coll Cardiol 2001;38(5): 1348–54.
3. Ducas R, Ariyarajah V, Philipp R, et al. The presence of ST elevation in lead aVR predicts significant left main coronary artery stenosis in cardiogenic shock resulting from myocardial infarction: the Manitoba cardiogenic shock registry. Int J Cardiol. November 27, 2011. [Epub ahead of print].
4. Kosuge M, Kimura K, Ishikawa T. Combined prognostic utility of ST segment in lead aVR and troponin T on admission in non ST segment elevation acute coronary syndromes. Am J Cardiol 2006;97(3):334–9.
5. Barrabes JA, Figueras J, Moure C, et al. Prognostic value of lead aVR in patients with a first non ST-segment elevation acute myocardial infarction. Circulation 2003;108(7):814–9.
6. Brady WJ, Erling B, Pollack M, et al. Electrocardiographic manifestations: acute posterior wall myocardial infarction. J Emerg Med 2001;20(4): 391–401.
7. Rokos IC, French WJ, Mattu A, et al. Appropriate cardiac cath lab activation: optimizing electrocardiogram interpretation and clinical decision-making for acute ST-elevation myocardial infarction. Am Heart J 2010;160(6):995–1003.e8.
8. Zafari AM. Myocardial infarction. Emedicine Online. 2011. Available at: http://emedicine.medscape.com/ article/155919-overview. Accessed February, 2012.
9. Mattu A, Brady WJ, Perron AD, et al. Prominent R wave in lead V1: electrocardiographic differential diagnosis. Am J Emerg Med 2001;19(6):504–13.
10. Zema MJ. Electrocardiographic tall R waves in the right precordial leads. J Electrocardiol 1990;23(2): 147–56.
11. Somers MP, Brady WJ, Bateman DC, et al. Additional electrocardiographic leads in the ED chest pain patient. Am J Emerg Med 2003;21(7):563–73.
12. Zalenski RJ, Cooke D, Rydman R, et al. Assessing the diagnostic value of an ECG containing leads V4R, V8, and V9: the 15 lead ECG. Ann Emerg Med 1993;22(5):786–93.
13. Zalenski RJ, Rydman RJ, Sloan EP, et al. Value of posterior and right ventricular leads in comparison to the standard 12 lead electrocardiogram in evaluation of ST-segment elevation in suspected acute myocardial infarction. Am J Cardiol 1997;79(12):1579–85.

14. Wung SF, Drew BJ. New electrocardiograpghic criteria for posterior wall acute myocardial ischemia validated by a percutaneous transluminal coronary angioplasty model of acute myocardial infarction. Am J Cardiol 2001;87(8):970–4.

15. de Winter RJ, Verounden NJ, Wellens HJ, et al. A new ECG sign of proximal LAD occlusion. N Engl J Med 2008;359(19):2071–3.

16. Goldberger AL. Hyperacute T waves revisited. Am Heart J 1982;104(4):888–90.

17. Verounden NJ, Koch KT, Peters RJ, et al. Persistent precordial "hyperacute" T-waves signify proximal left anterior descending artery occlusion. Heart 2009; 95(20):1701–6.

18. de Zwaan C, Bar FW, Wellens HJ, et al. Characteristic electrocardiographic pattern indicating a critical stenosis high in left anterior descending artery. Am Heart J 1982;103(4):730–6.

19. Rhinehardt J, Brady WJ, Perrod AD, et al. Electrocardiographic manifestations of Wellens' syndrome. Am J Emerg Med 2002;20(7):638–43.

20. Tandy TK, Bottomy DP, Lewis JG. Wellens' syndrome. Ann Emerg Med 1999;33(3):347–51.

21. de Zwaan C, Bar FW, Janssen JH, et al. Angiographic and clinical characteristics of patients with unstable angina showing an ECG pattern indicating critical narrowing of the proximal LAD coronary artery. Am Heart J 1989;117(3):657–65.

22. Tatli E, Aktoz M. Wellens' syndrome: the electrocardiographic finding that is seen as unimportant. Cardiol J 2009;16(1):73–5.

23. Fibrinolytic Therapy Trialists' (FTT) collaborative group. Indications for fibrinolytic therapy in suspected acute myocardial infarction: collaborative overview of early mortality and major morbidity results from all randomized trials of more than 1000 patients. Lancet 1994;343(8893):311–22.

24. Hindman MC, Wagner GS, JaRo M, et al. The clinical significance of bundle branch block complicating acute myocardial infarction. Circulation 1978;58(4):679–88.

25. Hamby RI, Weissman RH, Prakash MN, et al. Left bundle branch block: a predictor of poor left ventricular function in coronary artery disease. Am Heart J 1983;106(3):417–77.

26. Antman EM, Anbe DT, Armstrong PW, et al. ACC/AHA guidelines for the management of patients with ST-elevation myocardial infarction – executive summary: a report of the American College of Cardiology/American Heart Association Task Force on Practice Guidelines (writing committee to revise the 1999 guidelines for the management of patients with acute myocardial infarction). J Am Coll Cardiol 2004;44(3):590–636.

27. Yeo KK, Li S, Amsterdam EA, et al. Comparison of clinical characteristics, treatments and outcomes of patients with ST-elevation acute myocardial. Am J Cardiol 2012;109(4):497–501.

28. Kontos MC, Aziz HA, Chau VQ, et al. Outcomes in patients with chronicity of left bundle-branch block with possible acute myocardial infarction. Am Heart J 2011;161(4):698–704.

29. Chang AM, Shofer FS, Tabas JA, et al. Lack of association between left bundle-branch block and acute myocardial infarction in symptomatic ED patients. Am J Emerg Med 2009;27(8):916–21.

30. Sgarbossa EB, Pinski SL, Barbagelata A, et al. Electrocardiographic diagnosis of evolving acute myocardial infarction in the presence of left bundle-branch block. GUSTO-1 (Global Utilization of Streptokinase and Tissue Plasminogen Activator for Occluded Coronary Arteries) Investigators. N Engl J Med 1996;334(8):481–7.

31. Al-Faleh H, Fu Y, Wagner G, et al. Unraveling the spectrum of left bundle branch block in acute myocardial infarction: insights from the assessment of the safety and efficacy of a new Thrombolytic (ASSENT 2 and 3) trials. Am Heart J 2006;151(1):10–5.

32. Jain S, Ting HT, Bell M, et al. Utility of left bundle branch block as a diagnostic criterion for acute myocardial infarction. Am J Cardiol 2011;107(8):1111–6.

33. Larson DM, Menssen KM, Sharkey SW, et al. "False-positive" cardiac catheterization laboratory activation among patients with suspected ST-segment elevation myocardial infarction. JAMA 2007; 298(23):2754–60.

34. Rosner MH, Brady WJ. The electrocardiographic diagnosis of acute myocardial infarction in patients with ventricular paced rhythms. Am J Emerg Med 1999;17(2):182–5.

35. Sgarbossa EB, Pinski SL, Gates KB, et al. Early electrocardiographic diagnosis of acute myocardial infarction in the presence of ventricular paced rhythm. Am J Cardiol 1996;77(5):423–4.

Electrocardiographic Patterns Mimicking ST Segment Elevation Myocardial Infarction

Peter Pollak, MD[a], William Brady, MD[b],*

KEYWORDS

- Electrocardiogram • ECG • ST segment elevation • STEMI • Mimic

KEY POINTS

- The 12-lead surface electrocardiogram (ECG) is inexpensive, portable, and transmittable; it remains the cornerstone of prompt diagnosis of and primary indication for the management of ST elevation myocardial infarction (STEMI).
- Although the ECG is reasonably reliable, it remains an imperfect diagnostic tool. Some patients do present with classic symptoms and findings; however, approximately 60% to 80% of patients with ST segment elevation on the presenting ECG are ultimately found to not be associated with STEMI.
- In certain difficult cases, a patient's ECG can resemble STEMI yet manifest ST segment elevation from a non–acute coronary syndrome entity, the so-called *STEMI mimics*. In other situations, the patient's ECG makes it difficult or impossible to determine whether STEMI is present, the so-called *STEMI confounders*; these *confounders* to STEMI diagnosis are also *mimickers* of AMI.
- The ultimate goal with both the STEMI mimics and the confounders is to maximize rapid, accurate diagnosis while avoiding delays in treatment of alternative causes of ST segment elevation.

INTRODUCTION

Cardiovascular disease is the leading cause of death worldwide. In fact, 7 million patients present annually to emergency departments in the United States with symptoms concerning for myocardial ischemia.[1] Prompt reperfusion in the setting of ST segment elevation myocardial infarction (STEMI) can dramatically reduce the associated mortality and morbidity. Unfortunately, the benefit of reperfusion therapies in acute myocardial infarction (AMI) decays quickly over time. Improvements in care systems, such as the door-to-balloon initiative and the American Heart Association's Mission Lifeline have altered the landscape of STEMI management over the past decade, minimizing delays to reperfusion and significantly improving outcomes. These systems require the rapid mobilization of large teams of practitioners and resources, involve not insignificant risk to patients, and rely heavily on the clinician to quickly and accurately determine whether an electrocardiographic finding represents acute closure of a coronary artery and related STEMI. The 12-lead surface electrocardiogram (ECG) is inexpensive, portable, and transmittable; it remains the cornerstone of the prompt diagnosis of and the primary indication for management of STEMI. Although reasonably reliable, the ECG remains an imperfect diagnostic tool. Some patients do present with classic symptoms and findings; however, approximately 60% to 80% of patients with ST segment elevation on the presenting ECG ultimately are found to not be associated with STEMI.[2,3] Refer to **Fig. 1** for a depiction of the

[a] Division of Cardiovascular Medicine, Department of Medicine, University of Virginia School of Medicine, Lee Street, Charlottesville, VA 22908, USA; [b] Departments of Emergency Medicine and Medicine, University of Virginia School of Medicine, Lee Street, Charlottesville, VA 22908, USA
* Corresponding author.
E-mail address: wb4z@virginia.edu

Cardiol Clin 30 (2012) 601–615
http://dx.doi.org/10.1016/j.ccl.2012.07.012
0733-8651/12/$ – see front matter © 2012 Elsevier Inc. All rights reserved.

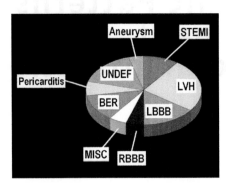

Fig. 1. Causes of ST segment elevation in adult patients with chest pain. BER, benign early repolarization; LBBB, left bundle branch block; LVH, left ventricular hypertrophy; MISC, miscellaneous; RBBB, right bundle branch block; UNDEF, undefined.

causes of ST segment elevation in adult patients with chest pain.[2,3]

In certain difficult cases, a patient's ECG can resemble STEMI, yet manifest ST segment elevation from a non–acute coronary syndrome (ACS) entity, the so-called *STEMI mimics*. In other situations, the patient's ECG makes it difficult or impossible to determine whether STEMI is present, the so-called *STEMI confounders*; these *confounders* to STEMI diagnosis are also *mimickers* of AMI.

All such cases can leave a practitioner wondering whether to initiate reperfusion therapy, either via administration of a fibrinolytic agent or activation of STEMI alert process, in essence, whether to expose patients to both the benefits and the risks of fibrinolysis or invasive coronary angiography. In some cases, the astute clinician can detect an alternative diagnosis masquerading as an STEMI. Failure to recognize these mimics can lead to inappropriate use of resources, exposure of patients to unnecessary risk, and increased rather than decreased morbidity and mortality. The ultimate goal with both the STEMI mimics and the confounders is to maximize rapid, accurate diagnosis while avoiding delays in the treatment of alternative causes of ST segment elevation. Because the risk of cerebral hemorrhage from fibrinolysis is not insignificant, careful consideration of the ECG, looking for the STEMI mimics, is required in patient-care situations in which primary percutaneous coronary intervention (PCI) is not an option. More importantly, fibrinolysis given in the setting of certain STEMI mimics, such as acute myopericarditis, is associated with high mortality.

Although each of the conditions discussed here is unique, a common issue that must not be overlooked is the interpretation of the ECG within the context of the patient's presentation; in other words, does the patient look like he or she is experiencing a STEMI? The STEMI mimics and confounders more often imitate the ECG findings of AMI than the clinical syndrome, so the patient *with* ST segment elevation but *without* a convincingly clinical picture of STEMI should prompt the provider to suspect a non-AMI presentation. At times, these diagnoses are very challenging, which will understandably impact the rapid application of reperfusion therapy and likely increase the door-to-therapy time.

STEMI MIMICKING PATTERNS
Myocarditis and Myopericarditis

Inflammation of the pericardium and heart muscle is a common cause of chest pain with ST segment elevation. Seventy-three percent of patients diagnosed with acute myopericarditis will have ST segment elevation on initial ECG.[4] Additionally, 44% of patients with chest pain and positive troponin but who do not have obstructive coronary disease by angiography demonstrate evidence of myocarditis by cardiac magnetic resonance imaging (MRI) using late gadolinium enhancement to reveal areas of myocardial necrosis in a noncoronary distribution (ie, midwall or subepicardial rather than subendocardial).[5]

Myocarditis affects patients of all ages and has a wide spectrum of clinical severity, ranging from incidental chest discomfort to fulminant heart failure with cardiogenic shock. The term *myocarditis* refers to an inflammatory process of the heart muscle (as reflected by the presence of biomarkers and ECG changes), whereas *pericarditis* refers to isolated inflammation of the lining around the heart. The pericardium is electrically silent, thus, when patients present with a clinical picture suggestive of pericarditis and demonstrate ST segment changes, the myocardium is also affected. Frequently, inflammation involves both components, hence, the term *myopericarditis* is used.

The cause is not frequently elucidated, but a viral cause is thought to be most common, with a minority of cases stemming from toxins or autoimmune processes. Patients may remember a prodrome of viral illness in the previous week or two. The pain is classically pleuritic in nature and changes in severity with position (sitting forward or lying back).

Biomarkers of myocardial necrosis, such as troponin and creatinine kinase, are positive in the setting of myocarditis, although they may be negative in the setting of pure pericarditis. The absolute value of troponin elevation is associated with the extent of myocardial cell injury but only very roughly correlates with clinical severity. A rub on cardiac auscultation is a highly specific but very insensitive physical examination finding and is frequently absent when even a small effusion is present.[6] Although a small pericardial effusion is not uncommon, it is quite rare for pericarditis to present with cardiac tamponade.

The electrocardiogram (**Figs. 2** and **3**) generally evolves in patients with myocarditis/myopericarditis, yet this evolution occurs less rapidly than that seen with STEMI; thus, serial ECGs, which demonstrate changes in the ST segment and T-wave morphologies over minutes, are frequently useful in making the distinction. ST segment elevation in multiple coronary distributions, especially when seen in patients who are clinically stable, favors inflammation over STEMI in large part because patients who simultaneously occlude multiple coronary arteries typically present with shock or death.[7] The presence of ST segment depression is less likely with myocarditis/myopericarditis (with the exception of lead AVR); when present, ST segment depression likely represents reciprocal ST segment depression and suggests STEMI. The presence of PR segment depression

in leads with ST segment elevation as well as PR segment elevation in lead AVR favors inflammation over STEMI. It is possible for myocarditis to be isolated anatomically in a single coronary artery distribution, leaving distinction from STEMI more challenging. In cases involving a coexistent pericardial effusion, electrical alternans and/or diminished electrical forces of the QRS complex can also be seen.

Early Repolarization (Also Known as Benign Early Repolarization)

Benign early repolarization (BER) is a normal variant electrocardiographic pattern; it manifests as ST segment elevation at the J point, predominantly in the precordial leads. It is frequently present in the general population, particularly in younger patients and male gender. BER is associated with young athletic men and is seen across all races; it has been linked to the black race, although some have disputed this association. It is not itself a pathologic finding and has not been

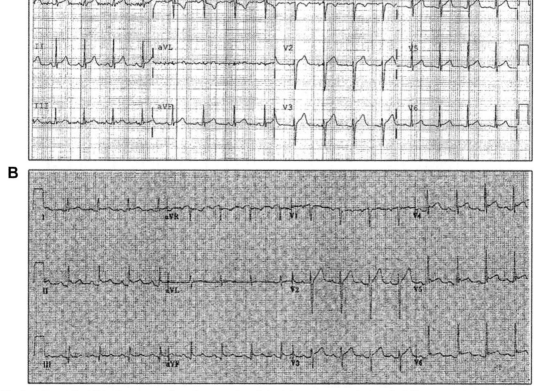

Fig. 2. Myopericarditis: Two examples of myopericarditis. (*A*) Myopericarditis with diffuse ST segment elevation. (*B*) Myopericarditis with diffuse ST segment elevation and PR segment changes (depression in leads II, III, aVF, and V6 and elevation in lead aVR).

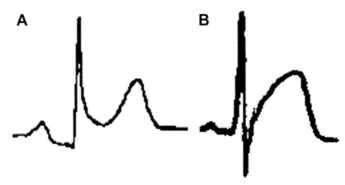

Fig. 3. Myopericarditis versus STEMI. (*A*) ST segment elevation with PR segment depression of myopericarditis. (*B*) STEMI.

tied to a disease process; for unknown reasons, BER is seen frequently in patients with chest pain who have used cocaine.

The electrocardiographic description (**Figs. 4** and **5**) of BER focuses on ST segment elevation with the following associated features: ST segment elevation with an upward concavity of its initial portion, notching or slurring of the terminal QRS complex (the J point), prominent T waves that are symmetric and concordant with the QRS complex (except in leads V1-V2), widespread distribution of ST segment elevation, and relative temporal stability of the pattern. The degree of ST segment elevation, beginning at the J-point elevation, is usually less than 3.0 mm, with a range of 0.5 to 5.0 mm. The ST segment elevation morphologically seems as if the ST segment has been evenly lifted upwards from the isoelectric baseline at the J point with preservation of the normal concavity of the initial, up-sloping portion of the ST segment. The J point itself is frequently notched or irregular in contour and is considered highly suggestive of BER. Prominent T waves are seen and are of large amplitude, slightly asymmetric morphology, and concordant with the QRS complex; the height of the T waves in BER ranges from approximately 6.5 mm in the precordial distribution to 5.0 mm in the limb leads. The ST segment and T-wave abnormalities of BER are most often seen in leads V1 to V4. At times, coexistent changes are also seen in leads II, III, AVF, V5, and V6; importantly, BER-related changes noted only in the limb leads are unusual and likely result from some other pathologic process, such as STEMI. Lastly, the chronic nature of the ST segment elevation is helpful in the

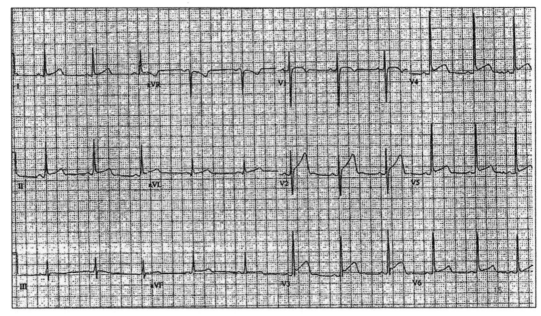

Fig. 4. Benign early repolarization with widespread, concave ST segment elevation.

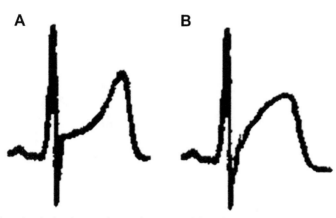

Fig. 5. ST segment elevation in benign early repolarization (*A*) and STEMI (*B*).

diagnosis of BER. The ST segment and T-wave abnormalities seen in BER will change very slowly over time with a diminution of ST segment elevation over decades; STEMI-related changes, on the other hand, evolve over minutes to hours.

Previous Infarction with Ventricular Aneurysm

The presence of ST segment elevation on ECG in patients with known prior myocardial infarction presents a special diagnostic challenge; these patients have known coronary disease and remain at an increased risk of recurrent STEMI. Patients who have had a past myocardial infarction can present with the various mechanical complications and have lingering ST segment elevation that has not resolved. Other patients, after a past myocardial infarction with remodeling, can present with persistent ST segment elevation attributable to aneurysmal dilatation of the infarcted segment of myocardium. In the prereperfusion era, rates of

left ventricular (LV) aneurysm approached 10%, but they have decreased dramatically since the introduction of fibrinolysis and mechanical reperfusion. Approximately one-quarter of patients with persistent ST segment elevation following STEMI will have an LV aneurysm as determined by echocardiography.[8]

When considered together, the patients' history of present illness, past medical history, and prior ECG are the most useful tools to identify LV aneurysm and distinguish the ST segment elevation from that of STEMI. Patients should be able to clarify whether they had a prior heart attack and to what degree their current presentation is similar or dissimilar. In this case, the bedside echocardiogram is generally unhelpful because the preexisting wall motion abnormality is difficult to distinguish from a new one.

The most frequent electrocardiographic manifestation (**Figs. 6** and **7**) of ventricular aneurysm is ST segment elevation, most often in the anterior

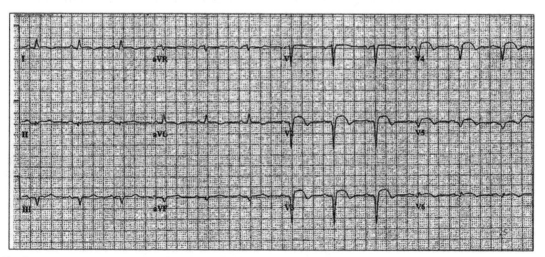

Fig. 6. LV aneurysm. ST segment elevation in leads V1 to V5 along with Q waves and T-wave inversion.

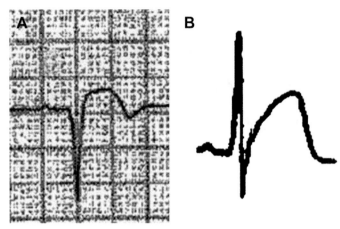

Fig. 7. ST segment elevation in LV aneurysm (*A*) versus STEMI (*B*).

distribution; inferior and lateral aneurysms are also encountered. The 12-lead electrocardiogram demonstrates ST segment elevation of varying morphologies and magnitudes, ranging from obvious, convex ST segment elevation to minimal, concave elevations. Pathologic Q waves are usually observed in leads with ST segment elevation. Inverted T waves of minimal magnitude are also seen in these same leads. Of course, a comparison with a past ECG since the myocardial infarction, if available, can determine if any change has occurred. Reciprocal ST segment depression is usually not present and this is helpful in distinguishing aneurysm from true STEMI. Lastly, the performance of serial ECGs can be invaluable, with dynamic changes suggesting STEMI and the absence of evolution suggesting aneurysm.

Coronary Vasospasm (Prinzmetal Angina)

Coronary vasospasm presents along a wide spectrum of disease severity, ranging from intermittent chest pain (so-called variant angina) to clinically severe STEMI equivalents with concomitant heart failure and ventricular fibrillation. It is exceptionally common among patients presenting to emergency departments with chest pain syndromes. The Clopidogrel and Acetyl Salicylic Acid in Bypass Surgery for Peripheral ARterial Disease (CASPAR) trial found 49% of patients presenting with acute chest pain who did not have a culprit lesion by angiography did have coronary vasospasm by acetylcholine challenge.[9] Coronary vasospasm can occur in patients across a broad demographic without clear gender or race associations; moreover, it can occur along the length of any of the coronary arteries. Coronary vasospasm is associated with tobacco, cocaine use, and ergonovine derivatives and can occur in both atherosclerotic

as well as angiographically normal vessels. There is a form of coronary vasospasm caused by allergic histamine release, called Kounis syndrome.[10] The final diagnosis of coronary vasospasm is made in the heart catheterization laboratory. Prior use of provocation tests with acetylcholine and methylergonovines has largely fallen out of favor.

Because acute coronary vasospasm can lead to near complete cessation of blood flow in the affected coronary artery, its presentation and pathophysiology parallels STEMI with the important distinction of absent vessel thrombosis. Rapid response to nitrates is a hallmark of coronary vasospasm. Treatment of normotensive patients with ST segment elevation remains a useful strategy to identify those with rapidly resolving syndromes when vasospasm is more likely. When considering reperfusion treatment, it is important to consider the possibility of coronary vasospasm.

The association of coronary vasospasm with cocaine (and other amphetamines) ingestion presents another challenge. Cocaine is both vasospastic as well as thrombogenic, leaving users at an increased risk of both mechanisms of coronary flow obstruction and resultant infarction. In patients with a clear amphetamine toxidrome (eg, hypertension, agitation, and so forth) as well as ST segment elevation, it is prudent to treat the patients with intravenous benzodiazepines and oral or topical nitrates with repeat performance of the ECG to determine if persistent ST segment elevation is present. It must be stressed that STEMI remains the working diagnosis and, if unable to demonstrate resolution of the ST segment elevation within a short period of time, reperfusion therapy should follow. Refer to **Figs. 8** and **9** for a depiction of ST segment elevation as seen in coronary vasospasm.

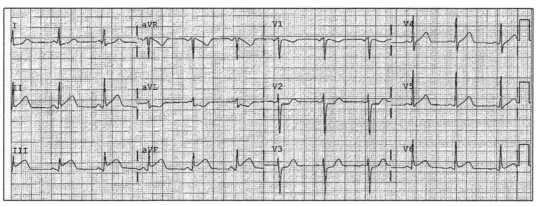

Fig. 8. Coronary vasospasm: ST segment elevation in the inferior leads along with ST segment depression in leads aVL, V2, and V3. This patient presented with chest pain and was ultimately diagnosed with coronary vasospasm (Prinzmetal angina). This form of ST segment elevation is indistinguishable from that seen in STEMI.

Other Non-STEMI ST Segment Elevation Syndromes

Takotsubo cardiomyopathy (apical ballooning syndrome)

Apical ballooning syndrome (ABS) is a recently identified disease in cardiology. In its short history, it has had different names, including *Takostubo cardiomyopathy* and the *broken heart syndrome*, and it falls along the spectrum of acute stress-induced cardiomyopathies. Although the name and classic presentation involve dyskinesis at the LV apex, multiple variations, including basal and midcavitary dyskinesis, have also been reported. The clinical presentation of ABS is frequently indistinguishable from ACS and is well known to mimic STEMI.[11] Patients can present with the full spectrum of chest pain equivalents from vague atypical chest pain to severe chest pain with acute heart failure and malignant dysrhythmia.

The spectrum of ECG findings is likewise varied, from minimal abnormality to profound anterior ST segment elevation (**Fig. 10**). In its most common apical form, the ECG changes are limited to the anterior precordial leads, reflecting apical location of injury. The inferior leads can also be involved, reflecting inferoapical injury. Because the history and ECG and even echocardiogram can be indistinguishable from true AMI, the diagnosis of ABS is made in the heart catheterization laboratory following diagnostic angiography.

Brugada syndrome and idiopathic ventricular fibrillation

The Brugada pattern includes right bundle branch block (RBBB) (both incomplete and complete) with ST segment elevation in leads V1 to V3; the natural history of this syndrome is sudden cardiac death. Brugada syndrome was first described as a clinical entity in 1992 to explain the observation that a particular cohort of patients prone to ventricular fibrillation despite structurally normal hearts had a distinct ECG pattern.[12] Since its first description,

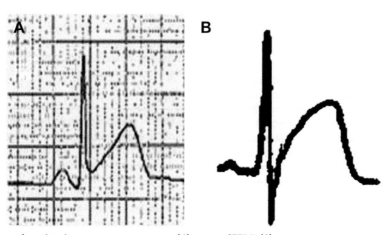

Fig. 9. ST segment elevation in coronary vasospasm (*A*) versus STEMI (*B*).

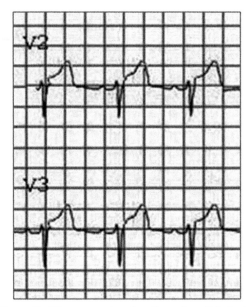

Fig. 10. ST segment elevation in Takotsubo cardiomyopathy.

a great deal has been learned about this relatively rare inherited disease. It occurs in approximately 5 out of 100 000 people across all nationalities, has an autosomal-dominant inheritance pattern, and a male predominance (~70%).[13] Three subtypes have been described, with subtle variations in the shape of the ST segment. The underlying mechanism, resulting from a gene mutation, is a sodium channel loss of function.[14]

Clinically, the disease can present at any age, but the mean age of sudden death is 41 years. The characteristic ECG findings (**Fig. 11**) are dynamic and may vary from one ECG to the next. Chest pain is not part of the Brugada syndrome; however, syncope is a significant poor prognostic marker. The natural history includes cardiac arrest resulting from polymorphic ventricular tachycardia and/or ventricular fibrillation. The disease and ECG findings can be exacerbated by multiple medications as well as conditions that alter myocardial membrane electrical stability (eg, fever, hypokalemia, ischemia, bradycardia, and increased autonomic tone). Vaughan Williams class Ic antiarrhythmic medications (eg, flecainide and procainamide) are potent sodium channel blockers and are clinically used to elicit the Brugada pattern in suspected cases. A large number of medications in addition to sodium channel blockers have been reported to elicit a Brugadalike pattern on ECG. The significance of these findings to a particular patient remains unclear.

Hyperkalemia
As the serum potassium concentration increases, changes occur in ECG that can mimic ACS,

including STEMI.[15] The elevation of the ST segment occurs following peaking of the T wave and widening of the QRS complex, suggesting high serum potassium concentrations. Although the accompanying ST segment elevation may be most impressive in a single region, the ECG changes of hyperkalemia are present throughout the limb and precordial leads.

Postelectrical cardioversion/defibrillation
Following transthoracic electrical cardioversion or defibrillation, the ECG can manifest ST segment elevation, among other abnormalities. ST segment elevation has been noted following both cardioversion for atrial as well as ventricular tachyarrhythmias in up to 20% of patients. Additionally, ST segment deviation occurs following countershock by internal cardioverter-defibrillator in 25% of patients.[16] The ST segment elevation is transient and resolves within minutes but can be profound, as much as 5 mm.[17] Although impressive and alarming, this finding has not been associated with evidence of ongoing myocardial injury or additional adverse sequelae.[18]

Hypothermia and Osborn waves
Prominent J-point elevations, also known as Osborn waves, are a common finding in patients who are hypothermic.[19] When profound, the ST segment can be elevated, mimicking STEMI. Other findings include bradycardia and motion artifact. The mechanism and clinical implications of the Osborn wave remain unclear, but it is a transient finding that resolves with normothermia. Osborn waves can occur with either therapeutic hypothermia or accidental hypothermia.[20]

STEMI Confounding Patterns

The confounder electrocardiographic patterns are those ECG entities that markedly reduce the electrocardiogram's ability to detect changes related to ACS, not because the findings mimic STEMI but because the condition obscures the detection of ST segment elevation. The commonly confounding patterns include left bundle branch block (LBBB), ventricular paced rhythms, and LV hypertrophy.

LBBB

LBBB is the most classic example of a confounder and is exceptionally common in the evaluation of patients with chest pain. This pattern is linked very closely with ischemic heart disease in that the development of LBBB is associated with significant heart disease; it also identifies a population at an increased risk for STEMI, acute cardiovascular complication, and poor outcome.[21] The LBBB pattern on the ECG includes an elevated

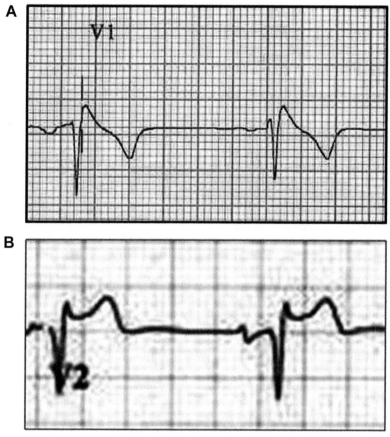

Fig. 11. Two forms of ST segment elevation as seen in the Brugada syndrome. (*A*) Convex form. (*B*) Concave (saddle-type) form.

ST segment at baseline making it impossible to use the standard STEMI criteria for ST segment elevation. The issue is further complicated by the fact that LBBB itself is a risk factor for cardiac death in that a new LBBB can be the presenting ECG pattern in a proximal left anterior descending coronary artery (LAD) occlusion, thus a new LBBB pattern ECG in patients with a compatible clinical scenario is considered a *STEMI equivalent.* Unfortunately, the rate of patients with AMI who present with new LBBB remains so small the mere presence of new or presumed new LBBB does not itself confer an increased risk of AMI.[22] Moreover, although LBBB is associated with a poor prognosis for patients with chest pain, the diagnostic utility of its presence alone has been shown to be weak with respect to the diagnosis of AMI.[23]

Two recurring scenarios illustrate the difficulty of correctly identifying AMI in patients with LBBB. The first is patients with an intermediate risk story and a previously undiagnosed or unrecognized LBBB. The question, then, is this: should this new LBBB be considered a STEMI? In considering the answer to this important question, it is instructive to recall

the mechanism through which AMI causes a new LBBB infarction of that portion of the conduction system related to LAD occlusion proximal to the first septal perforator branch. Given the proximal location of the occlusion in the LAD, these AMIs involve a larger area of ischemic heart muscle and tend to have more severe presentations and hemodynamic compromise. It is likewise less common for the new LBBB to be the ECG finding of AMI in patients with an otherwise nonthreatening clinical presentation; in other words, these patients with AMI tend to be rather ill on presentation, with a toxic appearance, pulmonary congestion, and compromised perfusion.

The second clinical scenario occurs when patients with known LBBB present with acute chest pain, potentially suggestive of AMI; the clinical challenge is focusing on the possible presence of AMI. This situation is the most appropriate application of the criteria Sgarbossa and colleagues[24] derived from the Global Utilization of Streptokinase and Tissue Plasminogen Activator for Occluded Coronary Arteries (GUSTO) trial. These criteria are based on the finding that STEMI, when presenting in the setting of LBBB, often seems different than the LBBB at baseline. Of course, an understanding of the ECG in the LBBB presentation is important. Such an understanding allows the clinician to recognize the expected findings of LBBB and, thus, the inappropriate findings that are associated with AMI, not only those described by Sgarbossa and colleagues but also other abnormalities. The 12-lead ECG (**Figs. 12** and **13**) in patients with LBBB records the abnormal ventricular activation as it moves from right to left, producing a broad, mainly negative QS or rS complex in lead V1. In lead V6, late intrinsicoid deflection is noted, resulting in a positive, monophasic R wave; similar structures are frequently found in leads I and aVL. Poor R wave progression or QS complexes are noted in the right to mid precordial leads, rarely extending beyond leads V4 or V5. QS complexes may also be encountered in leads III and aVF. The anticipated or expected ST segment–T-wave configurations are discordant, directed opposite from the terminal portion of the QRS complex, and called QRS complex–T-wave axes discordance. As such, leads with either QS or rS complexes may have markedly elevated ST segments, mimicking AMI. Leads with a large monophasic R wave demonstrate ST segment depression. The T wave, especially in the right to midprecordial leads, has a convex upward shape or a tall, vaulting appearance, similar to the hyperacute T wave of early myocardial infarction. The T waves in leads with the monophasic R wave are frequently inverted. Loss of this normal QRS complex–T-wave axes discordance in patients with LBBB may imply an acute process, such as AMI. An inspection of the ECG in patients with LBBB must be performed,

looking for a loss of this QRS complex–T-wave axes discordance.

Patients with known LBBB presenting with a clinical presentation potentially suggestive of AMI is the most appropriate application of the criteria Sgarbossa and colleagues[24] derived from the GUSTO trial. These criteria are based on the finding that STEMI, when presenting in the setting of LBBB, often seems different than the LBBB at baseline. Unfortunately, although the most accepted and widely used clinical criteria for diagnosis of AMI in LBBB, the Sgarbossa criteria suffer from low sensitivity of 36% while retaining a relatively robust specificity of 96% in the validation cohort. The most appropriate course in these cases, then, is to proceed most briskly in patients meeting the Sgarbossa criteria (with a score of 3 or more) and, in those who do not, relying on the pretest probability based on history and clinical risk to determine the overall risk of AMI. This rule states that 3 specific ECG criteria (**Fig. 14**, **Table 1**) are independent predictors of AMI in patients with LBBB. The ECG criteria suggesting a diagnosis of AMI, ranked with a scoring system based on the probability of such a diagnosis, include (1) ST segment elevation greater than 1 mm, which was concordant with the QRS complex (score of 5); (2) ST segment depression greater than 1 mm in leads V1, V2, or V3 (score of 3); and (3) ST segment elevation greater than 5 mm, which is discordant with the QRS complex (score of 2). A total score of 3 or more suggests that patients are likely experiencing an AMI based on the ECG criteria. With a score less than 3, the electrocardiographic diagnosis is less assured, requiring

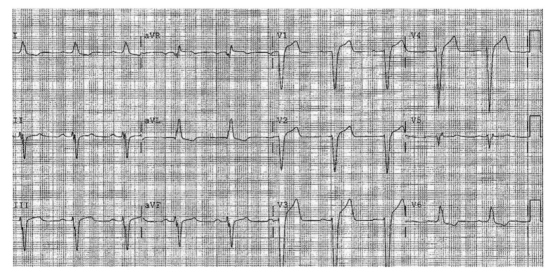

Fig. 12. ST segment and T-wave changes seen in the normal appearing left bundle branch block.

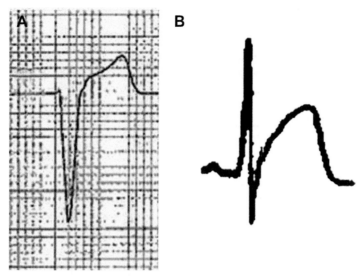

Fig. 13. ST segment elevation as seen in LBBB (*A*) versus STEMI (*B*).

additional evaluation. This clinical prediction instrument supports the contention that a detailed knowledge of the associated, or anticipated, ST segment–T-wave changes resulting from the abnormal ventricular conduction of the LBBB is a must. Such an understanding of the ECG in LBBB consequently allows the clinician to recognize the unanticipated morphologies that may be suspicious for AMI.

LV Hypertrophy

LV hypertrophy (LVH) pattern is one of the most common clinical pathologic findings on the

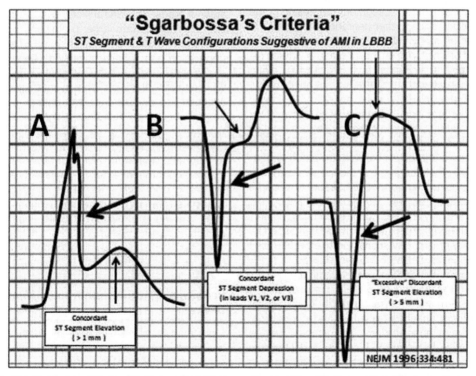

Fig. 14. The Sgarbossa criteria. (*A*) Concordant ST segment elevation. (*B*) Concordant ST segment depression limited to leads V1, V2, and V3. (*C*) Excessive discordant ST segment greater than 5 mm. Note that the relationship of the major, terminal portion of the QRS complex (*thick arrow*) and the initial portion of the ST segment (*thin arrow*) is key determinant in the consideration of the Sgarbossa criteria.

Table 1
The Sgarbossa criteria

Odds Rations Supporting AMI and Prediction Scores for Independent Electrocardiographic Criteria		
Criterion	Odds Ratio (95% CI)	Score
ST segment elevation ≥1 mm concordant with QRS complex	25.2 (11.6–54.7)	5
ST segment depression ≥1 mm in lead V1, V2, or V3	6.0 (1.9–19.3)	3
ST segment elevation ≥5 mm & discordant with QRS complex	4.3 (1.8–10.6)	2

Abbreviation: CI, confidence interval.

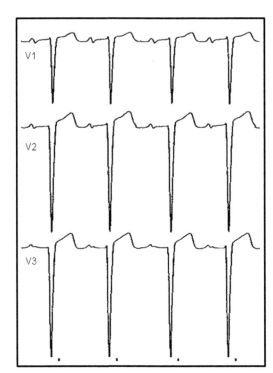

Fig. 15. ST segment elevation in leads V1 to V3 as seen in the LVH with strain pattern.

electrocardiogram. Although 50% of the adult population diagnosed with hypertension will have LVH by echocardiogram, only 20% of those will have characteristic ECG findings of LVH. Indeed, the presence of LVH does carry a worse prognosis for a given patient, and the presence of concomitant downsloping ST segment depression, the strain appearance further degrades prognosis.[25]

There are many criteria for determining LVH by ECG, all of which rely on the increase in voltage reflected by the increased myocardial mass along with either leftward axis or left atrial abnormality. Unfortunately, all ECG criteria suffer from relatively poor performance characteristics (sensitivity approximately 50% and specificity approximately 80%) when validated against LV mass calculated by echocardiography or cardiac computed tomography (CT).[26] Although the detection of underlying, anatomic LVH is important with respect to patient management, in this particular instance, the authors are only addressing the secondary repolarization abnormalities caused by LVH, in essence, the ST segment deviations (both elevation and depression) as well as T-wave inversions.

Approximately 80% of patients with the LVH by voltage (**Figs. 15** and **16**) pattern demonstrate the strain pattern; the strain pattern includes significant ST segment changes (elevation and depression) and T-wave abnormalities (prominent T waves and T-wave inversion). ST segment elevation in the setting of LVH is almost exclusively seen in the anterior distribution (leads V1 to V4). ST segment elevation is encountered in this distribution along with prominent T waves; the ST segment elevation can reach up to 5 mm in height in the

anterior leads. The lateral leads (leads I, aVL, V5, and V6) demonstrate large, prominent, positively oriented QRS complexes with marked ST segment depression and T-wave inversion. Although the strain pattern can also be seen inferiorly, inferior ST segment elevation should not quickly be ascribed to LVH. The LVH with pattern is associated with poor R-wave progression, most commonly producing a QS pattern; these complexes are located in leads V1, V2, and V3; furthermore, a leftward axis and left atrial abnormality add credence to ST segment elevation stemming from LVH. The ST segment elevation associated with LVH is generally unchanging over time, making a previous ECG for comparison particularly useful. Serial ECGs are similarly useful because there should be no evidence of evolving changes unless there is active ischemia.

Ventricular Paced Pattern from Implanted Device

More than 2 million people in the United States have an implanted pacemaker or internal cardioverter-defibrillator. Because a paced ventricular rhythm causes bundle-branch block morphology, it produces many of the same diagnostic limitations as LBBB described earlier. Moreover, patients with implanted cardiac devices

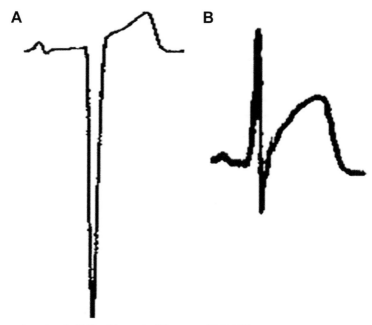

Fig. 16. ST segment elevation in LVH with strain (*A*) versus STEMI (*B*).

tend to be older and are more likely to have underlying heart disease.

Ventricular pacing leads can be placed in the apex of the right ventricle causing a left bundle pattern or on the surface of the LV either in a coronary vein or in an epicardial location causing more of a RBBB type of pattern. Patients with LV pacing leads frequently have such units placed for cardiac resynchronization therapy as part of the treatment

of heart failure. Patients presenting with a paced rhythm may or may not be dependent on their pacemaker to maintain a perfusing ventricular rate. It can be tempting to pause pacing and analyze the morphology of the underlying rhythm, but this is unreliable because of T-wave memory wherein the myocyte repolarization vector remains despite the change in depolarization vector.[27] Sgarbossa and colleagues[28] have investigated

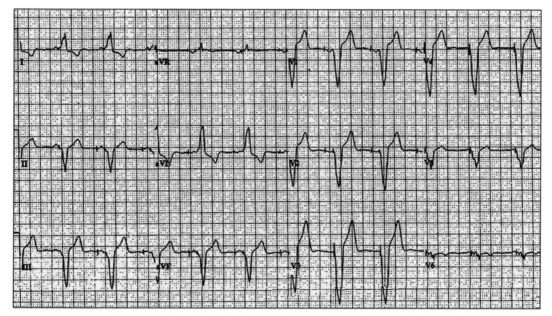

Fig. 17. ST segment elevation in the ventricular paced pattern.

A   **B**

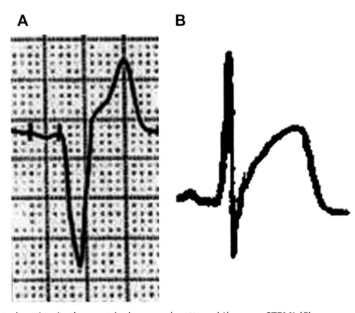

Fig. 18. ST segment elevation in the ventricular paced pattern (A) versus STEMI (B).

the utility of applying their criteria to patients with an LBBB caused by paced rhythm and found very poor sensitivity and modest specificity; in a very basic sense, they found similar findings as noted in the ECG diagnosis of AMI in the setting of LBBB. Refer to **Figs. 17** and **18** for a depiction of the ST segment changes seen in the ventricular paced pattern.

The RBBB has long been recognized as a high-risk feature in the presentation of AMI; in fact, it has been noted that the presence of a new RBBB on presentation with AMI significantly increases 30-day mortality.[29] Current guidelines require ST segment elevation be present with RBBB for the diagnosis of STEMI; further, the longstanding maxim has been the presence of RBBB does not alter the detection of ST elevation. However, this notion has been challenged by those who point out T-wave inversions in the anterior leads of patients with RBBB can impair the detection of more subtle ST segment changes; also, severe proximal coronary occlusions can be associated with new RBBB with hemiblock and, thus, do not demonstrate typical ST segment elevation.[30–35] Patients with a clinically worrisome presentation and new bundle branch block (both left and right) should be carefully considered for AMI because the benefit of early reperfusion therapy is quite high in these patients.

REFERENCES

1. Niska R, Bhulya F, Xu J. National Hospital Ambulatory Medical Care Survey: 2007 emergency department summary. Natl Health Stat Report 2010;26:1–32.
2. Brady WJ. Electrocardiographic ST segment elevation: the diagnosis of AMI by morphologic analysis of the ST segment. Acad Emerg Med 2001;8:961–7.
3. Brady WJ. Electrocardiographic ST segment elevation in emergency department chest pain centers: etiology responsible for the ST segment abnormality. Am J Emerg Med 2001;19:25–8.
4. Bruce M, Spodick D. Atypical electrocardiogram in acute pericarditis: characteristics and prevalence. J Electrocardiol 1980;13:61–6.
5. Codreanu A. Detection of myocarditis by contrast-enhanced MRI in patients presenting with acute coronary syndrome but no coronary stenosis. J Magn Reson Imaging 2007;25:957–64.
6. Spodick D. Acute pericarditis. JAMA 2003;289:1150–3.
7. Pollak P. Multiple culprit arteries in patients with ST segment elevation myocardial infarction referred for primary percutaneous coronary intervention. Am J Cardiol 2009;104:619–23.
8. Galiuto L. Functional and structural correlates of persistent ST elevation after acute myocardial infarction successfully treated by percutaneous coronary intervention. Heart 2007;93:1376–80.
9. Ong P. Coronary artery spasm as a frequent cause of acute coronary syndrome. J Am Coll Cardiol 2008;52:523–7.
10. Kounis N. Kounis syndrome (allergic angina and allergic myocardial infarction): a natural paradigm? Int J Cardiol 2006;110:7–14.
11. Prasad A, Lerman A, Rihal C. Apical ballooning syndrome (Tako-Tsubo or stress cardiomyopathy): a mimic of acute myocardial infarction. Am Heart J 2008;155:408–17.

12. Brugada P. Right bundle branch block, persistent ST segment elevation and sudden cardiac death: a distinct clinical and electrocardiographic syndrome. J Am Coll Cardiol 1992;20:1391–6.

13. Benito B. Gender differences in clinical manifestations of Brugada syndrome. J Am Coll Cardiol 2008;52:1567–73.

14. Antzelvitch C. Brugada syndrome: report of the second consensus conference. Circulation 2005; 111:659–70.

15. Simon B. Pseudomyocardial infarction and hyperkalemia: a case report and subject review. J Emerg Med 1988;6:511–5.

16. Gurevitz O. ST-segment deviation following implantable cardioverter defibrillator shocks: incidence, timing, and clinical significance. Pacing Clin Electrophysiol 2002;25:1429–32.

17. Van Gelder IC. Incidence and clinical significance of ST segment elevation after electrical cardioversion of atrial fibrillation and atrial flutter. Am Heart J 1991;121:51–6.

18. Kok LC. Transient ST elevation after transthoracic cardioversion in patients with hemodynamically unstable ventricular tachyarrhythmia. Am J Cardiol 2000;85:878–81.

19. Antzelevitch C. J wave syndromes. Heart Rhythm 2010;7:549–58.

20. Noda T. Prominent J wave and ST segment elevation: serial electrocardiographic changes in accidental hypothermia. J Cardiovasc Electrophysiol 2003;14:223.

21. Schneider JF. Newly acquired left bundle-branch block: the Framingham Study. Ann Intern Med 1979; 90(3):303–10.

22. Chang AM. Lack of association between left bundle-branch block and acute myocardial infarction in symptomatic ED patients. Am J Emerg Med 2009; 27(8):916–21.

23. Jain S. Utility of left bundle branch block as a diagnostic criterion for acute myocardial infarction. Am J Cardiol 2011;107:1111–6.

24. Sgarbossa E. Electrocardiographic diagnosis of evolving acute myocardial infarction in the presence of left bundle branch block. N Engl J Med 1996;334: 481–7.

25. Sullivan J. Left ventricular hypertrophy: effect on survival. J Am Coll Cardiol 1993;22:508–13.

26. Hancock EW. AHA/ACCF/HRS recommendation for the standardization and interpretation of the electrocardiogram: part V: electrocardiogram changes associated with cardiac chamber hypertrophy. J Am Coll Cardiol 2009;53:992–1002.

27. Rosenbaum M. Electrotonic modulation of the T wave and cardiac memory. Am J Cardiol 1982;50: 213–23.

28. Sgarbossa E. Early electrocardiographic diagnosis of acute myocardial infarction in the presence of ventricular paced rhythm. Am J Cardiol 1996;77: 423–4.

29. Scheinman M. Clinical and anatomic implications of intraventricular conduction blocks in acute myocardial infarction. Circulation 1972;46:753–60.

30. Widimsky P. Primary angioplasty in acute myocardial infarction with right bundle branch block: should new onset right bundle branch block be added to future guidelines as an indication for reperfusion therapy? Eur Heart J 2012;33(1):86–95.

31. Kamp T. Myocardial infarction, aortic dissection, and thrombolytic therapy. Am Heart J 1994;128: 1234–7.

32. Luo JL. Type A aortic dissection manifesting as acute myocardial infarction: still a lesson to learn. Acta Cardiol 2009;64:499–504.

33. Ohlmann P. Diagnostic and prognostic value of circulating d-dimers in patients with acute aortic dissection. Crit Care Med 2006;34:1358–64.

34. Falterman T. Pulmonary embolism with ST segment elevation in leads V1 to V4: case report and review of the literature regarding electrocardiographic changes in acute pulmonary embolism. J Emerg Med 2001;21:255–61.

35. Fasullo S. An unusual presentation of massive pulmonary embolism mimicking septal acute myocardial infarction treated with tenecteplase. J Thromb Thrombolysis 2009;27:215–9.

Acute Coronary Syndromes
From the Emergency Department to the Cardiac Care Unit

Neville F. Mistry, MD, Mark R. Vesely, MD*

KEYWORDS

- Acute coronary syndrome • Risk stratification • Rapid assessment • Reperfusion therapy

KEY POINTS

- Despite novel diagnostic and therapeutic modalities, the combination of history, physical examination, and electrocardiographic analysis remains the cornerstone of management for acute coronary syndromes (ACS). Initial steps in care should include recognition of possible ACS with subsequent risk stratification.
- Providing excellent care to patients with ACS is a team effort. Coordination of care from the emergency department to the cardiac care unit requires input from the patient, nurses and ancillary care staff, the emergency physicians, and cardiology consultants. Clear communication between these individuals is of the utmost importance, especially in the case of ST-elevation myocardial infarction, which represents a medical emergency.
- Hospitals should have systems of care in place to ensure compliance with guidelines. Monitoring compliance with guidelines as well as clinical outcomes has the potential to ensure excellent care.

INTRODUCTION

Acute coronary syndromes (ACS) represent a spectrum of disease including unstable angina (UA), non-ST-segment elevation myocardial infarction (NSTEMI) and ST-elevation myocardial infarction (STEMI) (**Table 1**). This continuum of presentations reflecting obstructive disease of the coronary arteries represents a significant burden of morbidity and mortality in the United States. Conservative estimates suggest that in 2007 alone there were more than 1 million hospital discharges with a diagnosis of ACS.[1]

Over the last 20 years, the management of ACS has evolved through the findings of several large, randomized clinical trials. Advancements have included novel cardiac biomarkers, novel antiplatelet agents and anticoagulants, and numerous refinements in percutaneous revascularization. In response to the rapid advancements in ACS management, the American College of Cardiology (ACC) and American Heart Association (AHA) have published several guidelines for care. Guideline-recommended care is not performed in up to 25% of cases and such care is associated with significantly increased in-hospital mortality.[2] Adherence to guidelines is associated with significant improvement in patient outcomes.[3,4] Thus the accurate and timely diagnosis of ACS and subsequent initiation of guideline-based therapy are critical in providing excellent care. Hospital performance in meeting ACS guidelines is now closely monitored through Medicare core measures and various other initiatives.

In evaluating patients with potential ACS, emergency physicians must determine (1) whether a patient's signs and symptoms reflect ACS and (2) the likelihood of an adverse clinical outcome

The authors have nothing to disclose.
Department of Medicine, Division of Cardiology, University of Maryland School of Medicine, 110 South Paca Street, 7th Floor, Baltimore, MD 21201, USA
* Corresponding author.
E-mail address: mvesely@medicine.umaryland.edu

cardiology.theclinics.com

Table 1
The spectrum of ACS

ACS	Pathophysiology	Initial Treatment
UA	Nonocclusive thrombus in an epicardial coronary vessel with associated ischemia but no evidence of infarction	Aspirin Heparin, LMWH, bivalirudin Thienopyridine, β-blockade
NSTEMI	Nonocclusive thrombus in an epicardial coronary vessel with associated infarction	Aspirin Heparin, LMWH, bivalirudin Thienopyridine β-blockade *consider GP IIB/IIIA inhibitor
STEMI	Occlusive thrombus in an epicardial coronary vessel with transmural ischemia	Aspirin Urgent reperfusion via thrombolysis or primary PCI

Abbreviations: LMWH, low-molecular-weight heparin; PCI, percutaneous coronary intervention.

from ACS (risk assessment). These 2 assessments are critical in guiding therapy toward the initial goals of relieving discomfort related to ischemia, assessing and correcting hemodynamic abnormalities, and choosing a management strategy. Appropriate completion of these assessments in patients with ACS should include history and physical examination findings, electrocardiographic (ECG) analysis, and cardiac biomarker results.

The first clinical decision point is determining if a patient with suspect ACS is having a STEMI (**Table 2**). These patients need emergent reperfusion, either via primary percutaneous revascularization or thrombolysis. In the case of primary percutaneous revascularization, system-based protocols are recommended to minimize time to reperfusion and are discussed in detail by Gupta and colleagues elsewhere in this issue. Once STEMI is excluded, therapy should proceed down a common pathway for initial treatment of UA and NSTEMI. Prompt contact with a cardiology care provider is important to guide decisions regarding antiplatelet and anticoagulant therapies. Although serum cardiac biomarkers are commonly used to clarify the diagnosis of ACS, therapy should not be delayed for the results of serum cardiac biomarker levels from the chemistry laboratory. Barriers to prompt delivery of therapy include delays in patient presentation and a lack of recognition of ACS in patients without a complaint of chest pain.[5,6]

RISK ASSESSMENT

Most therapies for acute coronary syndromes, whether drugs or interventional procedures, possess both risks and benefits that must be considered. In intermediate-risk and high-risk patients the benefits of aggressive therapies typically outweigh the risks. On the other hand, in low-risk patients the benefits of these therapies may be minimal and the risks substantial.[7] The goal of risk assessment is to deliver appropriate therapies to strata of patients at low, intermediate, and high risk. In the case of ACS, significant adverse events typically evaluated in risk models include mortality, new or recurrent infarction, need for urgent revascularization, and the development of heart failure.

Table 2
Criteria for STEMI

Diagnostic ECG Criteria for STEMI	Additional ECG Findings (Supportive but not Diagnostic of Myocardial Infarction)
New ST-segment elevation at the J point ≥0.2 mV in men (0.15 mV in women) in leads V2 and V3. ≥2 contiguous leads should be involved	Hyperacute T-waves often precede ST-elevation
New ST-segment elevation at the J point ≥0.1 mV in leads other than V2 or V3. ≥2 contiguous leads should be involved	Reciprocal ST-segment depressions
New left bundle branch block	Development of pathologic Q-waves can be seen as the infarction progresses

Data from Thygesen K, Alpert JS, White HD, et al. Universal definition of myocardial infarction. Eur Heart J 2007;28:2525.

Risk stratification systems (RSSs) can be a helpful tool in treating patients with ACS by estimating risk of adverse events and guiding therapeutic decisions. These models have the potential to improve compliance with guidelines. Important considerations in using an RSS include the relevance of a scoring system to the patient being evaluated, ease of use, and accuracy. Most risk scoring systems for ACS are based on a point system. One of the simplest and most widely used RSSs for ACS is the TIMI (Thrombolysis in Myocardial Infarction) risk score for UA and NSTEMI. This score, developed from a cohort in the TIMI 11B trial, has been validated in multiple patient populations.[8,9] The TIMI score for UA/NSTEMI assigns 1 point for each of the following risk factors:

1. Age 65 years or older
2. Aspirin use within the last 7 days
3. Known coronary artery stenosis 50% or greater
4. 3 or more coronary artery disease (CAD) risk factors (family history of CAD, hypertension, hyperlipidemia, diabetes, and smoking)
5. Severe angina (at least twice within 24 hours)
6. Increased creatine kinase-MB (CK-MB) or troponin levels
7. ST-segment deviation 0.05 mV or greater.

TIMI risk scores correlate well with 14-day, 30-day, and 1-year outcomes.[10] Rates of a composite end point including death, new or recurrent myocardial infarction (MI), and urgent revascularization secondary to recurrent ischemia at 14 days ranged from 4.7% for those with TIMI scores of 0 to 1 to 40.9% for those with TIMI scores of 6 to 7 (**Table 3**). Therapies shown to have statistical

benefit in intermediate-risk and high-risk patients (TIMI score ≥3) include glycoprotein (GP) IIb/IIIa inhibitors, low-molecular-weight heparin (as opposed to unfractionated heparin), and an early invasive strategy toward revascularization.[11–13] Thus the TIMI score represents a well-validated, simple risk assessment model that can be used to guide management. One caveat of the TIMI score is that in the interest of simplicity, all risk factors are assumed to contribute equal risk. In practice, positive troponins likely reflect a high-risk patient population because this group is known to benefit from aggressive therapies, including IIB/IIIA inhibitors and an early invasive strategy toward revascularization.[12,13]

An alternative risk model for patients presenting with non-ST elevation ACS is the 23-variable PURSUIT (Platelet Glycoprotein IIb/IIIa in Unstable Angina: Receptor Suppressor Using Integrilin Therapy Trial) model, which has shown usefulness in predicting 30-day mortality.[14] The Global Registry of Acute Coronary Events (GRACE) RSS is another alternative which assesses risk across the entire spectrum of ACS, including UA, NSTEMI, and STEMI.[15] Both the GRACE and PURSUIT RSSs are more difficult to determine at the bedside than the TIMI score. RSSs all have limitations and complete evaluation of ACS requires the integration of history, physical examination, ECG, and laboratory findings.

PATIENT HISTORY

In evaluating patients with possible ACS, a rapid, focused history should be taken. The goal of this history is to establish the likelihood of ACS in a prompt fashion and to prevent delays in the initiation of therapy. Because the traditional risk factors for CAD are not strongly predictive of acute ischemia, special attention must be paid to the presenting symptoms.[16] In 1 study, the only historical factors that increased likelihood of ACS were diabetes and a family history of CAD in men. Both of these risk factors conferred only a 2-fold relative risk for ischemia.[17] In comparison, chest discomfort, ST-segment abnormalities, and T-wave abnormalities conferred increased risks of 12-fold, 9-fold, and 5-fold, respectively, in the same study. Most patients presenting with ACS have a chief complaint of chest discomfort[18]; however, any combination of chest discomfort, dyspnea, diaphoresis, and nausea can be representative of angina. Many patients do not describe their symptom as frank chest pain but rather as chest pressure, tightness, or a squeezing sensation.

Although the differential diagnosis for chest discomfort is large, the high prevalence of CAD

Table 3
Implications of TIMI score for non-ST-segment ACS

TIMI Score	Composite End Point at 14 d (%)[a]	Risk Level
0–1	4.7	Low
2	8.3	Low
3	13.2	Intermediate
4	19.9	Intermediate
5	26.2	High
6–7	40.9	High

[a] Composite end point includes all-cause mortality, new/recurrent MI, and severe recurrent ischemia requiring revascularization.

Data from Antman EM, Cohen M, Bernink PJ, et al. The TIMI risk score for unstable angina/non-ST elevation MI: a method for prognostication and therapeutic decision making. JAMA 2000;284(7):835.

mandates that ACS be a prime consideration in any patient presenting with this symptom. The level of discomfort does not necessarily correlate with the severity of ischemia. Some patients do not even experience chest discomfort and, rather, present with isolated jaw, neck, arm, or back pain. Discomfort related to exertion or associated with nausea or diaphoresis raises concern for ACS. Perhaps the most important anginal equivalent is dyspnea, the chief complaint in up to 16% of patients presenting with ACS.[18] Response to nitroglycerin or antacids does not aid in the diagnosis of ACS.[19,20] In patients with a history of coronary disease, comparison between their current symptoms and previous angina/MI can be helpful. In patients with stable angina, ACS should be suspected if episodes of angina are more severe, if symptoms are prolonged, or if symptoms occur with less exertion or at rest.

Features that are traditionally deemed to be uncharacteristic of ACS including pleuritic pain, discomfort of brief duration (a few seconds), and discomfort reproduced with palpation do not exclude ACS. One study reported that 13% of patients with partially pleuritic chest pain had acute ischemia.[21] Similarly, 7% of patients with pain fully reproducible by palpation were found to have acute ischemia.

Other important details to consider in the history include relevant allergies such as those to aspirin, heparin, intravenous (IV) contrast dye, and thienopyridines. Because antiplatelet and anticoagulant therapies are mainstays of ACS treatment, patients should be asked about any issues with bleeding. In addition, patients should be queried about the use of phosphodiesterase inhibitors such as sildenafil, tadalafil, or vardenafil, because recent use of these drugs may preclude the use of nitrates.

PHYSICAL EXAMINATION

The physical examination contributes to the management of ACS in several ways. First, it can assist in identifying precipitating causes of ischemia, including but not limited to severe hypertension, severe tachycardia, and thyrotoxicosis. Cardiovascular comorbidities such as valvular regurgitation, arrhythmias, ventricular septal defects, and heart failure can often be detected on physical examination before the results of imaging modalities. The physical examination can also identify alternative diagnoses, including but not limited to pneumonia, pleural effusion, aortic dissection, acute pericarditis, and pericardial tamponade (**Table 4**).

The initial examination should be brief, focused on hemodynamic parameters and the cardiopulmonary examination. It should include auscultation of the heart and lungs, measurement of jugular venous pressure, and evaluation of lower extremity pulses and edema. In patients with a clinical history concerning for aortic dissection, the blood pressure in both arms should be assessed. A rapid neurologic examination is also recommended, especially in patients who may receive thrombolytics.

In evaluating patients with ACS, particular attention must be paid to patients with possible cardiogenic shock. Hypothermia, hypotension, and a low pulse pressure may all be signs of cardiogenic shock, which should be recognized as a medical emergency.[22] These patients may also present with evidence of end-organ hypoperfusion, such as altered mental status, oliguria, and jaundice.

IMAGING AND ADDITIONAL TESTING
ECG

The ECG is indispensable in the evaluation and management of patients with ACS. ACC/AHA

Table 4
Physical examination findings in patients without ACS with chest discomfort

Examination Finding	Alternative Diagnosis
Markedly disparate blood pressure in right vs left arm	Aortic dissection
S3, increased jugular venous pressure, edema	Congestive heart failure (which can be a consequence of ACS)
Irregular heart rhythm	Atrial fibrillation or other rhythm with variable block
Murmur	Valvular heart disease (which can be a consequence of ACS)
Crackles, diminished breath sounds, egophony	Pneumonia
Pericardial friction rub	Pericarditis
Wheezing with decreased air movement	Bronchospasm caused by asthma, chronic obstructive pulmonary disease

guidelines suggest that 12-lead ECGs should be evaluated by experienced emergency department (ED) physicians within 10 minutes of patient arrival to the ED.[23] ECGs performed in the field by emergency medical services personnel can assist in triaging patients with STEMIs to hospitals with primary percutaneous coronary intervention (PCI) capabilities. In addition to the diagnosis of STEMI (see **Table 2**), the ECG can aid in the management of ACS by:

- Suggesting ischemia in patients whose symptoms are ambiguous
- Identifying alternative diagnoses that may mimic ACS, such as pericarditis and arrhythmias
- Improving risk stratification in patients with suspected ACS, as seen in the TIMI score for UA/NSTEMI
- Showing recurrent ischemia

ECG findings strongly suggestive of ischemia in the setting of suspected UA/NSTEMI include:

- Transient ST-segment changes 0.05 mV (0.5 mm) or greater that develop during a symptomatic episode[23]
- T-wave inversions 0.2 mV (2 mm) or greater

Although ECGs are helpful in the diagnosis and management of ACS, sensitivity and specificity can vary widely based on the criteria used for interpretation and the selected patient population. One study reported that specificity can vary from 21% to 95% and sensitivity from 61% to 99% based on the stringency of criteria used to evaluate ACS.[24] Thus the implications of ECG findings must be interpreted in a Bayesian fashion, accounting for the likelihood of ACS given all data applicable to the patient. Physicians should not hesitate to obtain a second opinion if there are concerns regarding interpretation of an ECG. Additional caveats of the ECG in evaluating ACS include:

- The standard 12-lead ECG has limited ability to assess for ischemia in the posterior basal or lateral walls, corresponding with the left circumflex coronary distribution. Posterior ECG leads, V7-V9, can aid in the diagnosis of ischemia in this territory. Up to 4% of patients with MI show ST elevations isolated to these leads and such patients should be treated as STEMIs.[25,26] Posterior ECG leads should be considered in all patients with suspected ACS, especially those with ST-segment depression in V1 and V2.
- Standard 12-lead ECGs have a limited ability to assess for right ventricular infarction.

Right-sided ECGs can assist in the diagnosis of right ventricular involvement in inferior MI by showing ST elevation in leads RV4-6. The presence of right ventricular infarction can have significant implications for clinical management.
- ST-segment elevations can be seen in the absence of ischemia in the following common circumstances: bundle branch blocks, pericarditis, left ventricular hypertrophy, repolarization abnormalities, and ventricular aneurysm.
- A single ECG is a temporally limited assessment for ischemia. Thus, repeat ECGs can increase diagnostic yield and should be obtained with changes in clinical status such as recurrent or worsening chest discomfort. Patients with suspected ACS are at risk for malignant arrhythmias and should be monitored on telemetry.

Chest Radiograph

A chest roenterogram can assist in the diagnosis and management of ACS in the following ways:

- Identification of noncardiac causes of chest discomfort or dyspnea, such as pneumonia, pleural effusion, or pneumothorax
- Showing pulmonary edema as a complication of ACS
- Suggestion of aortic dissection by the presence of a widened mediastinum. Aortic dissections can involve the coronary arteries and can present as STEMIs

Cardiac Biomarkers

The development of novel cardiac biomarkers has revolutionized ACS. Ideal qualities of a biomarker include cardiac specificity, rapid release in the setting of myocardial injury, and a strong correlation with the extent of myocardial damage. Cardiac troponin I and T have now largely replaced CK-MB and myoglobin as the biomarkers of choice in ACS. Highly reproducible and highly sensitive troponin I and T assays are readily available. In 2007, the AHA released an expert consensus document that redefined MI, incorporating troponin measurement.[27,28] In the case of STEMI, reperfusion therapy (either thrombolytics or primary PCI) should not be delayed pending the results of troponin levels.

An increased troponin level above the 99th percentile of normal measurements is now defined to represent myocyte necrosis.[23] However, a single increased troponin level does not discriminate between nonischemic and ischemic causes.

Thus, increased troponin level alone is insufficient to diagnose NSTEMI. Rather, the troponin level must be assessed in a clinical context that integrates history, physical examination, and ECG findings. Increased troponin level is sometimes seen 8 to 12 hours after the onset of symptoms, and thus serial measurements are often necessary to diagnose NSTEMI. The presence of a positive troponin identifies a high-risk cohort of patients with ACS who benefit from aggressive therapies such as low-molecular-weight heparin (as opposed to unfractionated heparin), GP IIb/IIIa inhibitors, and an early invasive strategy toward revascularization.[11–13] Forty-two-day mortality increases with troponin I in patients with ACS from 1.0% for those with a troponin I 0.4 ng/mL or less to 7.5% for those with levels 9.0 ng/mL or greater. CK-MB has a shorter half-life than troponin and has been traditionally used for the diagnosis of reinfarction and periprocedural MI in the setting of cardiac catheterization or coronary artery bypass grafting.[23]

Treatment

Specific strategies for STEMI

The primary goal of treatment in STEMI is reperfusion. In hospitals with the capability to perform PCI, primary PCI is the preferred strategy for reperfusion. When compared with thrombolysis, primary PCI is associated with lower rates of intracranial hemorrhage and recurrent infarction.[29] Prompt recognition of STEMI and activation of the cardiac catheterization team are critical. All patients undergoing primary PCI should receive aspirin 162 to 325 mg orally and a thienopyridine. The choice of thienopyridine, anticoagulation strategy (low-molecular-weight heparin, unfractionated heparin, or bivalirudin), and IIB/IIIA inhibitor should be based on prespecified protocols or after close discussion with the interventional cardiologist. Patients presenting between 12 and 24 hours after onset of symptoms should be referred for primary PCI if evidence of heart failure, hemodynamic instability, malignant arrhythmias, or persistent ischemic symptoms is present.[30]

In centers in which primary PCI is unavailable or is delayed more than 90 minutes, then administration of thrombolytics is the therapy of choice for STEMI. Patients presenting within 12 hours of symptom onset are candidates for lytic therapy provided no contraindications are present (**Table 5**). The door-to-needle time (ie, from presentation to administration of thrombolytics) should be less than 30 minutes.[30] Patients receiving thrombolytics should be loaded with clopidogrel (300–600 mg orally) and treated with an anticoagulant but should not routinely receive GP IIB/IIIA inhibitors.[30–32] After administration of fibrinolytics, transfer to a PCI-capable center is recommended. This transfer provides availability of rescue PCI should the thrombolytic therapy not be effective.

Aspirin

Aspirin inhibits cyclooxygenase 1 in platelets, which results in reduced production of thromboxane A_2. Platelet aggregation is thus decreased. Clinical trials of aspirin in ACS ranging from UA to STEMI have consistently shown clinical benefit.[23,30,33,34] In all patients with suspected ACS, 162 to 325 mg

Table 5
Thrombolytics used for reperfusion in STEMI

Thrombolytic Agent	Special Attributes	Dosage
Alteplase	Recombinant tissue-type plasminogen activator. Fibrin-specific	15 mg IV x 1, followed by 30 min of 0.75 mg/kg (maximum dose 50 mg), then 60 min of 0.5 mg/kg (maximum 35 mg)
Streptokinase	Low cost. Likely less effective than alteplase but has a lower incidence of intracranial hemorrhage. Benefit of concomitant anticoagulation is not well proved	1.5 million units over 60 min
Tenecteplase	As effective as alteplase but with a lower incidence of bleeding	Dosing is weight-based. A single IV bolus is given
Reteplase	Less fibrin-selective than alteplase but with a longer half-life	10 units IV bolus followed by another 10 units IV bolus (after 30 min)

Absolute contraindications to thrombolysis include previous intracranial hemorrhage, known cerebral vascular lesion, known intracranial malignancy, ischemic stroke within 3 months, suspected aortic dissection, active bleeding, and closed head or facial trauma within the last 3 months.

of nonenteric coated aspirin should be administered. Adverse side effects of aspirin include bleeding and allergic reactions. Patients with a significant aspirin allergy should receive a thienopyridine as a substitute, with an initial loading dose followed by a maintenance dose.

Nitrates

Although nitrates are not known to reduce mortality in ACS, they can relieve chest discomfort. ACC/AHA guidelines suggest that sublingual nitroglycerin 0.4 mg should be administered every 5 minutes in patients with ongoing chest discomfort for a maximum of 3 doses.[30] After 3 doses, one should consider the need for IV nitroglycerin. Adverse effects of nitroglycerin include hypotension and headache. In patients with right ventricular infarction, nitrates are generally avoided secondary to concern that decreased right ventricular preload may result in hemodynamic compromise.

Thienopyridines

In the absence of a contraindication, patients with suspected ACS should be treated with dual antiplatelet therapy, including aspirin and a thienopyridine. Thienopyridines reduce platelet aggregation by blocking the 2PY12 adenosine diphosphate (ADP) receptor. The initial thienopyridines on the market in the United States included ticlopidine and clopidogrel. Ticlopidine use has largely been supplanted by clopidogrel because of significant risks of neutropenia and thrombotic thrombocytopenic purpura.

Clopidogrel has been well studied in the spectrum of ACS. In STEMI, clopidogrel has shown efficacy, whether a primary PCI or fibrinolytic approach is taken.[32,35] In non-ST elevation ACS, clopidogrel use is associated with a reduction in a composite end point of death from cardiovascular causes, nonfatal MI, and stroke.[36] This benefit is strongest in patients undergoing PCI, with a 30% reduction in the composite end point.[37] The benefit seen from clopidogrel use began in the first few hours after presentation, and thus early administration is critical. To quickly reach therapeutic activity, it is now recommended that patients with ACS be loaded orally with clopidogrel, 300 to 600 mg. Clopidogrel resistance has been documented and may reflect variations in enzymes that metabolize the drug as well as polymorphisms in the ADP receptor itself.[38-40] Patients with reduced responsiveness to clopidogrel are at increased risk of ischemic events.[41] The major adverse effect of clopidogrel is increased bleeding.

Prasugrel is a newer thienopyridine with more potent platelet inhibition than clopidogrel. Prasugrel has been studied in ACS and was found to have superior reduction in clinical ischemic events when compared with clopidogrel.[42] The reduction in a composite end point of death because of cardiovascular causes, nonfatal MI, and nonfatal stroke came at the expense of increased bleeding. Patients with a history of transient ischemic attack or stroke, patients aged 75 years or older, and patients with a body weight of less than 60 kg derived no net benefit from prasugrel and had higher rates of bleeding. The US Food and Drug Administration (FDA) has provided a warning against the use of prasugrel in patients aged 75 years or older and has established previous transient ischemic attack or stroke as a contraindication to prasugrel use. In the TRITON TIMI-38 (Trial to Assess Improvement in Therapeutic Outcomes by Optimizing Platelet Inhibition with Prasugrel–Thrombolysis in Myocardial Infarction) study, the largest trial of prasugrel in ACS, most patients received prasugrel after diagnostic coronary angiography. Thus, data on the use of prasugrel on presentation are limited. The 2011 American College of Cardiology Foundation/AHA guidelines state that a 60-mg loading dose of prasugrel on presentation followed by 10 mg daily is reasonable in patients with UA/NSTEMI for whom PCI is planned, the bleeding risk is low, and coronary artery bypass grafting is considered unlikely.[43] Prasugrel has not been studied in the setting of thrombolytic use, and thus clopidogrel remains the thienopyridine of choice in this application.

Ticagrelor is a novel P2Y12 ADP receptor antagonist that was recently approved by the FDA. Unlike the thienopyridines, ticagrelor has a rapid onset of action and binds reversibly to the ADP receptor. A large, randomized clinical trial found that ticagrelor, when compared with clopidogrel, was associated with a significant reduction in a composite end point of death from cardiovascular causes, MI, or stroke in patients with ACS.[44] There was no significant difference in the rates of major bleeding between the clopidogrel and ticagrelor arms.

Anticoagulants

Heparins and direct thrombin antagonists reduce the conversion of fibrinogen into fibrin, limiting clot formation. Unfractionated heparin has been a mainstay of therapy for ACS. Although no trials have assessed the clinical benefit of heparin in the dual antiplatelet therapy era of ACS treatment, older trials reported reductions in refractory angina and progression from UA to NSTEMI.[45,46] Adverse reactions to heparin include increased major bleeding and heparin-induced thrombocytopenia. Drawbacks of unfractionated heparin include abundant binding to plasma proteins, with consequent variable dosing and the inability to inactivate thrombin within a clot. Advantages of heparin over its alternatives include easy monitoring of effect through partial thromboplastin time and activated clotting time and the ability to reverse anticoagulation with protamine.

Low-molecular-weight heparins such as enoxaparin and fondaparinux inactivate factor Xa but have a less pronounced effect on thrombin. Their anticoagulant effect is believed to be more predictable than unfractionated heparin. Enoxaparin is the best-studied low-molecular-weight heparin in ACS. Studies addressing the clinical efficacy of enoxaparin compared with unfractionated heparin reveal reduced rates of recurrent ischemia along with lower rates of composite end points, including death, MI, and urgent revascularization.[9,12] Subgroup analysis suggested that high-risk patients, particularly those with positive troponins, derived the largest benefit from enoxaparin. Enoxaparin use with GP IIB/IIIA inhibitors is not associated with improvement in death or nonfatal MI and is associated with an increased risk of major bleeding.[47]

Bivalirudin is a direct thrombin inhibitor that has been studied extensively in ACS. When used in patients with non-ST elevation ACS, bivalirudin was noninferior to the combination of heparin and a GP IIB/IIIA inhibitor in preventing ischemic events and death.[48,49] In addition, rates of bleeding were lower for bivalirudin than the heparin + GP IIB/IIIA inhibitor combination. Similar efficacy was noted when bivalirudin was studied in STEMI.[50] The benefit of reduced bleeding is especially relevant to patients aged 75 years or older, who are at significant risk for this complication.[51] Patients treated with bivalirudin (as opposed to heparin ± GP IIB/IIIA inhibitor) who are to undergo PCI should be treated with a thienopyridine at least 2 hours before coronary intervention.[52]

β-blockers

β-blockers have several beneficial effects in the setting of ACS, including reduction in oxygen demand through reduced heart rate and inotropy, increased coronary perfusion by reducing heart rate and lengthening diastole, and prevention of arrhythmias. Multiple trials in the prethrombolysis era showed a mortality benefit in favor of β-blocker use.[53,54] The ideal timing and route of administration for β-blockers remains unclear. Data in the modern era of dual antiplatelet therapy and percutaneous revascularization are limited. The COMMIT/CCS2 trial randomly assigned patients with ST-elevation ACS to placebo or metoprolol (5 mg IV x 3 doses then long-acting metoprolol at 200 mg daily).[55] In this study, there was no significant reduction in a composite end point (death, reinfarction, cardiac arrest) or in mortality with metoprolol. An increased frequency of cardiogenic shock was noted in patients who were hemodynamically compromised. Thus early IV β-blockade in hemodynamically tenuous patients should be avoided. The ACC/AHA guidelines from 2007 recommend β-blockers be initiated orally in the absence of heart failure within the first 24 hours of presentation.[23] Cardioselective β-blockers without intrinsic sympathomimetic activity are generally preferred.

GP IIB/IIIA inhibitors

GP IIB/IIIA inhibitors inhibit the final common pathway of platelet aggregation. The efficacy of this class of drugs during PCI and in high-risk patients with UA and NSTEMI has been well established. The bulk of trials validating GP IIB/IIIA use predated the routine use of dual antiplatelet therapy with aspirin and a thienopyridine. A more recent trial with early thienopyridine administration revealed no statistically significant improvement in a composite end point of all-cause mortality, MI, and recurrent ischemia requiring revascularization for patients treated with eptifibatide before PCI.[56] In addition, there was increased bleeding in patients treated with upstream eptifibatide. Thus routine use of GP IIB/IIIA inhibitors in patients who are treated with thienopyridine and aspirin therapies is not encouraged. The benefits of triple-antiplatelet therapy must be weighed against the significant risk of bleeding.

Disposition

After stabilization and initiation of ACS treatment, physicians in the ED must address the issue of disposition. Patients treated with thrombolytics as well as those with hemodynamic instability, active anginal symptoms, ventricular arrhythmias, and new-onset heart failure in the setting of ACS should all be triaged to a specialized cardiac care unit (CCU). Patients with STEMIs are usually taken directly to the cardiac catheterization laboratory and then to the CCU. Patients who are intermediate to high risk, including all patients with positive cardiac enzymes, should be admitted to a telemetry unit for monitoring and further observation. Cardiology evaluation of these patients is critical. Low-risk patients with negative biomarkers, no recurrence of chest discomfort, and suspected noncardiac chest pain can be evaluated in the outpatient setting provided follow-up is available within 72 hours. Such patients should be carefully instructed to return to the ED immediately if symptoms recur.

SUMMARY AND FUTURE DIRECTIONS

The diagnosis and management of ACS have evolved rapidly over the last 20 years, largely under the guidance of large clinical trials. Despite novel diagnostic and therapeutic modalities, the combination of history, physical examination, and ECG analysis remains the cornerstone of management. Initial steps in care should include recognition of possible ACS with subsequent risk stratification. The risks of any therapy for ACS should be weighed against the clinical benefit. Risk assessment tools can identify patient populations who benefit from specific therapies. In the future, prospective clinical trials should incorporate risk assessment models to confirm that use of these tools results in improved patient outcomes.

Providing excellent care to patients with ACS is a team effort. Coordination of care from the ED to the CCU requires input from the patient, nurses and ancillary care staff, the emergency physicians, and cardiology consultants. Clear communication between these individuals is of the utmost importance, especially in the case of STEMI, which represents a medical emergency.

Evidence-based practice and adherence to guidelines have repeatedly been shown to reduce mortality in patients with ACS.[3,4] Hospitals should have systems of care in place to ensure compliance with guidelines. In addition, monitoring compliance with guidelines as well as clinical outcomes has the potential to ensure excellent care. Data registries designed to monitor adherence to guidelines, clinical outcomes, and complications have been developed. Participation in such registries allows hospitals and physicians to receive feedback on their performance and subsequently modify their practice habits.

The future of ACS management is promising. Novel antiplatelet and anticoagulant therapies are being developed. Genetic assays designed to guide therapy may eventually become a cornerstone of ACS management. Stem cells represent another area of inquiry with promising applications in ACS. With the development of these new therapies comes the responsibility of identifying the patient populations who benefit from them.

REFERENCES

1. Roger VL, Go AS, Lloyd-Jones DM, et al. Heart disease and stroke statistics–2011 update: a report from the American Heart Association. Circulation 2011;123:e18–209.
2. Fox KA, Steg PG, Eaglke KA, et al. GRACE investigators. Decline in rates of death and heart failure in acute coronary syndromes, 1999-2006. JAMA 2007;297:1892–900.
3. Peterson ED, Roe MT, Lytle BL, et al. The association between care and outcomes in patients with acute coronary syndromes: national results from CRUSADE. J Am Coll Cardiol 2004;43:406A.
4. Peterson ED, Parsons LS, Pollack CV, et al. Variations in AMI care quality across 1085 hospitals and its association with hospital mortality rates. Circulation 2002;106:II-722.
5. Goff DC Jr, Feldman HA, McGovern PG, et al. Prehospital delay in patients hospitalized with heart attack symptoms in the United States: the REACT trial. Rapid Early Action for Coronary Treatment (REACT) Study Group. Am Heart J 1999;138:1046–57.
6. Canto JG, Shlipak MG, Rogers WJ. Prevalence, clinical characteristics, and mortality among patients with myocardial infarction presenting without chest pain. JAMA 2000;283:3223–9.
7. Patel M, Dehmer GJ, Hirshfeld JW, et al. ACCF/SCAI/STS/AATS/AHA/ASNC/HFSA/SCCT 2012 Appropriate use criteria for coronary revascularization focused update. J Am Coll Cardiol 2012;59(9):857–81.
8. Vesley MR, Keleman MD. Cardiac risk assessment: matching intensity of therapy to risk. Cardiol Clin 2006;24:67–78.
9. Sabatine MS, Antman EM. The thrombolysis in myocardial infarction risk score in unstable angina/non-ST-segment elevation myocardial infarction. J Am Coll Cardiol 2003;41:89S.
10. Antman EM, Cohen M, Bernink PJ, et al. The TIMI risk score for unstable angina/non-ST segment elevation: a method for prognostication and therapeutic decision making. JAMA 2000;284:835–42.
11. Morrow DA, Antman EM, Snapinn SM, et al. An integrated clinical approach to predicting the benefit of tirofiban in non-ST elevation acute coronary syndromes. Application of the TIMI Risk Score for UA/NSTEMI in PRISM-PLUS. Eur Heart J 2002;23:223–9.
12. Cohen M, Demers C, Gurfinkel EP, et al. A comparison of low-molecular-weight heparin with unfractionated heparin for unstable coronary artery disease. Efficacy and Safety of Subcutaneous Enoxaparin in Non-Q-Wave Coronary Events Study Group. N Engl J Med 1997;337:447.
13. Cannon CP, Weintraub WS, Demopoulos LA, et al. Comparison of early invasive and conservative strategies in patients with unstable coronary syndromes treated with the glycoprotein IIb/IIIa inhibitor tirofiban. N Engl J Med 2001;344:1879.
14. Boersma E, Pieper KS, Steyerberg EW, et al. Predictors of outcome in patients with acute coronary syndromes without persistent ST-segment elevation. Results from an international trial of 9461 patients. The PURSUIT Investigators. Circulation 2000;101:2557.

15. Granger CB, Goldberg RJ, Dabbous O, et al. Predictors of hospital mortality in the global registry of acute coronary events. Arch Intern Med 2003; 163:2345.

16. Jayes RLJ, Beshansky JR, D'agostino RB, et al. Do patients' coronary risk factor reports predict acute cardiac ischemia in the emergency department? A multicenter study. J Clin Epidemiol 1992;45:621–6.

17. Jayes R, Larsen G, Beshansky J, et al. Physician electrocardiogram reading in the emergency department: accuracy and effect on triage decisions: findings from a multicenter study. J Gen Intern Med 1992;7:387–92.

18. Pope J, Ruthazer R, Beshansky J, et al. Clinical features of emergency department patients presenting with symptoms of acute cardiac ischemia: a multicenter study. J Thromb Thrombolysis 1998;6:63–74.

19. Henrikson CA, Howel EE, Bush DE, et al. Chest pain relief by nitroglycerin does not predict active coronary artery disease. Ann Intern Med 2003;139:979–86.

20. Swap CJ, Nagurney JT. Value and limitations of chest pain history in the evaluation of patients with suspected acute coronary syndromes. JAMA 2005; 294:2623–9.

21. Lee T, Cook E, Weisberg M, et al. Acute chest pain in the emergency room: identification and examination of low-risk patients. Arch Intern Med 1985;145:65–9.

22. Holmes DR Jr, Berger PB, Hochman JS, et al. Cardiogenic shock in patients with acute ischemic syndromes with and without ST-segment elevation. Circulation 1999;100:2067–73.

23. Anderson JL, Adams CD, Antman EM, et al. ACC/ AHA 2007 Guidelines for the management of patients with unstable angina/non-ST-elevation myocardial infarction–executive summary. J Am Coll Cardiol 2007;50:652–726.

24. Selker HP, Zalenski RJ, Antman EM, et al. An evaluation of technologies for identifying acute cardiac ischemia in the emergency department. Ann Emerg Med 1997;29:1–87.

25. Matetzky S, Freimark D, Feinberg MS, et al. Acute myocardial infarction with isolated ST-segment elevation in posterior chest leads V7-V9: "hidden" ST-segment elevation revealing acute posterior infarction. J Am Coll Cardiol 1999;34:748–53.

26. Matetzky S, Freimark D, Chouraqui P, et al. Significance of ST segment elevations in posterior chest leads V7 to V9 in patients with acute inferior myocardial infarction: application for thrombolytic therapy. J Am Coll Cardiol 1998;31:506–11.

27. Thygesen K, Alpert JS, White HD, et al. Universal definition of myocardial infarction. Circulation 2007; 116:2634–53.

28. Antman EM, Tanasijevic MJ, Thompson B, et al. Cardiac-specific troponin I levels to predict the risk of mortality in patients with acute coronary syndromes. N Engl J Med 1996;335:1342–9.

29. Keeley EC, Boura JA, Grines CL. Primary angioplasty versus intravenous thrombolytic therapy for acute myocardial infarction: a quantitative review of 23 randomised trials. Lancet 2003;361(9351):13.

30. Antman EM, Anbe DT, Armstrong PW, et al. ACC/AHA guidelines for the management of ST-elevation myocardial infarction: a report of the American College of Cardiology/American Heart Association Task Force on Practice Guidelines. Circulation 2004; 110(9):e82.

31. Antman EM, Hand M, Armstrong PW, et al. 2007 focused update of the ACC/AHA 2004 guidelines for the management of patients with ST-elevation myocardial infarction: a report of the American College of Cardiology/American Heart Association Task Force on Practice Guidelines. J Am Coll Cardiol 2008;51(2):210–47.

32. Sabatine MS, Cannon CP, Gibson CM, et al. Addition of clopidogrel to aspirin and fibrinolytic therapy for myocardial infarction with ST-segment elevation. N Engl J Med 2005;352:1178–89.

33. Theroux P, Ouimet H, McCans J, et al. Aspirin, sulfinpyrazone or both in unstable angina: results of a Canadian multicenter trial. N Engl J Med 1985; 313:1369–75.

34. Antithrombotic Trialists' Collaboration. Collaborative meta-analysis of randomized trials of antiplatelet therapy for prevention of death, myocardial infarction, and stroke in high risk patients. BMJ 2002; 324(7330):141.

35. Chen ZM, Jiang LX, Xie JX, et al. Addition of clopidogrel to aspirin in 45,852 patients with acute myocardial infarction: randomized placebo-controlled trial. Lancet 2005;366(9497):1607–21.

36. Yusuf S, Zhao F, Mehta SR, et al. Effects of clopidogrel in addition to aspirin in patients with acute coronary syndromes without ST-segment elevation. N Engl J Med 2001;345(7):494.

37. Mehta SR, Yusuf S, Peters RJ, et al. Effects of pretreatment with clopidogrel and aspirin followed by long-term therapy in patients undergoing percutaneous coronary intervention: the PCI-CURE study. Lancet 2001;358:527–33.

38. Gurbel PA, Mahla E, Antonino MJ, et al. Response variability and the role of platelet function testing. J Invasive Cardiol 2009;21(4):172.

39. Cairns JA, Eikelbloom J. Clopidogrel resistance: more grist for the mill. J Am Coll Cardiol 2008;51(20):1935.

40. Serebruany VL, Steinhubl SR, Berger PB, et al. Variability in platelet responsiveness to clopidogrel among 544 individuals. J Am Coll Cardiol 2006;48: 2584–91.

41. Matetzky S, Shenkman B, Guetta V, et al. Clopidogrel resistance is associated with increased risk of recurrent atherothrombotic events in patients with acute myocardial infarction. Circulation 2004;109: 3171–5.

42. Wiviott SD, Braunwald E, McCabe CH, et al. Prasugrel versus clopidogrel in patients with acute coronary syndromes. N Engl J Med 2007;357:2001–15.

43. Wright RS, Anderson JL, Adams CD. 2011 ACCF/AHA focused update of the guidelines for the management of patients with unstable angina/non-ST-elevation myocardial infarction. J Am Coll Cardiol 2011;57:1920–59.

44. Wallentin L, Becker RC, Budaj A, et al. Ticagrelor versus clopidogrel in patients with acute coronary syndromes. N Engl J Med 2009;361:1045–57.

45. Theroux P, Ouimet H, McCans J, et al. Aspirin, heparin, or both to treat acute unstable angina. N Engl J Med 1988;319(17):1005.

46. Theroux P, Waters D, Qiu S, et al. Aspirin versus heparin to prevent myocardial infarction during the acute phase of unstable angina. Circulation 1993; 88(5 Part 1):2045.

47. Ferguson JJ, Califf RM, Antman EM, et al. Enoxaparin vs. unfractionated heparin in high-risk patients with non-ST-segment elevation acute coronary syndromes managed with an intended early invasive strategy: primary results of the SYNGERGY randomized trial. JAMA 2004;292(1):45.

48. Stone GW, McLaurin BT, Cox DA, et al. Bivalirudin for patients with acute coronary syndromes. N Engl J Med 2006;355(21):2203.

49. Stone GW, White HD, Ohman EM, et al. Bivalirudin in patients with acute coronary syndromes undergoing percutaneous coronary intervention: a subgroup analysis from the Acute Catheterization and Urgent Intervention Triage strategy (ACUITY) trial. Lancet 2007;369(9565):907.

50. Stone GW, Witzenbichler B, Guagliumi G, et al. Bivalirudin during primary PCI in acute myocardial infarction. N Engl J Med 2008;358(21):2218.

51. Lopes RD, Alexander KP, Manoukian SV, et al. Advanced age, antithrombotic strategy, and bleeding in non-ST-segment elevation acute coronary syndromes: results from the ACUITY (Acute Catheterization and Urgent Intervention Triage Strategy) trial. J Am Coll Cardiol 2009;53(12):1021.

52. Kastrati A, Neumann FJ, Mehilli J, et al. Bivalirudin versus unfractionated heparin during percutaneous coronary intervention. N Engl J Med 2008;359(7):688.

53. The MIAMI Trial Research Group. Metoprolol in acute myocardial infarction. Am J Cardiol 1985; 56(14):10G–4G.

54. Randomised trial of intravenous atenolol among 16,027 cases of suspected acute myocardial infarction: ISIS-1. First International Study of Infarct Survival Collaborative Group. Lancet 1986;2(8498): 57–66.

55. Chen ZM, Pan HC, Chen YP, et al. Early intravenous then oral metoprolol in 45,852 patients with acute myocardial infarction: randomized placebo-controlled trial. Lancet 2005;366(9497):1622.

56. Giugliano RP, White JA, Bode C, et al. Early versus delayed, provision eptifibatide in acute coronary syndromes. NEJM 2009;3650:2176–90.

Reperfusion Strategies and Systems of Care in ST-Elevation Myocardial Infarction

Tapan Godiwala, MD, Mukta Srivastava, MD,
Anuj Gupta, MD*

KEYWORDS

- ST-elevation myocardial infarction • Systems of care • Percutaneous coronary intervention
- Thrombolysis • Reperfusion

KEY POINTS

- Primary percutaneous coronary intervention (PCI) should be performed within 90 minutes of hospital contact. Centers without PCI should consider thrombolysis if PCI-related time delay exceeds 60 minutes.
- If primary PCI cannot be performed, a pharmacoinvasive strategy should be considered, especially in patients with high risk ST-elevation myocardial infarction (STEMI).
- Numerous interventions have been identified that streamline the care of STEMI patients, and these should be targets for improving the delivery of timely and efficacious reperfusion therapy for STEMI patients.
- Regional systems of STEMI care improve door-to-balloon times and clinical outcomes in STEMI patients, and require the integration of emergency medical services, emergency departments, cardiologists, transport systems, and catheterization laboratories.

INTRODUCTION

The global burden of coronary heart disease continues to increase, driven primarily by an increasing incidence in the developing world. However, in the United States the incidence of acute myocardial infarction (MI), especially those with ST elevation, has continued to decrease. The rates of ST-elevation MI (STEMI) have decreased from 133 cases per 100,000 person-years in 1999 to 50 cases per 100,000 person-years in 2008.[1] Concurrently, mortality from acute infarction has improved significantly over the last 2 decades. Vital to this success has been the development of novel therapeutic regimens and the implementation of national guidelines regarding the efficient and timely access to coronary reperfusion. In 2006 the American College of Cardiology launched the D2B Alliance, a campaign describing strategies to reduce systems delay in the care of STEMI patients.[2] As a result, median door-to-balloon times declined 32 minutes, from 96 to 64 minutes, between 2005 and 2010.[3]

It is paramount that all team members from emergency medical services (EMS), nursing, emergency physicians, and cardiologists understand the treatment options available and the most efficient method of delivering them. This article reviews the available data on the selection of reperfusion strategies and systems-of-care models.

BACKGROUND

Primary percutaneous coronary intervention (PCI) is the preferred reperfusion strategy when it can

Disclosures: None.
Department of Cardiology, University of Maryland, 110 South Paca Street, 7th Floor, Baltimore, MD 21201, USA
* Corresponding author.
E-mail address: agupta@medicine.umaryland.edu

cardiology.theclinics.com

be performed in a timely fashion. A meta-analysis of 10 trials comparing balloon angioplasty with fibrinolytics found a significant difference in mortality of 4.4% versus 6.5% and a reduction in mortality or infarction of 7.2% versus 11.9%.[4] Given the ability to treat complications such as dissections and reduce acute recoil, it seemed plausible that the use of intracoronary stents would also improve outcomes over fibrinolytics. The DANAMI-2 and PRAGUE-2 trials bore out this conclusion. In DANAMI-2, 1572 patients were randomized to primary PCI versus alteplase. The majority of study participants presented to referral centers without PCI capability, thus requiring transfer of a large proportion of patients randomized to the interventional arm to a PCI center. The composite end point of death, reinfarction, or stroke at 30 days occurred significantly less with primary PCI, driven largely by reinfarction rates.[5] In the PRAGUE-2 trial, patients were again randomized to thrombolytic therapy versus primary PCI, with transfer as necessary. Mortality at 30 days was significantly better with immediate transfer, at a rate of 6% versus 15.3% with thrombolysis.[6]

These trials confirmed the superiority of primary PCI in comparison with fibrinolysis, as well as the feasibility of transfer. However, both were performed in countries with systems of care capable of facilitating rapid transfer. The median time from randomization to treatment was 90 minutes in those transferred from a non–PCI-capable facility in the DANAMI-2 trial.[5] Nallamothu and Bates[7] showed that the 4- to 6-week mortality benefit from primary PCI is lost with a PCI-related time delay of greater than 60 minutes. PCI-related time delay is defined as the difference between the door-to-balloon time and the door-to-needle time. Based on these and other data, transfer strategies target a 60-minute maximal delay in transfer to a primary PCI center in addition to the standard 90-minute door-to-balloon time (**Fig. 1**).

RESCUE PCI

Failed fibrinolysis is classically defined as hemodynamic or electrical instability, persistent chest pain, or failure to achieve at least a 50% reduction in ST elevation in the lead with maximal elevation at 90 minutes. In the REACT trial, 427 patients with STEMI who failed thrombolytics defined by less than 50% resolution in ST elevation at 90 minutes were randomized to repeat thrombolysis, PCI, or conservative management. The primary composite end point of death, reinfarction, stroke, or severe heart failure within 6 months occurred significantly less in those who underwent PCI. PCI remains the recommended management strategy for those who have failed thrombolysis.[8] The American College of Cardiology and American Heart Association (ACC/AHA) has given a Class IIa indication for rescue PCI in patients who are unstable, have ongoing ischemia, or have evidence of reperfusion failure on electrocardiography (ECG) with a large territory of myocardium at risk.[9]

FACILITATED AND PHARMACOINVASIVE REPERFUSION STRATEGIES

Initial investigations into angioplasty after intravenous fibrinolysis were disappointing at best. Multiple studies have failed to show additional benefit with balloon angioplasty alone after fibrinolysis. In one such study, 386 patients underwent coronary angiography after receiving tissue plasminogen activator and were randomized to immediate angioplasty or elective angioplasty after 7 to 10 days, if a severely stenotic vessel was found on angiography. No difference in reocclusion rates, systolic function, or degree of wall-motion abnormalities in the infarct zone were seen with early angioplasty.[10] With the advent of new more potent antithrombotic regimens in combination with the development of intracoronary stents, interest in PCI after fibrinolysis was rejuvenated. Two disparate strategies of combining fibrinolysis with PCI have been studied.

These 2 treatment strategies on the surface appear similar; however, the rationale and timing of PCI are different. Facilitated PCI involves pretreatment of all patients with glycoprotein (GP) IIb/IIIa inhibitors or thrombolytics before PCI. These patients are eligible for primary PCI and receive pharmaceutical agents to begin

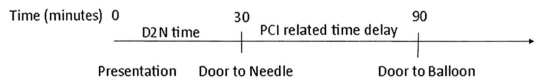

Fig. 1. The accepted time intervals between presentation and thrombolysis (door to needle; D2N) or primary PCI (door to balloon) are depicted. The difference between the door-to-balloon and door-to-needle time is the PCI-related time delay.

recanalization of the infarct-related artery before intervention. A pharmacoinvasive strategy plans for early (but not emergent) PCI after thrombolysis in those who are ineligible for primary PCI owing to time delay. These patients receive pharmaceutical agents as their primary reperfusion strategy, with PCI used as an adjunct to maintain vessel patency while potentially avoiding the difficulties with recent fibrinolytic administration, namely increased bleeding and paradoxically increased platelet activation.

The first strategy, termed facilitated PCI, involves full-dose or half-dose fibrinolytic therapy with or without a GP IIb/IIIa inhibitor followed by immediate PCI. The ASSENT-4 PCI trial randomized patients to primary PCI versus full-dose tenecteplase and PCI. Enrollment was ceased early because of a higher mortality in the facilitated PCI group (6% vs 3%). The primary end point of death, congestive heart failure, or shock within 90 days was met in 19% of patients assigned to facilitated PCI versus 13% in the primary PCI arm.[11] In the FINESSE trial, patients with STEMI who presented 6 hours or less after the onset of symptoms received abciximab plus half-dose reteplase–facilitated PCI, abciximab-facilitated PCI, or primary PCI. There was no statistically significant difference in the composite end point of death, ventricular fibrillation rates 48 hours after randomization, cardiogenic shock, and heart failure during the first 90 days between the 3 groups. Of interest, the abciximab and half-dose reteplase–facilitated PCI group fared no better despite a higher rate of ST-segment resolution.[12] A meta-analysis of 17 facilitated PCI trials showed an increased rate of death, nonfatal reinfarction, target vessel revascularization, and major bleeding with facilitated PCI compared with primary intervention.[13]

The second studied approach, a pharmacoinvasive strategy, involves administering pharmacologic agents (ie, fibrinolytics and/or GPIIb/IIIa inhibitors) at a non–PCI-capable facility followed by transfer for urgent PCI. Multiple studies including the GRACIA-1,[14] SIAM-III,[15] CARESS-in-AMI,[16] and TRANSFER-AMI[17] trials have confirmed the benefit of early PCI after fibrinolysis. CARESS-in-AMI randomized 600 STEMI patients with high-risk features who all received abciximab, heparin, half-dose reteplase, and acetylsalicylic acid (ASA) to immediate PCI versus rescue-only PCI. A significant reduction in all-cause mortality, reinfarction, and refractory myocardial ischemia within 30 days was seen with immediate transfer and PCI.[16] In the TRANSFER-in-AMI trial, 1059 high-risk patients who presented to a non–PCI-capable hospital were randomized to immediate PCI versus standard care (rescue or late PCI). All patients received standard-dose tenecteplase, ASA, and either unfractionated heparin or enoxaparin. Once again the composite end point occurred significantly more in those who did not receive early PCI.[17]

A large proportion of patients in the major facilitated PCI trials presented to centers that were PCI capable and received thrombolytics despite a short expected door-to-balloon time. The median difference between door-to-lytic time and door-to-balloon time was 90 minutes in the FINESSE trial, compared with 240 minutes in the TRANSFER-AMI trial. The longer interval between lytics and PCI in a pharmacoinvasive strategy could have theoretically decreased the risk of bleeding complications. Furthermore, thrombolytics were given at a median of 165 minutes after symptom onset in FINESSE versus 113 minutes in TRANSFER-AMI.[12,17] The delayed administration of thrombolytics in the facilitated trials may have reduced any incremental benefit of thrombolytics preceding PCI. Finally, the use of potent antiplatelet agents such as clopidogrel and GP IIb/IIIa inhibitors was limited in the earlier facilitated trials. It has been shown that platelet activity after thrombolysis is increased.[18] The lack of antiplatelet therapy may have limited the potential benefit of early PCI with a facilitated approach.

The 2009 ACC/AHA guidelines give a Class IIa indication for transferring those with anterior or high-risk inferior STEMI to a PCI-capable facility for intervention after thrombolysis. A Class I indication is given to those with heart failure of Killip Class III or more, hemodynamically compromising ventricular rhythms, or cardiogenic shock.[19] The Should We Emergently Revascularize Occluded Coronaries for Cardiogenic Shock (SHOCK) trial specifically addressed the issue of left ventricular failure–mediated shock during MI. Early revascularization did not confer a mortality benefit at 30 days; however, at 6 and 12 months a statistically significant mortality benefit was seen.[20] At least half of those randomized to early revascularization received thrombolytics, giving credence to the addition of early transfer for PCI in cardiogenic shock.

SELECTING A REPERFUSION STRATEGY

The selection of a reperfusion strategy depends on the time from symptom onset, patient factors, and the systems of care in place. The adage that "time is myocardium" is especially true when fibrinolysis is an option in patient management. When fibrinolysis was compared with placebo, most of the benefit seen was in those presenting within 2 hours of symptoms, with the incremental benefit falling off significantly beyond this time point. For every 1000 MIs, 65 lives will be saved by thrombolytics if treated within the first hour of symptoms, compared with 29 lives if treated within the first 3 to 6 hours of symptom onset.[21] It is during these critical early hours that thrombus has yet to completely organize and fibrinolysis is maximally effective.

Patient related factors that should be taken into account are age and coronary territory involved. An analysis of the National Registry of Myocardial Infarction stratified these risk factors. Those patients younger than 65 years with anterior MI lost a survival benefit with PCI at 40 minutes of PCI-related time delay. Conversely, those older than 65 with nonanterior MI retained a benefit with primary PCI even with a 168-minute PCI-related time delay. This analysis also confirmed that thrombolysis began to lose efficacy after 2 hours, increasing the acceptable PCI-related time delay in all subgroups.[22] Younger patients and those with anterior MI should be triaged to thrombolysis if systems for rapid transfer are not in place.

The systems of care in place in local communities are the only modifiable factors that directly affect decisions on reperfusion strategy. The AHA continues to advocate for the regional development of systems of care in the management of STEMI. Data are available from multiple United States and International community-based systems.

CURRENT STATE OF TREATMENT

Despite validation of mortality and morbidity benefits of early reperfusion therapy with either fibrinolytic therapy or PCI in STEMI, the delivery of appropriate and timely therapy for acute MI remains suboptimal. Approximately 25% of nearly 5000 acute-care hospitals in the United States have PCI capabilities, with even fewer equipped with round-the-clock PCI capabilities.[23] Up to 20% of STEMI patients have contraindications to fibrinolytic therapy, further challenging timely institution of reperfusion therapy. National initiatives have effected significant progress in door-to-balloon times at PCI-capable hospitals in recent years. The most contemporary, comprehensive, and nationally representative investigation of changes in door-to-balloon times in the United States reported an increase in the percentage of patients that achieved door-to-balloon times within less than 90 minutes from 44% to 91%.[2] This finding is in comparison to only one-third of patients receiving primary PCI within 90 minutes in 2002.[2] Of note, declines in median times were greatest among groups that previously had the highest median door-to-balloon times including women, African Americans, and patients older than 75 years.[2] However, patients requiring interfacility transfer for primary PCI remain a limitation to universally achieving benchmark door-to-balloon times. In an analysis by Wang and colleagues[23] of hospitals participating in the ACC National Cardiovascular Data Registry Catheterization PCI (ACC NCDR CathPCI) from 2005 to 2007, 25% of STEMI patients presented to a non–PCI-capable hospital. Median door-to-balloon times for patients requiring interhospital transfer was 149 minutes, with only 9.7% of patients achieving door-to-balloon times of less than 90 minutes.[23] These data suggest the need for systemized improvement of timely care of STEMI patients presenting to non-PCI-capable hospitals and those requiring interfacility transfer.

BARRIERS TO OPTIMIZED CARE FOR STEMI PATIENTS

Barriers to achieving rapid and efficacious reperfusion therapy exist at several levels in the continuum of care of STEMI patients. There is a lack of awareness amongst the lay community of the symptoms of acute heart attacks and the importance of seeking attention in a timely fashion. Delay to seeking medical attention because of denial, a "wait-and-see" approach, and reluctance to burden the medical system have been targeted by community-based public-awareness interventions with suboptimal efficacy in reducing time from symptom onset to first medical contact. At present, 76% of STEMI patients arrive at the hospital via self-transport or by family and friends. Prehospital ECGs have been shown to reduce door-to-needle and door-to-balloon times, but are underutilized and performed on fewer than 10% of STEMI patients. Community protocols that direct EMS to transport patients to the nearest hospital rather than the nearest PCI-capable hospital, and transport patients between non–PCI-capable hospitals and PCI-capable facilities via a "next available ambulance" route rather than a 9-1-1 system of activation, further handicap timely reperfusion. Lack of standardized algorithms that delineate reperfusion options, as well as protocols for administration of adjunctive therapies for STEMI care for emergency department (ED) physicians before transfer to a catheterization laboratory, also impose delays on STEMI treatment. Single-call catheterization laboratory activation systems improve door-to-balloon times but are not implemented across all PCI-capable hospitals. Finally, financial considerations pose barriers to ideal care because reimbursement patterns often adversely affect non–PCI-capable hospitals when STEMI patients are transferred directly from EDs.[24]

BARRIERS TO OPTIMIZED CARE FOR PATIENTS REQUIRING TRANSFER FOR PRIMARY PCI

Door-in-door-out (DIDO) time is defined as the time from arrival of a STEMI patient at a non–PCI-capable facility to the patient being discharged and en-route to a PCI-capable facility.[25] DIDO time is a metric for quality improvement for optimizing regional and statewide networks for STEMI care, which reflects the efficiency of a STEMI-referral hospital's ability to coordinate care and transfer and accounts for 75% of total reperfusion time for patients requiring interfacility transfer for primary PCI.[24] A national benchmark of less than 30 minutes for DIDO time has been recommended by the 2008 ACC/AHA Clinical Performance Measures for Acute Myocardial Infarction.[26] In a review of 14,821 patients with STEMI transferred to receiving centers for primary PCI in the ACTION Registry—Get With the Guidelines, median DIDO time was 68 minutes, with only 11% of patients achieving the benchmark DIDO time of less than 30 minutes.[24]

Larger-volume centers with larger volumes of PCI transfer demonstrate greater improvements in DIDO times, reflecting that larger-volume acute PCI hospital centers have broader networks of regional referral hospitals and have standardized transportation and treatment protocols that lead to fewer system-based delays. The lack of monitoring agencies with data feedback allowing identification of delays in the system and evaluation of interventions implemented for efficacy limit improvements in this metric in smaller-volume centers. Modification of the infrastructure at a community and regional level and across emergency services, EDs, cardiology teams, and catheterization laboratories requires significant financial and personnel investment, building an additional barrier to improving performance. Initiatives for improvement are hindered by competing interests between STEMI-referring hospitals and STEMI-receiving hospitals. Finally, a lack of accountability for improving patient care by any of multiple agencies involved in the care of an STEMI patient leads to a built-in component of inertia in the system. Maturation of regional STEMI care-delivery systems requires that quality-assessment programs and reimbursement strategies reflect performance in terms of patient outcomes instead of centering on individual hospitals.[24]

INITIATIVES FOR IMPROVEMENT

The importance of door-to-balloon times is reflected in its inclusion as a core quality measure collected and reported by the Centers for Medicare and Medicaid Service and the Joint Commission on Accreditation of Health Care Organizations. In a study by Bradley and colleagues,[27] a multivariate analysis was performed of 28 strategies identified to reduce door-to-balloon times across 365 hospitals, with 6 strategies found to be significantly associated with faster reperfusion times: catheterization-laboratory activation by emergency medicine physicians; implementation of a single-call catheterization laboratory activation system; activation of the catheterization laboratory before patient arrival via EMS; requiring catheterization laboratory staff to arrive within 20 minutes of being paged; having an attending cardiologist always on site; and having staff in the ED and catheterization laboratory use real-time data feedback to implement improvements in the system.[27] An investigation sponsored by the National Heart, Lung, and Blood Institute examined how top-performing hospitals achieve guideline-recommended door-to-balloon times and identified several themes including commitment to an explicit door-to-balloon goal, innovative protocols for transfer, flexibility in refining standardized protocols, data feedback to monitor progress, and an organizational culture fostering perseverance to attain the initiative goals.[27,28]

The D2B: An Alliance for Quality was conceived in 2006 as an organized effort by the ACC in partnership with the AHA as well as 37 other organizations to improve the timeliness of primary PCI in STEMI patients by advocating these previously identified strategies to improve reperfusion time. Further goals of the Alliance are to generate knowledge about the best methods of dispersing and translating new health care research into standards of care. The Alliance has been successful in uniting a broad-based coalition of practitioners to improve door-to-balloon times, integrating evidence-based strategies and improving the care of STEMI patients. Improvement in door-to-balloon times for patients requiring hospital transfer for primary PCI, more effective use of prehospital ECG capability, and improving time from symptom onset to presentation at a hospital have been identified by the Alliance as areas warranting further focus and improvement.[2] Integration of these evaluated strategies involving all components of regional STEMI systems can effect direct improvements on door-to-balloon times and DIDO times (**Fig. 2**).

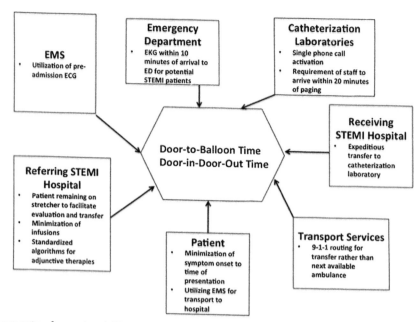

Fig. 2. Components of a regional STEMI program and interventions at each level that affect door-to-balloon times and door-in-door-out times.

MODELS OF CARE

The RACE trial represents one of the largest and most extensive regional systems for the reperfusion of STEMI developed in the United States, and was implemented in North Carolina across 65 of 100 acute-care hospitals in the area. By coalescing and coordinating EMS, EDs, and catheterization laboratories, the interventions promoted by the RACE initiative increased the frequency of reperfusion and substantially reduced time to treatment across 65 hospitals. The greatest improvements were noted in the decrease in interfacility transfer times for PCI.[29] Of note, despite improvements in time to reperfusion therapy, a mortality benefit following intervention was not noted, although trial design was not intended to examine mortality or evaluate treatment regimens.[30]

The RACE investigators focused on EMS, EDs, hospital networks, and their associated communication and transportation systems to institute a more efficient and effective STEMI protocol. Numerous simplifications to the reperfusion and transfer process were introduced. Continuous infusions were minimized, decreasing previously identified delays related to need for changing tubing and pumps between transfers; patients were left on transfer stretchers to minimize bed transfers and facilitate rapid evaluation and transfer; receiving PCI facilities accepted patients for transfer without delays for ensuring bed availability after intervention; and transportation relied on

local ambulances rather than helicopters or mobile critical care units. One controversial measure introduced included implementing algorithmic reperfusion plans for EMS and EDs to follow, thereby avoiding delays resulting from indecision and the time required to individualize a treatment plan. A predetermined algorithm-directed approach to reperfusion resulted in rapid, coordinated treatment and expedient patient disposition. A final important intervention was the introduction of a regional coordinator, funded by the RACE program and the PCI hospitals, whose role was to facilitate regional and statewide collaboration by overseeing all aspects of intervention from PCI hospital catheterization activation systems, ED and EMS STEMI plans, and regional education of EMS, nursing, and other personnel.[29]

Successful regional models have been implemented by the Minneapolis Heart Institute, with a similar strategy of improving interfacility transfer times and standardized protocols for therapy by EMS and EDs. Further emphasis is placed on measures to provide feedback and continuous improvements to the regional system. An additional component of the Minneapolis Heart Institute is prioritizing communication between cardiologists treating STEMI patients and their primary care physicians who will follow these patients on discharge.[31]

Regional systems in Europe for STEMI care have had success in improving patient outcomes as well. Distances between tertiary medical centers and community hospitals in Europe are substantially shorter than in the United States, facilitating the development of regional care systems.[32] In the PRAGUE Study, conducted in the 1990s in the Czech Republic and enrolling 300 patients presenting to non–PCI-capable hospitals, time from arrival at a non–PCI-capable hospital to a PCI center was 67 minutes, with an average travel time of 35 minutes.[33] Furthermore, widely socialized health care systems in Europe eliminate bureaucratic delays in health care delivery. National networks have been established in Denmark as well as in Prague.[32]

C-PORT

The Atlantic Cardiovascular Patient Outcomes Research Team (C-PORT) trial addressed the safety of primary PCI in community hospitals without surgical backup. In C-PORT, 451 thrombolytic-eligible patients with STEMI who presented within 12 hours of symptoms were randomized to primary PCI versus tissue plasminogen activator at 11 centers without cardiac surgery or full PCI programs. A composite end point of major adverse cardiac events occurred significantly less with primary PCI than with thrombolytic therapy.[34] These data have been used to support the expansion of primary PCI programs into community hospitals that do not necessarily have cardiothoracic surgery backup, thereby improving access to the preferred reperfusion strategy.

SYSTEM LIMITATIONS

Using time to reperfusion as a single quality measure overlooks other important evaluations of a system of care for STEMI patients, such as the process of patient selection. For example, this measure does not reflect the false positives or patients referred for emergent PCI who ultimately do not have a coronary occlusion, or false negatives, STEMI patients who are missed. In a review by Larson and colleagues[35] of 1335 patients referred over 3.5 years for an STEMI, 14% had no clear culprit coronary lesion and 9.5% had no significant coronary disease. Although a certain number of these patients may have had coronary spasm or highly suggestive ECGs and thus were appropriate for referral for diagnostic angiography, a nontrivial percentage was referred for catheterization potentially without sufficient evaluation. Thus the impetus for attaining a rapid door-to-balloon time must be balanced with adequate prereferral evaluation to result in an acceptable false-positive and false-negative rate. To this end, regional STEMI systems must be open to continued internal reviews for outcome measures, including not only times to reperfusion therapy but also other aspects of patient care for STEMI presentations.

SUMMARY

Primary PCI remains the preferred reperfusion strategy when performed within 90 minutes. In addition, those patients presenting to a non–PCI-capable facility should have a PCI-related time delay of less than 60 minutes. It is reasonable to allow for longer PCI-related time delays in older patients, those with low-risk STEMI, and those presenting at more than 3 hours after symptom onset. If primary PCI cannot be performed in a timely manner, a pharmacoinvasive strategy seems to be advantageous. A reasonable pharmacoinvasive strategy would include full-dose thrombolytics followed by dual antiplatelet therapy and anticoagulation with PCI performed 2 to 6 hours later. Patients deemed high risk by CARESS-in-AMI and TRANSFER-AMI criteria (previous MI, left bundle-branch block, extensive ST elevation, Killip class >2, and so forth) have a Class IIa indication for transfer, with all others a Class IIb for transfer after thrombolysis.[16,17,19]

The ACC's D2B Alliance has successfully integrated evidence-based therapy and has united practitioners with the common goal of decreasing door-to-balloon times. All communities should implement a system of care for STEMI that involves EMS, EDs, non–PCI-capable facilities, and PCI hospitals. Models such as those tested in North Carolina and Minneapolis lend themselves to the development of efficient, safe, and evidence-based treatment algorithms. Just as important as the development of a local STEMI care system is the continual evaluation and quality control to identify systems problems.

Continued public education, improved access to primary PCI or a pharmacoinvasive strategy, and the development of local systems of care for STEMI will undoubtedly lead to further reductions in reperfusion times with potential reductions in mortality.

REFERENCES

1. Yeh RW, Sidney S, Chandra M, et al. Population trends in the incidence and outcomes of acute myocardial infarction. N Engl J Med 2010;362: 2155–65.
2. Krumholz HM, Bradley EH, Nallamothu BK, et al. A campaign to improve the timeliness of primary percutaneous coronary intervention. Door-to-balloon: an alliance for quality. JACC Cardiovasc Interv 2008;1:97–104.

3. Krumholz HM, Herrin J, Miller L. Improvements in door-to-balloon time in the United States, 2005 to 2010. Circulation 2011;124:1038–45.

4. Weaver WD, Simes RJ, Betru A. Comparison of primary coronary angioplasty and intravenous thrombolytic therapy for acute myocardial infarction: a quantitative review. JAMA 1997;278(23): 2093–108.

5. Andersen HR, Nielsen TT, Rasmussen K, et al, DANAMI-2 Investigators. A comparison of coronary angioplasty with fibrinolytic therapy in acute myocardial infarction. N Engl J Med 2003;349:733–42.

6. Widimský P, Budesínský T, Vorác D, et al, 'PRAGUE' Study Group Investigators. Long distance transport for primary angioplasty versus immediate thrombolysis in acute myocardial infarction. Final results of the randomized national multicentre trial—PRAGUE-2. Eur Heart J 2003;24:94–104.

7. Nallamothu BK, Bates ER. Percutaneous coronary intervention versus fibrinolytic therapy in acute myocardial infarction: is timing (almost) everything? Am J Cardiol 2003;92:824–6.

8. Gershlick AH, Stephens-Lloyd A, Hughes S, et al. Rescue angioplasty after failed thrombolytic therapy for acute myocardial infarction. N Engl J Med 2005; 353:2758–68.

9. Antman EM, Hand M, Armstrong PW, et al. 2007 focused update of the ACC/AHA 2004 guidelines for the management of patients with ST-elevation myocardial infarction: a report of the American College of Cardiology/American Heart Association task force on practice guidelines. J Am Coll Cardiol 2008;51:210–47.

10. Topol EJ, Califf RM, George BS, et al. A randomized trial of immediate versus delayed elective angioplasty after intravenous tissue plasminogen activator in acute myocardial infarction. N Engl J Med 1987; 317(10):581–8.

11. Assessment of the Safety and Efficacy of a New Treatment Strategy with Percutaneous Coronary Intervention (ASSENT-4 PCI) Investigators. Primary versus tenecteplase-facilitated percutaneous coronary intervention in patients with ST-segment elevation acute myocardial infarction (ASSENT-4 PCI): randomised trial. Lancet 2006;367:569–78.

12. Ellis SG, Tendera M, de Belder MA, et al. Facilitated PCI in patients with ST-elevation myocardial infarction. N Engl J Med 2008;358:2205–17.

13. Keeley EC, Boura JA, Grines CL. Comparison of primary and facilitated percutaneous coronary interventions for ST-elevation myocardial infarction: quantitative review of randomised trials. Lancet 2006;367:579–88.

14. Fernandez-Aviles F, Alonso JJ, Castro-Beiras A, et al. Routine invasive strategy within 24 hours of thrombolysis versus ischaemia-guided conservative approach for acute myocardial infarction with ST-segment elevation (GRACIA-1): a randomised controlled trial. Lancet 2004;364:1045–53.

15. Scheller B, Hennen B, Hammer B, et al. Beneficial effects of immediate stenting after thrombolysis in acute myocardial infarction. J Am Coll Cardiol 2003;42(4):634–41.

16. Di Mario C, Dudek D, Piscione F, et al. Immediate angioplasty versus standard therapy with rescue angioplasty after thrombolysis in the Combined Abciximab Reteplase Stent Study in Acute Myocardial Infarction (CARESS-in-AMI): an open, prospective, randomised, multicentre trial. Lancet 2008;371:559–68.

17. Cantor WJ, Fitchett D, Borgundvaag B, et al. Routine early angioplasty after fibrinolysis for acute myocardial infarction. N Engl J Med 2009;360:2705–18.

18. Gurbel PA, Serebruany VL, Shustov AR, et al. Effects of reteplase and alteplase on platelet aggregation and major receptor expression during the first 24 hours of acute myocardial infarction treatment. GUSTO-III Investigators. Global use of strategies to open occluded coronary arteries. J Am Coll Cardiol 1998;31:1466–73.

19. Kushner F, Hand M, Smith S, et al. 2009 focused updates: ACC/AHA guidelines for the management of patients with ST-elevation myocardial infarction. J Am Coll Cardiol 2009;54:2205–41.

20. Hochman JS, Sleeper LA, Webb JG, et al. Early revascularization in acute myocardial infarction complicated by cardiogenic shock. N Engl J Med 1999;341(9):625–34.

21. Boersma E, Maas AC, Deckers JW, et al. Early thrombolytic treatment in acute myocardial infarction: reappraisal of the golden hour. Lancet 1996; 348(9030):771–5.

22. Pinto DS, Kirtane AJ, Nallamothu BK, et al. Hospital delays in reperfusion for ST-elevation myocardial infarction: implications when selecting a reperfusion strategy. Circulation 2006;114:2019–25.

23. Wang TY, Peterson ED, Ou FS, et al. Door-to-balloon times for patients with ST-elevation myocardial infarction requiring inter-hospital transfer for primary percutaneous coronary intervention. Am Heart J 2011;161(1):76–83.

24. Jacobs A, Antman E, Faxon D, et al. Development of systems of care for ST-elevation myocardial infarction patients: executive summary. Circulation 2007; 116:217–30.

25. Wang T, Nallamothu B, Krumholz H, et al. Association of door-in to door-out time with reperfusion delays and outcomes among patients transferred for primary percutaneous coronary intervention. JAMA 2011;305(24):2540–7.

26. Krumholz HM, Anderson JL, Bachelder BL, et al. ACC/AHA 2008 performance measures for adults with ST-elevation and non-ST elevation myocardial infarction: a report of the American College of Cardiology/American Heart Association Task Force on

Performance Measures (Writing Committee to develop performance measures for ST-elevation and non-ST-elevation myocardial infarction) developed in Collaboration With the American Academy of Family Physicians and American College of Emergency Physicians Endorsed by the American Association of Cardiovascular and Pulmonary Rehabilitation, Society for Cardiovascular Angiography and Interventions, and Society of Hospital Medicine. J Am Coll Cardiol 2008;52:2046–99.

27. Bradley E, Herrin J, Wang Y, et al. Strategies for reducing the door-to-balloon time in acute myocardial infarction. N Engl J Med 2006;355(22):2308–20.

28. Bradley E, Curry L, Webster T, et al. Achieving rapid door-to-balloon times: how top hospitals improve complex clinical system. Circulation 2006;113:1079–85.

29. Jollis J, Roettig M, Aluko A, et al. Implementation of a statewide system for coronary reperfusion for ST-segment elevation myocardial infarction. JAMA 2007;298(20):2371–80.

30. Glickman S, Greiner M, Lin L, et al. Assessment of temporal trends in mortality with implementation of a statewide ST-segment elevation myocardial infarction (STEMI) regionalization program. Ann Emerg Med 2012;59(4):243–252.e1.

31. Henry T, Sharkey S, Burke N, et al. A regional system to provide timely access to percutaneous coronary intervention for ST-elevation myocardial infarction. Circulation 2007;116:721–8.

32. Faxon D. Development of systems of care for ST-elevation myocardial infarction patients: current state of ST-elevation myocardial infarction care. Circulation 2007;116:e29–32.

33. Widimisky P, Groch L, Zelizko M, et al. Multicenter randomized trial comparing transport to primary angioplasty vs immediate thrombolysis vs combined strategy for patients with acute myocardial infarction presenting to a community hospital without a catheterization laboratory: the PRAGUE Study. Eur Heart J 2000;21:823–31.

34. Aversano T, Aversano LT, Passamani E, et al. Thrombolytic therapy vs primary percutaneous coronary intervention for myocardial infarction in patients presenting to hospitals without on-site cardiac surgery. JAMA 2002;287(15):1943–51.

35. Larson D, Menssen K, Sharkey S, et al. False-positive cardiac catheterization laboratory activation among patients with suspected ST-segment elevation myocardial infarction. JAMA 2007;298(23): 2754–60.

Cooling the Fire
Resuscitated Sudden Death

Semhar Z. Tewelde, MD[a], Michael E. Winters, MD[b],*

KEYWORDS

- Postcardiac arrest syndrome • Postcardiac arrest management • Therapeutic hypothermia
- Return of spontaneous circulation • Sudden cardiac death

KEY POINTS

- Sudden cardiac death (SCD) occurs when the electrical impulses in the heart become disorganized, causing the heart to suddenly stop beating. Approximately 383,000 out-of-hospital cardiac arrests occur annually.
- Return of spontaneous circulation (ROSC) is the resumption of perfusing cardiac activity after cardiac arrest; cardiopulmonary resuscitation and defibrillation increase the probability of ROSC.
- Postcardiac arrest syndrome ensues after ROSC and is the compilation of a systemic-reperfusion response, myocardial dysfunction, brain injury, and the underlying precipitating pathology.
- Postcardiac arrest management necessitates optimizing oxygenation, ventilation, and hemodynamics; initiating therapeutic hypothermia; and performing early cardiac catheterization.
- Comatose out-of-hospital survivors of SCD should be rapidly cooled within the first 8 hours following ROSC to a target temperature between 32° and 34°C for 12 to 24 hours.

INTRODUCTION

Out-of-hospital cardiac arrest (OHCA) is a leading cause of death among adults in the United States.[1,2] Despite significant advances in medical research and emergency cardiac care, the survival rate for patients with OHCA who regain spontaneous circulation remains a dismal 8%.[1] Surprisingly, survival rates vary widely across the United States, ranging from 2% to 35%, and differ depending on the patient's location when the arrest occurs.[3] Despite the publication of postcardiac arrest guidelines for the management of OHCA patients by the American Heart Association (AHA), there continues to be considerable variation in postcardiac arrest care.[4] Postcardiac arrest care is intricate and requires a multidisciplinary approach, with a prospective plan, monitoring, and continuous reassessment by every health care professional involved in the patient's care. This article discusses recent advances in the understanding of patients with the postcardiac arrest syndrome (PCAS) and provides management recommendations for the care of patients with return of spontaneous circulation (ROSC) following OHCA. Specific emphasis is placed on optimizing oxygenation, ventilation, and hemodynamics; initiating therapeutic hypothermia; and performing early cardiac catheterization. With this information, the provider managing patients with ROSC from OHCA can minimize morbidity and improve patient outcomes.

POSTCARDIAC ARREST SYNDROME

PCAS is a composite of pathophysiologic processes that occur during cardiac arrest, defined by the period of systemic ischemia and the

Disclosures: The authors have no relevant financial interests to disclose.
[a] Department of Emergency Medicine, University of Maryland Medical Center, 110 South Paca Street, 6th Floor, Suite 200, Baltimore, MD 21201, USA; [b] Emergency Medicine/Internal Medicine/Critical Care Program, University of Maryland School of Medicine, 110 South Paca Street, 6th Floor, Suite 200, Baltimore, MD 21201, USA
* Corresponding author.
E-mail address: mwint001@umaryland.edu

subsequent reperfusion that occurs after ROSC. PCAS comprises 4 distinct processes: systemic ischemic-reperfusion response, myocardial dysfunction, brain injury, and the underlying precipitating pathology.[3]

Systemic Ischemic-Reperfusion Syndrome

Cardiac arrest results in the cessation of the delivery of oxygen and metabolic substrates and the elimination of toxic metabolites. Deprivation of oxygen to vital organs results in the conversion of aerobic to anaerobic cellular metabolism. Cardiopulmonary resuscitation (CPR) attempts to reverse this process, but provides only a meager increase in oxygen delivery and cardiac output. Ironically, reperfusion after ROSC exacerbates existing damage through "the oxygen paradox."[5,6] Toxic substrates produced during the initial ischemic event are distributed into the circulation, further propagating organ dysfunction. The cascade of immunologic pathways causes a systemic circulatory response syndrome that mimics sepsis.[6,7]

Analogous to the pathophysiology of sepsis, the systemic ischemic-reperfusion syndrome results in an increase in the circulating levels of cytokines and inflammatory mediators (eg, interleukin-6 and tumor necrosis factor), thereby producing tissue hypoxia and lactic acidosis.[8,9] This process is followed by the recruitment of neutrophils and growth factors, such as platelet-derived and vascular endothelial growth factor, which increase capillary permeability, resulting in intravascular volume depletion. Additional proinflammatory molecules assist in the formation of microthrombi, creating a coagulopathic milieu and further impairing tissue perfusion. These insults activate the fight-or-flight mechanism, releasing cortisol into the circulation. Unfortunately, after resolution of the acute phase of the PCAS the initial surge of cortisol dwindles, which may hasten cardiovascular collapse through a relative adrenal insufficiency.[10,11] Once thought to be protective, the theory of "endotoxin tolerance" has been proved to be detrimental by initiating immune dysfunction and increasing susceptibility to infection.[5]

The amalgam of impaired oxygen delivery, circulatory compromise, procoagulation, relative adrenal suppression, and increased susceptibility to infection defines the systemic ischemic-reperfusion response. As demonstrated by early goal-directed therapy for the treatment of patients with septic shock, a targeted, systematic approach to counteract the cause, duration, and components of the systemic ischemic-reperfusion syndrome can limit the sequelae of the response.[12–14]

Myocardial Dysfunction

The leading cause of sudden cardiac death is heart disease.[3] Yet myocardial dysfunction seen after cardiac arrest is typically not secondary to acutely infarcted or scarred myocardium; rather, it is considered a true stunning phenomenon.[3,15] This finding is illustrated in several studies of patients with ROSC after OHCA, which reveal left ventricular dysfunction and a poor ejection fraction despite favorable coronary artery anatomy at the time of cardiac catheterization.[16,17] In fact, more than 50% of patients with myocardial dysfunction after cardiac arrest have no angiographic evidence of acute myocardial disease.[18]

Myocardial stunning classically occurs within the first 8 hours after ROSC and usually resolves within 24 to 48 hours.[18] During this time, the heart rate and blood pressure are extremely capricious and should be monitored closely. Any sign of poor systemic perfusion, such as hypotension, should prompt immediate initiation of vasoactive agents (**Table 1**). Rare cases of persistent myocardial dysfunction weeks after cardiac arrest have been described in the literature.[19]

Table 1
Vasopressor/inotropic agents

	Norepinephrine	Epinephrine	Dopamine	Dobutamine
Dosing	0.1–0.5 µg/kg/min	0.1–0.5 µg/kg/min	5–10 µg/kg/min	5–10 µg/kg/min
Indications	Severe hypotension and decreased systemic vascular tone	Severe hypotension (systolic <70 mm Hg), anaphylaxis with hemodynamic or respiratory distress	Hypotension especially if associated with symptomatic bradycardia	Diastolic or systolic dysfunction

Data from Nichol G, Aufderheide TP, Eigel B, et al. Regional systems of care for out-of-hospital cardiac arrest: a policy statement from the American Heart Association. Circulation 2010;121:709–29; and Nichol G, Soar J. Regional cardiac resuscitation systems of care. Curr Opin Crit Care 2010;16:223–30.

No specific mechanism has been identified as the cause of myocardial dysfunction following cardiac arrest. Many factors have been implicated, including chest compression, defibrillation, epinephrine, and the catecholamine surge in response to the PCAS.[16] Microvascular factors such as adenosine triphosphate depletion, increased calcium metabolism, oxygen free radical formation, and upregulation of heat-shock proteins have also been postulated to cause postarrest myocardial dysfunction.[20–22]

Brain Injury

Cardiac arrest results in global ischemia to the brain. Brain injury is the cause of death in approximately two-thirds of patients who initially survive OHCA and in one-fourth of patients who initially survive in-hospital cardiac arrest.[23,24] The morphologic characteristics of neuronal death after transient global brain ischemia are often not apparent for hours to days.[25] Numerous mechanisms have been identified by which neuronal injury occurs during the ischemia. The pivotal component in neuronal injury pathways is the mitochondrion, which triggers the release of oxygen free radicals and activates protease and inflammatory mediators.[25–27] Ultimately this results in neuronal cell death by either necrosis or apoptosis. Increasing evidence has shown that arterial hyperoxia (see later discussion) following ROSC after cardiac arrest may further increase neuronal injury.[28,29]

ROSC alters normal cerebrovascular autoregulation, impairing both cerebral blood flow and cerebral perfusion pressure (CPP). The conventional mean arterial perfusion pressure (MAP) target of 65 mm Hg might be inadequate to provide sufficient CPP in the postcardiac arrest period.[30] ROSC has also been associated with transient cerebral edema, as seen on computed tomography (CT) imaging of postcardiac arrest patients. The clinical significance of cerebral edema remains controversial.[31]

Precipitating Pathology

Prompt identification of the cause of cardiac arrest is critical to the management and prognostication of individual patient care. More than half of all causes of cardiac arrest are found in the heart.[19] Respiratory failure is cited as the second most common cause of cardiac arrest, accounting for roughly 35% of cases.[32] Other important causes of cardiac arrest include pulmonary embolism, sepsis, intracranial catastrophes, toxic ingestion, metabolic disorders, and environmental exposure.[32,33]

OPTIMIZING MECHANICAL VENTILATION
Ventilation

Most patients with ROSC following cardiac arrest are intubated and placed on mechanical ventilation (**Box 1**). For various reasons, these patients are at risk of developing the acute respiratory distress syndrome (ARDS). It is well established that patients with acute lung injury or ARDS should be ventilated initially using tidal volumes between 6 and 8 mL/kg of ideal body weight. This recommendation stems from a landmark article that demonstrated improved mortality rates in patients with ARDS who were ventilated with tidal volumes of 6 mL/kg compared with traditional tidal volume settings of 10 to 12 mL/kg.[34] To date, no studies have compared modes of mechanical ventilation or optimal tidal volume settings in postcardiac arrest patients. Nonetheless, current guidelines recommend ventilating the postcardiac arrest patient with initial tidal volumes between 6 and 8 mL/kg of ideal body weight.[4] In addition to low tidal volume settings, current guidelines also recommend measuring inspiratory plateau pressure, as an indicator of the potential for ventilator-induced lung injury.[4] Plateau pressures should be maintained below 30 cm H_2O. When plateau pressures rise above that level, the tidal volume should be decreased in 1-mL/kg increments until the plateau pressure falls below 30 cm H_2O or a tidal volume of 4 mL/kg is reached.[13,34]

Box 1
Optimizing mechanical ventilation

Initial Ventilator Settings

Low tidal volumes (TV) 6 to 8 mL/kg ideal body weight

Respiratory rate 10 to 12 beats/min

Positive end-expiratory pressure 5 cm H_2O

Lowest fraction of inspired oxygen to prevent oxygen toxicity (Fio_2) 60% or less

Goals

$Paco_2$ 40 to 45 mm Hg

$Petco_2$ 35 to 40 mm Hg

pH 7.3 to 7.4

Pao_2 ~100 mm Hg

S_pO_2 94% or greater

Plateau pressure 30 cm H_2O or less

Data from Nichol G, Aufderheide TP, Eigel B, et al. Regional systems of care for out-of-hospital cardiac arrest: a policy statement from the American Heart Association. Circulation 2010;121:709–29; and Nichol G, Soar J. Regional cardiac resuscitation systems of care. Curr Opin Crit Care 2010;16:223–30.

Equally as important as using low tidal volumes and following serial plateau pressure measurements is monitoring the arterial carbon dioxide concentration. Both hypocapnia (commonly caused by hyperventilation from aggressive bag-valve-mask ventilation) and hypercapnia (caused by low tidal volume settings) can be deleterious. There are currently no studies that have defined the ideal respiratory rate for mechanically ventilated postcardiac arrest patients. The current recommendation is to begin with a rate between 10 and 12 breaths per minute and titrate to maintain normocapnia, with the goal Pa_{CO_2} between 40 and 45 mm Hg.[4] Arterial CO_2 concentrations can be followed by either arterial blood gas analysis or end-tidal capnography ($PetCO_2$). An ideal $PetCO_2$ is between 35 and 40 mm Hg.[4] End-tidal capnography additionally provides the clinician with instantaneous feedback in the event that ventilatory changes or ventilator malfunctions occur.

Oxygenation

It is common practice to initially place patients with ROSC following cardiac arrest on 100% forced inspired oxygen. Nonetheless, there is mounting evidence to suggest that elevated levels of arterial oxygen concentration (hyperoxia) during reperfusion produce mitochondrial injury, cause the release of free radicals, and exacerbate neuronal damage.[26,28,35] In a recent trial, Kilgannon and colleagues[28] demonstrated increased in-hospital mortality rates for patients with hyperoxia (defined by the investigators as a Pa_{O_2} >300 mm Hg) compared with those with normoxia (defined as a Pa_{O_2} between 60 and 300 mm Hg). At present, the optimal Pa_{O_2} for postcardiac arrest patients is unknown. In light of recent evidence, current guidelines recommend titrating the fraction of inspired oxygen to target a Pa_{O_2} of approximately 100 mm Hg using arterial blood gas analysis or an oxygen saturation of at least 94% using continuous pulse oximetry.[4] Should the fraction of inspired oxygen remain above 60% (considered the threshold for developing oxygen toxicity), positive end-expiratory pressure (PEEP) can be increased in increments of 2 to 3 mm Hg to decrease the level of inspired oxygen. Increases in PEEP to reduce inspired oxygen concentrations, however, must be balanced with the potential deleterious effects of increases in intrathoracic pressure and impaired venous return.

HEMODYNAMIC OPTIMIZATION

Data regarding optimal hemodynamic targets in postcardiac arrest patients are scant (**Fig. 1**).

What is unmistakable is that hemodynamic instability is associated with a poor prognosis.[36] Postcardiac arrest hemodynamic optimization focuses on restoring intravascular volume, maintaining and monitoring adequate tissue perfusion and oxygenation, using adjunctive therapies in the most critically ill, and correcting the precipitating cause of the arrest.[36,37] A goal-directed approach to hemodynamic optimization in postcardiac arrest patients has been extrapolated from guidelines used in other critically ill patients, namely those with septic shock.[12,13]

Intravascular Volume Replacement and Monitoring

After ROSC, volume expansion with intravenous fluids is paramount to the restoration of intravascular volume and reperfusion of ischemic organs. Before initiating volume resuscitation, intravenous access is required and, in view of the fact that large quantities and a multitude of medications are given simultaneously, central venous access should be strongly considered. In addition, early placement of an arterial line should be considered for continuous measurement of MAP, as noninvasive measurements of blood pressure are inaccurate in hypotensive patients. MAP is a better physiologic estimate of true organ perfusion pressure and should be followed in lieu of systolic blood pressures. Although current guidelines recommend maintaining a MAP between 65 and 100 mm Hg, the ideal MAP goal for patients with ROSC following cardiac arrest has not been defined.[4] Several recent studies have observed improved outcomes with target MAPs ranging from 80 to 100 mm Hg.[38–40] There is no evidence to suggest that increasing the MAP to above 100 mm Hg improves outcomes and, in fact, this may be detrimental.[41]

The immune and inflammatory mediators of the PCAS result in massive volume depletion.[3] Isotonic fluids should be administered to restore and improve preload, thereby improving overall cardiac output and systemic perfusion.[42] Several liters of fluid may be required in the first 24 hours to achieve euvolemia. For patients who are candidates for therapeutic hypothermia, the early use of cold (4°C) isotonic fluids is recommended to achieve both volume and temperature targets.

Assessing volume status and determining which patients may be responsive to fluids are some of the most challenging aspects of caring for critically ill patients. Current guidelines for the management of select critical illnesses recommend targeting volume resuscitation to a central venous pressure (CVP) of 8 to 12 mm Hg for

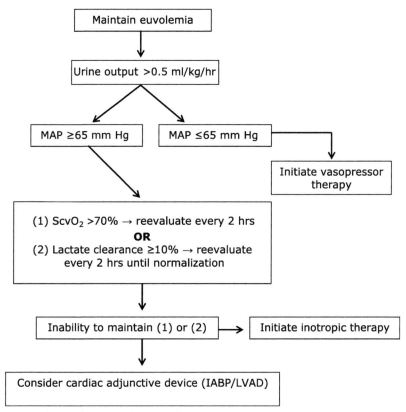

Fig. 1. Hemodynamic goals. MAP, mean arterial pressure; IABP, intra-aortic balloon pump; LVAD, left ventricular assist device. (*Data from* Nichol G, Aufderheide TP, Eigel B, et al. Regional systems of care for out-of-hospital cardiac arrest: a policy statement from the American Heart Association. Circulation 2010;121:709–29; and Nichol G, Soar J. Regional cardiac resuscitation systems of care. Curr Opin Crit Care 2010;16:223–30.)

nonintubated patients.[33,43] Despite this recommendation, there is no evidence to suggest that CVP is a reliable marker of volume status or fluid responsiveness. Dynamic markers of fluid responsiveness, such as measurement of respirophasic changes in diameter of the inferior vena cava using ultrasonography, arterial waveform analysis, and passive leg raising, are more accurate than CVP in the assessment of volume status and fluid responsiveness.

Vasopressor Therapy

If a MAP of at least 65 mm Hg cannot be maintained with intravenous fluids alone, a vasopressor agent should be administered (see **Table 1**). Current guidelines recommend the use of norepinephrine, epinephrine, or dopamine.[4] Of importance is that no studies to date have demonstrated superiority of any single vasopressor agent. In a recent trial, De Backer and colleagues[40] demonstrated that dopamine was associated with increased adverse events and a trend toward higher mortality when used in patients with cardiogenic shock.

Monitoring Tissue Perfusion

Vital-sign trends are unreliable in assessing the adequacy of organ perfusion. It is well known that patients with fairly normal vital signs can have poor perfusion and inadequate oxygen delivery. Therefore, current guidelines recommend measuring central venous oxygen saturation ($Scvo_2$) and lactate as markers of tissue perfusion.[4,44] $Scvo_2$ must be measured from a central venous catheter placed in the subclavian or internal jugular vein. The recommended target of $Scvo_2$ is greater than 70%.[4,12] Regarding lactate, there is no significant difference between arterial and venous samples; values greater than 2 mmol/L are considered abnormal. More important than a single lactate value is the trend in serial samples. In a recent study, Jones and colleagues[45] demonstrated decreased mortality rates for patients who had at least a 10% decrease (lactate clearance) in serial values. In similar studies, investigators found that lactate clearance was noninferior to $Scvo_2$ measurements in determining tissue perfusion.[46] Of importance, both

Scvo$_2$ and lactate can be affected by numerous variables, including renal and hepatic dysfunction and hypothermia. As a result, the authors believe it is reasonable to monitor both markers to assess tissue perfusion in postcardiac arrest patients. If the Scvo$_2$ is less than 70% and/or the trend in lactate values is unchanged or increasing despite adequate volume resuscitation with a MAP of less than 65 mm Hg, inotropic support to augment cardiac output should be initiated. Dobutamine reverses both diastolic and systolic dysfunction, and is considered by many to be the inotrope of choice in postcardiac arrest patients.[46,47]

Adrenal Insufficiency and Steroids

The PCAS is a massive physiologic stressor and is thought to cause a relative adrenal insufficiency.[48,49] Patients who are unable to ward off such an immune attack develop capillary permeability, have worsened vascular tone, suffer cardiovascular collapse, and have a higher mortality rate.[50] No current randomized control trials are investigating corticosteroid use in cardiac arrest survivors. The efficacy of corticosteroids remains controversial in septic-shock patients and in patients following cardiac arrest. Given the uncertain value of steroids, no recommendations have been made for or against such therapy at this time.

Mechanical Circulatory Support

Despite aggressive volume, vasopressor, and inotropic support, some postarrest patients remain gravely ill. In these patients, mechanical circulatory devices can be used as a temporizing measure until native hemodynamics are restored. Intra-aortic balloon pumps and left ventricular assist devices have proved to be effective in other critically ill patient populations.[51–55] Although the use of such devices should be considered, the routine placement of mechanical circulatory devices is not recommended because of inconsistent survival data.[4]

THERAPEUTIC HYPOTHERMIA

The research on therapeutic hypothermia dates back more than 50 decades (**Box 2**). However it was not until 2002, with the publication of one large randomized controlled trial and a smaller pseudorandomized trial, that therapeutic hypothermia was implemented as a critical component in postcardiac arrest care.[56,57] As a result of these landmark studies, the AHA incorporated therapeutic hypothermia into its guidelines for postresuscitation care.[4] Although the exact mechanisms remain unclear, therapeutic hypothermia is presumed to improve neurologic

---

Box 2
Therapeutic hypothermia

Induction

Immediate cooling

Target temperature 32° to 34°C

Ice-cold intravenous fluids, 30 mL/kg bolus

Surface cooling devices (ice packs/cooling blanket)

Endovascular cooling devices (no superiority)

Temperature-sensing devices (esophageal, bladder, or rectal probe)

Manage shivering with sedation with or without neuromuscular blockade if required

Maintenance

Continue temperatures 32° to 34°C for 12 to 24 hours

Monitor dysrhythmias (continuous cardiac monitoring)

Monitor electrolyte abnormalities (potassium, magnesium, calcium, and phosphate)

Monitor coagulation abnormalities (platelets, activated partial thromboplastin time, prothrombin time, fibrinogen, fibrin split products, and d-dimer)

Monitor hyperglycemia (consider cause, eg, sepsis)

Rewarming

Do not rapidly rewarm → portends worse outcomes

Rewarm at 0.25° to 0.5°C per hour

Monitor for dysrhythmias, electrolytes, and coagulation abnormalities

Data from Nichol G, Aufderheide TP, Eigel B, et al. Regional systems of care for out-of-hospital cardiac arrest: a policy statement from the American Heart Association. Circulation 2010;121:709–29; and Nichol G, Soar J. Regional cardiac resuscitation systems of care. Curr Opin Crit Care 2010;16:223–30.

---

recovery by decreasing cerebral metabolism, suppressing inflammatory cytokines, reducing the formation of oxygen free radicals, decreasing vascular permeability, and improving overall cerebral glucose metabolism.[58]

Patient Selection

The best available evidence demonstrates improved neurologic outcomes after hospital discharge for patients with OHCA secondary to pulseless ventricular tachycardia (VT) or ventricular fibrillation (VF).[59,60] Provided there are no absolute contraindications, therapeutic hypothermia should be induced in patients with ROSC after OHCA resulting from pulseless VT or VF.[4] Evidence of the efficacy of hypothermia in other cardiac rhythms (eg, asystole and pulseless electrical activity) and in-hospital cardiac arrest is less robust. Studies using historical controls along with observational cohorts have demonstrated conflicting results on the benefit of hypothermia in nonshockable rhythms.[61–63] Despite these limitations, current guidelines recommend the use of therapeutic hypothermia in all comatose survivors of cardiac arrest.[4] The AHA defines a "comatose survivor" as a patient who has a Glasgow Coma Scale score of less than 8 or lacks meaningful response to commands.[4]

Goals

Therapeutic hypothermia can be divided into 3 phases: induction, maintenance, and rewarming. For the comatose survivor of OHCA, therapeutic hypothermia should be initiated as soon as possible. Initiation of therapeutic hypothermia by prehospital care providers who have access to cooling pads or ice packs and can ensure no inadvertent rewarming of the patient has been shown to be safe.[64,65] Induction involves rapid cooling of the patient within the first 8 hours following ROSC to a target temperature between 32° and 34°C.[4] No mortality benefit has been seen at temperatures below 32°C. Induction can be accomplished by various methods. Ice packs on the head, neck, axilla, and groin, cooling blankets, and boluses of 30 mL/kg of cold (4°C) normal saline or Ringer lactate have been shown to be efficacious in reaching the target temperature.[66,67] More sophisticated techniques include nasogastric or bladder lavage with iced saline and endovascular cooling devices. There is no evidence to support the superiority of one method of cooling.[68] Accurate monitoring of core temperature during therapeutic hypothermia is essential. Conventional locations for monitoring temperature, namely, the mouth, the axilla, the tympanic membrane, and even the rectum, are not reliable during therapeutic hypothermia.[69] The preferred method of monitoring core temperature is via an esophageal or bladder probe.[4]

Dropping the core body temperature often produces shivering, which counteracts the goal of rapidly inducing hypothermia. Multiple combinations of sedative and analgesic agents can be used to halt shivering. The medications most often used for this purpose are propofol, dexmedetomidine, and fentanyl.[3] If shivering persists despite the aggressive use of sedatives and analgesics, administration of a neuromuscular blocking agent such as cisatracurium is indicated. The

neurologic examination may be altered by sedatives and analgesics, so short-acting boluses are preferred over long-acting medications. In addition to sedatives, analgesics, and neuromuscular blocking agents, magnesium can be used to control shivering, given its ability to reduce the shivering threshold and its lack of sedating qualities.[70]

The maintenance phase begins once core body temperature reaches 32° to 34°C. During this phase, a cooling method with continuous temperature monitoring and minimal temperature fluctuation is preferred, commonly referred to as a closed-feedback temperature-sensing loop. This goal is best achieved by a combination of internal and external cooling devices, as one method alone is not sufficient to ensure a stable core temperature. Based on consensus data, the recommended duration of therapeutic hypothermia is 12 to 24 hours,[4] after which, depending on institutional protocols, the rewarming phase begins. Current guidelines are based on consensus data and recommend that rewarming take place at a rate of 0.25° to 0.5°C per hour.[4] Rapid rewarming can significantly alter the body's metabolic and hemodynamic demands and may be detrimental to the patient.[70]

Complications

Postcardiac arrest therapeutic hypothermia is considered standard care for the patient with OHCA attributable to VF or pulseless VT. Potential complications of hypothermia include cardiac, hematologic, renal, endocrine, infectious, and metabolic derangements (**Box 3**).[71] Although hypothermia can cause complications, it is important to recognize that the benefit for many will outweigh the risk of developing complications. In fact, several studies have shown that hypothermia is well tolerated, and the proportions of complications in hypothermic patients are equivalent to those occurring in normothermic patients with ROSC following OHCA.[56,57,60]

CARDIAC CATHETERIZATION

Percutaneous coronary intervention (PCI) in postcardiac arrest survivors is an independent predictor of survival.[72] More than half of individuals who experience OHCA have atherosclerotic heart disease.[1,3] Many survivors of OHCA have nonspecific electrocardiographic abnormalities. A nondiagnostic electrocardiogram (ECG) is a poor predictor of cardiac ischemia, and for many survivors of OHCA has delayed urgent PCI.[19,72] Current guidelines recommend that all patients with evidence of ST-segment elevation myocardial infarction (STEMI) on a postarrest ECG be considered for emergent cardiac catheterization.[4] If PCI

Box 3
Potential complications of therapeutic hypothermia

Cardiac

Dysrhythmias

Increase systemic vascular resistance

Decreased cardiac output

Hematologic

Coagulopathy

Dysfunctional platelets

Renal

Diuresis

Hypovolemia

Electrolyte abnormalities (hypophosphatemia, hypokalemia, hypomagnesemia, hypocalcemia)

Endocrine

Insulin resistance and hyperglycemia

Infectious

Sepsis

Data from Nichol G, Aufderheide TP, Eigel B, et al. Regional systems of care for out-of-hospital cardiac arrest: a policy statement from the American Heart Association. Circulation 2010;121:709–29; and Nichol G, Soar J. Regional cardiac resuscitation systems of care. Curr Opin Crit Care 2010;16:223–30.

---

hypothermia and catheterization is associated with improved neurologic outcomes and overall survival rates.[74]

CRITICAL SUPPORTIVE THERAPY

During the postcardiac arrest resuscitation period, clinicians face many challenges in addition to optimizing oxygenation, ventilation, and hemodynamics, initiating therapeutic hypothermia, and early coronary revascularization (**Box 4**). These challenges are discussed in this section.

Dysrhythmias

Dysrhythmias emerge in some patients during the early postarrest period, and should be treated just as they would be in any other patient population. Current guidelines do not recommend the

---

Box 4
Critical supportive therapy

Dysrhythmias

12-lead electrocardiogram

Continuous cardiac monitoring

Ventricular tachycardia (VT) with hemodynamic instability → electrical therapy

VT with hemodynamic stability and normal QT interval → amiodarone or procainamide

Polymorphic VT with prolonged QT → magnesium sulfate

Seizures and Neuroimaging

Continuous electroencephalography in all comatose postcardiac arrest patients

No prophylactic antiepileptics without evidence of seizure activity

+ Seizure activity → benzodiazepines

After documented seizure, initiate antiepileptics (phenytoin, levetiracetam, or valproate)

Hyperglycemia

Moderate glycemic control with serum glucose levels of 144 to 180 mg/dL

Initiate insulin titration for glucose level exceeding above

Hyperthermia

Control pyrexia (>37°C) with antipyretics and cooling devices

Data from Nichol G, Aufderheide TP, Eigel B, et al. Regional systems of care for out-of-hospital cardiac arrest: a policy statement from the American Heart Association. Circulation 2010;121:709–29; and Nichol G, Soar J. Regional cardiac resuscitation systems of care. Curr Opin Crit Care 2010;16:223–30.

---

is not immediately available, thrombolytic therapy should be strongly considered.[4] In addition to postarrest STEMI patients, any patient with ROSC after OHCA and a nondiagnostic ECG should be considered for urgent catheterization.[1,3,4,19,72]

Patients who do not respond to aggressive volume resuscitation and vasopressors or inotropes have a lower survival rate. Given the prognosis, these patients are often not offered any adjunctive therapy. If quickly identified and considered for urgent cardiac catheterization, their labile native hemodynamics may respond to immediate cardiac augmentation. The revascularization of an acute arterial occlusion or the placement of a mechanical cardiac supportive device, such as an intra-aortic balloon pump or left ventricular assist device, may change the prognosis of patients in this subset.

Current evidence supports the use of therapeutic hypothermia for postarrest patients undergoing emergent PCI, but the cooling procedure should not delay immediate PCI when it is warranted.[72,73] Many hospital protocols continue therapeutic hypothermia while patients are in the cardiac catheterization suite. Simultaneous administration of empiric antidysrhythmic medications to all postarrest patients. If a patient experiences a dysrhythmia that results in hemodynamic compromise, electrical therapy should be applied. If the patient is hemodynamically stable and develops VT with a normal QT interval, either amiodarone or procainamide is an acceptable pharmacologic agent, but neither has been shown to improve the rate of survival to hospital discharge.[75] If the patient has a prolonged QT with polymorphic VT, the drug of choice is magnesium.[74]

Seizures

Up to 25% of postcardiac arrest patients have seizure activity.[76] Seizures are associated with poorer neurologic outcomes and an increased mortality rate.[77] As a result, current guidelines recommend that all comatose postcardiac arrest patients undergo continuous electroencephalographic monitoring.[4] If myoclonic seizure activity is observed, the drug of choice is a benzodiazepine.[76] Once seizure activity ends, administration of an antiepileptic medication, such as phenytoin, levetiracetam, or valproate, should be initiated.[78] Empiric treatment of all postarrest patients with antiepileptic medications is not warranted.

No specific neuroimaging recommendations are part of the postcardiac arrest guidelines. Several studies report that CT and magnetic resonance imaging illustrate cortical lesions and blurring of gray-white matter, respectively.[79,80] Whether these findings truly predict outcomes is debatable. Early imaging can provide valuable information regarding the cause of cardiac arrest (eg, structural lesion or intracranial hemorrhage) in a minority of patients. After stabilization and before transfer to the critical care unit, it is reasonable to obtain some form of neuroimaging.

Hyperglycemia

Hyperglycemia is common in critically ill patients, and has been associated with increased morbidity and mortality. Current guidelines for the postarrest patient recommend moderate glycemic control, with serum glucose values targeted between 144 and 180 mg/dL.[3] Consistent with similar critical care studies, strict glycemic control (maintaining glucose values between 80 and 110 mg/dL) has not improved the mortality rate but has increased the incidence of hypoglycemia.[79,80]

Hyperthermia

Current evidence demonstrates an association between pyrexia (>37°C) and poor survival after cardiac arrest.[81,82] If hyperthermia develops in the

postarrest patient, aggressive treatment with antipyretics and cooling techniques should be used.

SUMMARY

Management of the patient with ROSC following cardiac arrest is complex and challenging. Morbidity and mortality in patients can be improved by a systematic and comprehensive approach to therapy that includes optimizing oxygenation, mechanical ventilation, perfusion pressure, and oxygen delivery; initiating therapeutic hypothermia; and early cardiac catheterization. This comprehensive protocol, which initiates aggressive therapy in the emergency department and continues methodical goal-directed therapy in the cardiac critical care unit, has innumerable benefits for patients, physicians, and hospitals.

ACKNOWLEDGMENTS

This article was copyedited by Linda J. Kesselring, MS, ELS, the technical editor/writer in the Department of Emergency Medicine at the University of Maryland School of Medicine.

REFERENCES

1. Nichol G, Aufderheide TP, Eigel B, et al. Regional systems of care for out-of-hospital cardiac arrest: a policy statement from the American Heart Association. Circulation 2010;121:709–29.
2. Nichol G, Soar J. Regional cardiac resuscitation systems of care. Curr Opin Crit Care 2010;16:223–30.
3. Neumar RW, Nolan JP, Adrie C, et al. Post-cardiac arrest syndrome: epidemiology, pathophysiology, treatment, and prognostication. A consensus statement from the International Liaison Committee on Resuscitation (American Heart Association, Australian and New Zealand Council on Resuscitation, European Resuscitation Council, Heart and Stroke Foundation of Canada, InterAmerican Heart Foundation, Resuscitation Council of Asia, and the Resuscitation Council of Southern Africa); the American Heart Association Emergency Cardiovascular Care Committee; the Council on Cardiovascular Surgery and Anesthesia; the Council on Cardiopulmonary, Perioperative, and Critical Care; the Council on Clinical Cardiology; and the Stroke Council. Circulation 2008;118:2452–83.
4. Peberdy MA, Callaway CW, Neumar RW, et al. Part 9: post-cardiac arrest care: 2010 American Heart Association Guidelines for cardiopulmonary resuscitation and emergency cardiovascular care. Circulation 2010;122(18 Suppl 3):S768–86.
5. Adrie C, Adib-Conquy M, Laurent I, et al. Successful cardiopulmonary resuscitation after cardiac arrest

as a "sepsis-like" syndrome. Circulation 2002;106: 562–8.

6. Adrie C, Laurent I, Monchi M, et al. Postresuscitation disease after cardiac arrest: a sepsis-like syndrome? Curr Opin Crit Care 2004;10:208–12.

7. Karimova A, Pinsky DJ. The endothelial response to oxygen deprivation: biology and clinical implications. Intensive Care Med 2001;27:19–31.

8. Shoemaker WC, Appel PL, Kram HB. Role of oxygen debt in the development of organ failure sepsis, and death in high-risk surgical patients. Chest 1992;102: 208–15.

9. Shoemaker WC, Appel PL, Kram HB, et al. Hemodynamic and oxygen transport monitoring to titrate therapy in septic shock. New Horiz 1993;1:145–59.

10. Miller JB, Donnino MW, Rogan M, et al. Relative adrenal insufficiency in post-cardiac arrest shock is under-recognized. Resuscitation 2008;76:221–5.

11. Hékimian G, Baugnon T, Thuong M, et al. Cortisol levels and adrenal reserve after successful cardiac arrest resuscitation. Shock 2004;22:116–9.

12. Rivers EP. Early goal-directed therapy in severe sepsis and septic shock: converting science to reality. Chest 2006;129:217–8.

13. Rivers EP, Kruse JA, Jacobsen G, et al. The influence of early hemodynamic optimization on biomarker patterns of severe sepsis and septic shock. Crit Care Med 2007;35:2016–24.

14. Rivers EP, Martin GB, Smithline H, et al. The clinical implications of continuous central venous oxygen saturation during human CPR. Ann Emerg Med 1992;21:1094–101.

15. Laurent I, Monchi M, Chiche JD, et al. Reversible myocardial dysfunction in survivors of out-of-hospital cardiac arrest. J Am Coll Cardiol 2002;40: 2110–6.

16. Kern KB. Postresuscitation myocardial dysfunction. Cardiol Clin 2002;20:89–101.

17. Kern KB, Zuercher M, Cragun D, et al. Myocardial microcirculatory dysfunction after prolonged ventricular fibrillation and resuscitation. Crit Care Med 2008;36:S418–21.

18. Ruiz-Bailén M, Aguayo de Hoyos E, Ruiz-Navarro S, et al. Reversible myocardial dysfunction after cardiopulmonary resuscitation. Resuscitation 2005;66:175–81.

19. Spaulding CM, Joly LM, Rosenberg A, et al. Immediate coronary angiography in survivors of out-of-hospital cardiac arrest. N Engl J Med 1997;336: 1629–33.

20. El-Menyar AA. Postresuscitation myocardial stunning and its outcome: new approaches. Crit Pathw Cardiol 2004;3:209–15.

21. El-Menyar AA. Pathophysiology and hemodynamic of postresuscitation syndrome. Saudi Med J 2006; 27:441–5.

22. El-Menyar AA. The resuscitation outcome: revisit the story of the stony heart. Chest 2005;128:2835–46.

23. O'Leary MJ. Comment on "Mode of death after admission to an intensive care unit following cardiac arrest" by Laver et al. Intensive Care Med 2005;31:888.

24. Laver S, Farrow C, Turner D, et al. Mode of death after admission to an intensive care unit following cardiac arrest. Intensive Care Med 2004;30:2126–8.

25. Neumar RW. Molecular mechanisms of ischemic neuronal injury. Ann Emerg Med 2000;36:483–506.

26. Kuisma M, Boyd J, Voipio V, et al. Comparison of 30 and the 100% inspired oxygen concentrations during early post-resuscitation period: a randomised controlled pilot study. Resuscitation 2006;69:199–206.

27. White BC, Sullivan JM, DeGracia DJ, et al. Brain ischemia and reperfusion: molecular mechanisms of neuronal injury. J Neurol Sci 2000;179:1–33.

28. Kilgannon JH, Jones AE, Parriollo JE, et al. Relationship between supranormal oxygen tension and outcome after resuscitation from cardiac arrest. Circulation 2011;123:2717–22.

29. Kilgannon JH, Jones AE, Shapiro NI, et al. Association between arterial hyperoxia following resuscitation from cardiac arrest and in-hospital mortality. JAMA 2010;303:2165–71.

30. Sundgreen C, Larsen FS, Herzog TM, et al. Autoregulation of cerebral blood flow in patients resuscitated from cardiac arrest. Stroke 2001;32:128–32.

31. Torbey MT, Selim M, Knorr J, et al. Quantitative analysis of the loss of distinction between gray and white matter in comatose patients after cardiac arrest. Stroke 2000;31:2163–7.

32. Hess EP, Campbell RL, White RD. Epidemiology, trends, and outcome of out-of-hospital cardiac arrest of non-cardiac origin. Resuscitation 2007;72:200–6.

33. Kurkciyan I, Meron G, Sterz F, et al. Pulmonary embolism as a cause of cardiac arrest: presentation and outcome. Arch Intern Med 2000;160:1529–35.

34. Ventilation with lower tidal volumes as compared with traditional tidal volumes for acute lung injury and the acute respiratory distress syndrome. The Acute Respiratory Distress Syndrome Network. N Engl J Med 2000;342:13018.

35. Neumar RW. Optimal oxygenation during and after cardiopulmonary resuscitation. Curr Opin Crit Care 2011;17:236–40.

36. Gaieski DF, Band RA, Abella BS, et al. Early goal-directed hemodynamic optimization combined with therapeutic hypothermia in comatose survivors of out-of-hospital cardiac arrest. Resuscitation 2009; 80:418–24.

37. Carr BG, Matthew Edwards J, Martinez R, 2010 Academic Emergency Medicine consensus conference, Beyond Regionalization: Integrated Networks of Care. Regionalized care for time-critical conditions: lessons learned from existing networks. Acad Emerg Med 2010;17:1354–8.

38. Langhelle A, Nolan J, Herlitz J, et al. Recommended guidelines for reviewing, reporting, and conducting

research on post-resuscitation care: the Utstein style. Resuscitation 2005;66:271–83.

39. Langhelle A, Tyvoid SS, Lexow K, et al. In-hospital factors associated with improved outcome after out-of-hospital cardiac arrest. A comparison between four regions in Norway. Resuscitation 2003;56:247–63.

40. De Backer D, Biston P, Devriendt J, et al. Comparison of dopamine and norepinephrine in the treatment of shock. N Engl J Med 2010;362:779–89.

41. Mullner M, Sterz F, Binder M, et al. Arterial blood pressure after human cardiac arrest and neurologic recovery. Stroke 1996;27:59–62.

42. Pearse R, Dawson D, Fawcett J, et al. Early goal-directed therapy after major surgery reduces complications and duration of hospital stay. A randomised, controlled trial [ISRCTN38797445]. Crit Care 2005;9:R687–93.

43. Dellinger RP, Levy MM, Carlet JM, et al. Surviving Sepsis Campaign: international guidelines for management of severe sepsis and septic shock: 2008. Crit Care Med 2008;36:296–327.

44. Rivers EP, Rady MY, Martin GB, et al. Venous hyperoxia after cardiac arrest. Characterization of a defect in systemic oxygen utilization. Chest 1992;102:1787–93.

45. Jones AE, Shapiro NI, Trzeciak S, et al. Lactate clearance vs central venous oxygen saturation as goals of early sepsis therapy: a randomized clinical trial. JAMA 2010;303(8):739–46.

46. Cokkinos P. Post-resuscitation care: current therapeutic concepts. Acute Card Care 2009;11:131–7.

47. Vasquez A, Kern KB, Hilwig RW, et al. Optimal dosing of dobutamine for treating post-resuscitation left ventricular dysfunction. Resuscitation 2004;61:199–207.

48. Schultz CH, Rivers EP, Feldkamp CS, et al. A characterization of hypothalamic-pituitary-adrenal axis function during and after human cardiac arrest. Crit Care Med 1993;21:1339–47.

49. Kim JJ, Lim YS, Shin JH, et al. Relative adrenal insufficiency after cardiac arrest: impact on postresuscitation disease outcome. Am J Emerg Med 2006;24:684–8.

50. Pene F, Hyvernat H, Mallet V, et al. Prognostic value of relative adrenal insufficiency after out-of-hospital cardiac arrest. Intensive Care Med 2005;31:627–33.

51. Tennyson H, Kern KB, Hilwig RW, et al. Treatment of post resuscitation myocardial dysfunction: aortic counterpulsation versus dobutamine. Resuscitation 2002;54:69–75.

52. Prondzinsky R, Lemm H, Swyter M, et al. Intra-aortic balloon counterpulsation in patients with acute myocardial infarction complicated by cardiogenic shock: the prospective, randomized IABP SHOCK Trial for attenuation of multiorgan dysfunction syndrome. Crit Care Med 2010;38:152–60.

53. Christoph A, Prondizinsky R, Russ M, et al. Early and sustained haemodynamic improvement with levosimendan compared to intraaortic balloon counterpulsation (IABP) in cardiogenic shock complicating acute myocardial infarction. Acute Card Care 2008;10:49–57.

54. Chen EW, Canto JG, Parsons LS, et al. Relation between hospital intra-aortic balloon counterpulsation volume and mortality in acute myocardial infarction complicated by cardiogenic shock. Circulation 2003;108:951–7.

55. Barron HV, Every NR, Parsons LS, et al. The use of intra-aortic balloon counterpulsation in patients with cardiogenic shock complicating acute myocardial infarction: data from the National Registry of Myocardial Infarction 2. Am Heart J 2001;141:933–9.

56. Bernard SA, Gray TW, Buist MD, et al. Treatment of comatose survivors of out-of-hospital cardiac arrest with induced hypothermia. N Engl J Med 2002;346:557–63.

57. Hypothermia after Cardiac Arrest Study Group. Mild therapeutic hypothermia to improve the neurologic outcome after cardiac arrest. N Engl J Med 2002;346:549–56.

58. Polderman KH. Mechanisms of action, physiological effects, and complications of hypothermia. Crit Care Med 2009;37:S186–202.

59. Belliard G, Catez E, Charron C, et al. Efficacy of therapeutic hypothermia after out-of-hospital cardiac arrest due to ventricular fibrillation. Resuscitation 2007;75:252–9.

60. Castrejón S, Cortés M, Salto ML, et al. Improved prognosis after using mild hypothermia to treat cardiorespiratory arrest due to a cardiac cause: comparison with a control group. Rev Esp Cardiol 2009;62:733–41.

61. Don CW, Longstreth WT Jr, Maynard C, et al. Active surface cooling protocol to induce mild therapeutic hypothermia after out-of-hospital cardiac arrest: a retrospective before-and-after comparison in a single hospital. Crit Care Med 2009;37:3062–9.

62. Bro-Jeppesen J, Kjaergaard J, Horsted TI, et al. The impact of therapeutic hypothermia on neurological function and quality of life after cardiac arrest. Resuscitation 2009;80:171–6.

63. Dumas F, Grimaldi D, Zuber B, et al. Is hypothermia after cardiac arrest effective in both shockable and nonshockable patients?: insights from a large registry. Circulation 2011;123:877–86.

64. Kim F, Olsufka M, Longstreth WT Jr, et al. Pilot randomized clinical trial of prehospital induction of mild hypothermia in out-of-hospital cardiac arrest patients with a rapid infusion of 4 degrees C normal saline. Circulation 2007;115:3064–70.

65. Hammer L, Vitrat F, Savary D, et al. Immediate prehospital hypothermia protocol in comatose survivors

of out-of-hospital cardiac arrest. Am J Emerg Med 2009;27:570–3.

66. Larsson IM, Wallin E, Rubertsson S. Cold saline infusion and ice packs alone are effective in inducing and maintaining therapeutic hypothermia after cardiac arrest. Resuscitation 2010;81:15–9.

67. Jacobshagen C, Pax A, Unsöld BW, et al. Effects of large volume, ice-cold intravenous fluid infusion on respiratory function in cardiac arrest survivors. Resuscitation 2009;80:1223–8.

68. Arrich J, Holzer M, Herkner H, et al. Hypothermia for neuroprotection in adults after cardiopulmonary resuscitation. Cochrane Database Syst Rev 2009;(4):CD004128.

69. Akata T, Setoguchi H, Shirozu K, et al. Reliability of temperatures measured at standard monitoring sites as an index of brain temperature during deep hypothermic cardiopulmonary bypass conducted for thoracic aortic reconstruction. J Thorac Cardiovasc Surg 2007;133:1559–65.

70. Polderman KH, Herold I. Therapeutic hypothermia and controlled normothermia in the intensive care unit: practical considerations, side effects, and cooling methods. Crit Care Med 2009;37:1101–20.

71. Polderman KH. Application of therapeutic hypothermia in the ICU: opportunities and pitfalls of a promising treatment modality. Part 1: indications and evidence. Intensive Care Med 2004;30:556–75.

72. Wolfrum S, Pierau C, Radke PW, et al. Mild therapeutic hypothermia in patients after out-of-hospital cardiac arrest due to acute ST-segment elevation myocardial infarction undergoing immediate percutaneous coronary intervention. Crit Care Med 2008; 36:1780–6.

73. Batista LM, Lima FO, Januzzi JL Jr, et al. Feasibility and safety of combined percutaneous coronary intervention and therapeutic hypothermia following cardiac arrest. Resuscitation 2010;81:398–403.

74. Morrison LJ, Deakin CD, Morley PT, et al. Part 8: advanced life support: 2010 international consensus on cardiopulmonary resuscitation and emergency cardiovascular care science with treatment recommendations. Circulation 2010;122(16 Suppl 2): S345–421.

75. Kudenchuk PJ, Cobb LA, Copass MK, et al. Amiodarone for resuscitation after out-of-hospital cardiac arrest due to ventricular fibrillation. N Engl J Med 1999;341:871–8.

76. Hui AC, Cheng C, Lam A, et al. Prognosis following postanoxic myoclonus status epilepticus. Eur Neurol 2005;54:10–3.

77. Longstreth WT Jr, Nichol G, Van Ottingham L, et al. Two simple questions to assess neurologic outcomes at 3 months after out-of-hospital cardiac arrest: experience from the public access defibrillation trial. Resuscitation 2010;81:530–3.

78. Longstreth WT Jr, Fahrenbruch CE, Olsufka M, et al. Randomized clinical trial of magnesium, diazepam, or both after out-of-hospital cardiac arrest. Neurology 2002;59:506–14.

79. NICE-SUGAR Study Investigators, Finfer S, Chittock DR, Su SY, et al. Intensive versus conventional glucose control in critically ill patients. N Engl J Med 2009;360:1283–97.

80. Losert H, Sterz F, Roine RO, et al. Strict normoglycaemic blood glucose levels in the therapeutic management of patients within 12h after cardiac arrest might not be necessary. Resuscitation 2008; 76:214–20.

81. Takino M, Okada Y. Hyperthermia following cardiopulmonary resuscitation. Intensive Care Med 1991; 17:419–20.

82. Zeiner A, Holzer M, Sterz F, et al. Hyperthermia after cardiac arrest is associated with an unfavorable neurologic outcome. Arch Intern Med 2001;161: 2007–12.

Assessment and Management of Cardiogenic Shock in the Emergency Department

Thomas Klein, MD, Gautam V. Ramani, MD*

KEYWORDS

- Cardiogenic shock • Emergency department • Mechanical circulatory support • Heart failure
- Myocardial infarction

KEY POINTS

- Prompt diagnosis, expedient stabilization, initial medical management, and appropriate triage and consultation can drastically alter the course of cardiogenic shock.
- The most common cause of cardiogenic shock remains left ventricular failure complicating ST-elevation myocardial infarction.
- The use of bedside echocardiography in the emergency department allows the emergency physician to rapidly exclude cardiogenic shock from the differential diagnosis in undifferentiated shock patients with normal left ventricular ejection fraction and no structural cardiac abnormalities.
- In-hospital mortality from cardiogenic shock has decreased substantially over the past two decades, largely due to increased availability of percutaneous coronary intervention.
- Mechanical circulatory support, including short-term percutaneous left ventricular assist devices (LVADs) and intermediate-term surgically placed LVADs have expanded the capabilities of physicians to treat even the sickest of patients.

BACKGROUND

Trauma surgeons emphasize the Golden Hour, highlighting the critical importance of time in treating victims of penetrating and blunt trauma. Cardiologists are trained in the mantra "time is myocardium," emphasizing the role of rapid reperfusion therapy in patients suffering from ST-segment elevation myocardial infarction (STEMI). Although no such teaching exists for the management of cardiogenic shock (CS), successful treatment depends on rapid diagnosis and prompt initiation of therapy.

The overall management of shock has not changed appreciably in the past decade. Treatment is focused on maintaining blood volume, maximizing oxygen delivery to vital organs, and identifying and treating the underlying cause. For patients suffering from hypovolemic or distributive shock, correction of bleeding and fluid resuscitation are the cornerstones of therapy.

CS is unique among all other types of shock in that advances in mechanical circulatory support (MCS) have provided the clinician with several novel therapeutic options. Short-term percutaneous left ventricular assist devices (LVADs) and intermediate-term surgically placed LVADs have expanded the capabilities of physicians to treat even the sickest of patients. Despite these advances, the overall in-hospital mortality rate for these patients remains higher than 40%.[1,2]

Emergency department (ED) physicians are often the first providers to assess the CS patient, and comprise thereby a critical element in achieving a timely diagnosis and successful treatment. This review discusses the diagnosis and management of CS, focusing on the care within the ED.

Division of Cardiology, University of Maryland School of Medicine, 110 South Paca Street, Baltimore, MD 21202, USA
* Corresponding author.
E-mail address: gramani@medicine.umaryland.edu

Cardiol Clin 30 (2012) 651–664
http://dx.doi.org/10.1016/j.ccl.2012.07.004

cardiology.theclinics.com

DEFINITION OF CS

CS is defined as inadequate cardiac pumping function to meet the resting metabolic needs of the body despite adequate loading conditions. The clinical syndrome of CS has been described as: a systolic blood pressure (BP) of less than 90 mm Hg, or greater than 30 mm Hg below baseline BP, for at least 30 minutes, with signs of a reduced cardiac output (CO). Signs of reduced CO may be manifested as reduced urine output (<20 mL/h), impaired cognitive function, and evidence of peripheral vasoconstriction.[3] When hemodynamic data are available, the diagnosis is confirmed when cardiac index (CI) is less than 2.2 L/m² body surface area, and pulmonary capillary wedge pressure (PCWP) greater than 15 mm Hg.[4]

EPIDEMIOLOGY OF CS

Statistics reporting the incidence of CS must be interpreted with caution. The true incidence may be underestimated, as patients who die before arrival at hospital are not included in analyses. On the other hand, increased availability of percutaneous coronary intervention (PCI) and short-term MCS has resulted in more survivors following large myocardial infarctions. The incidence of CS complicating acute myocardial infarction (MI) is estimated at 3% to 9%.[1,2,5-7] Higher figures are reported (~9%) for patients who present with STEMI than for those who present with non–ST-segment elevation MI (NSTEMI).[2]

ETIOLOGY OF CS

Although left ventricular (LV) failure complicating acute STEMI is the most frequent cause of CS, mechanical complications of MI may present as CS. The SHOCK trial registry has provided the greatest insight into the various causes of CS and their respective outcomes. Predominant LV failure was the most common cause of CS, occurring in 78.5% of patients. Other causes included

severe mitral regurgitation (MR), ventricular septal rupture (VSR), isolated right ventricular (RV) failure, and cardiac tamponade, which occurred with decreasing frequency (**Fig. 1**). Patients with predominant LV failure complicating acute MI were more likely to have an anterior MI. Inferior MI was less often associated with LV failure, but associated with a greater risk of mechanical complications.[8]

Most patients who develop CS as a complication of acute MI do so following admission to the hospital. Cardiogenic shock at presentation of STEMI has been reported at 11% to 29%.[2,9] The average time to development of CS in the setting of STEMI has been reported as 7 to 10 hours, but is considerably longer for NSTEMI, with estimates ranging from 76 to 94 hours.[6-8]

CS can occur outside of the setting of acute MI (**Table 1**). This etiology may be more difficult to identify, as biomarker abnormalities and electrocardiogram (ECG) changes may not be as pronounced.

INITIAL ASSESSMENT

Establishing an accurate diagnosis for the hemodynamically unstable patient is critical. The initial evaluation of all patients presenting with suspicion of shock includes inspection for signs of tissue perfusion and assessment of volume status.

Physical examination is an invaluable, and often overlooked and underutilized tool in discriminating CS from other types of shock (**Table 2**). Alterations in mental status and oliguria are nonspecific and may accompany all subtypes of shock. Cardiac auscultation may reveal a third or fourth heart sound, or murmurs suggesting valvular heart disease or possible mechanical MI complication, although the absence of these findings does not exclude the diagnosis. The presence of cool extremities, a sign of peripheral vasoconstriction, may be helpful in differentiating CS from vasodilatory shock, where warm extremities and bounding pulses may be present.

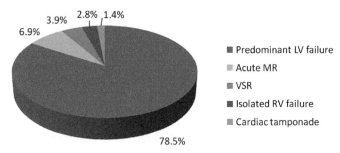

Fig. 1. Etiology of CS in the SHOCK Registry. (*Data from* Hochman JS, Buller CE, Sleeper LA. et al. Cardiogenic shock complicating acute myocardial infarction—etiologies, management and outcome: a report from the SHOCK Trial Registry. SHould we emergently revascularize Occluded Coronaries for cardiogenic shocK? J Am Coll Cardiol 2000;36(3 Suppl A):1063–70.)

Table 1
Non-MI etiology of cardiogenic shock

Mechanism	Underlying Cause
Primary pump failure	Progression of end-stage cardiomyopathy Acute myocarditis Tako-tsubo cardiomyopathy
Outflow obstruction	Aortic stenosis Mitral stenosis LV outflow tract obstruction (ie, hypertrophic cardiomyopathy)
Acute valvular regurgitation	Endocarditis Trauma Degenerative disease
Bradyarrhythmias	Sinus node dysfunction or conduction block with inadequate escape rhythm
Tachyarrhythmias	Supraventricular tachycardia (ie, atrial fibrillation, atrial flutter, paroxysmal supraventricular tachycardia) Ventricular tachycardia
Aortic dissection	Hemorrhagic pericardial effusion leading to tamponade MI (consider dissection into right coronary artery) Acute aortic regurgitation
Pericardial disease	Constriction Tamponade
Drug toxicity	Calcium-channel blocker β-Blocker

Additional physical examination findings in patients with CS or impending CS include pulmonary congestion, peripheral edema, and elevated jugular venous pressure (JVP). Patients with predominant RV involvement or cardiac tamponade may have clear lung fields. Small studies have shown that the differentiation of shock states based on physical examination alone is possible in the majority of patients.[10]

Examination of JVP forms the cornerstone of volume status assessment. Careful positioning of the patient maybe required, and in indeterminate cases the hepatojugular reflex should be elicited. If assessment of the jugular veins is limited by body habitus, central venous pressure (CVP) may be estimated with ultrasonography of the jugular vein. However, this technique, like estimated JVP by physical examination, tends to underestimate CVP.[11]

In patients with established HF who present with a decompensation, management is focused on 2 critical elements: assessment of tissue perfusion (warm vs cold) and assessment of volume status (wet vs dry). Such management has been shown to correlate with prognosis; patients who present as "cold/wet" have the highest risk of death or urgent transplantation.[12]

A severity-of-illness scoring system for patients with CS complicating acute MI has been proposed, which estimates in-hospital mortality, and may help with initial management and triage (**Table 3**). This scoring system has been validated with and without the incorporation of hemodynamic data.[13]

Table 2
Physical examination findings in states of shock

	Cardiogenic	Hypovolemic	Vasodilatory	Obstructive
Blood pressure	↓	↓	↓	↓
Heart rate	↑ (unless due to bradyarrhythmia)	↑	↑	↑
Jugular venous pressure	↑	↓	↓	↑
Extremities	Cool	Cool	Warm	Cool
Lung fields	Wet (unless due to RV failure)	Dry	Dry	Dry

Table 3
Predictors of mortality in cardiogenic shock

Clinical data	Advanced age
	Shock on admission
	Clinical evidence of end-organ hypoperfusion
	Anoxic brain injury
	Low systolic BP
	Prior coronary artery bypass grafting
	Noninferior MI
	Creatinine >1.9 mg/dL
Hemodynamic + clinical data	Age
	Clinical evidence of end-organ hypoperfusion
	Anoxic brain damage
	Stroke work
	LV ejection fraction <28%

Data from Sleeper LA, Reynolds HR, White HD, et al. A severity scoring system for risk assessment of patients with cardiogenic shock: a report from the SHOCK Trial and Registry. Am Heart J 2010;160(3):443–50.

The ECG may provide insight beyond the presence/absence of routine MI. ECG diagnosis of RV infarct (elevation in V4R) or posterior infarct ST-segment depression in V1, V2, and/or V3 in the presence of inferior MI portends an increased risk of complications and in-hospital mortality, and should be considered at triage.[14,15] Cardiac tamponade may also be suspected if low voltage, PR depression, or electrical alternans is present, though these signs are neither sensitive nor specific.[16]

Chest radiography (CXR) should be performed in all patients. It is important to note that the absence of congestion on an initial CXR does not exclude the diagnosis of acute decompensated heart failure.[17]

Laboratory abnormalities in patients with CS are omnipresent. Significant abnormalities on a complete blood count may be present in CS, although it is primarily obtained to exclude other causes of shock. While an elevated white blood cell (WBC) count accompanied by low BP may suggest the diagnosis of septic shock, it is important to consider that a potent inflammatory response in MI or CS can also cause a leukocytosis, and the presence of an elevated WBC count should not exclude the diagnosis of CS. An arterial blood gas should be obtained. Metabolic acidosis, or elevated lactate levels, suggests inadequate tissue perfusion requiring escalation of therapy, and hypoxia may dictate the need for additional ventilatory support. Liver enzyme abnormalities may be due to decreased forward flow to the liver, from passive congestion, or both, manifesting as elevated levels of transaminases, bilirubins, or alkaline phosphatase. In fact, the predominant complaint of a patient in CS may be epigastric pain from liver congestion. Coagulation-factor abnormalities may be present, and may be particularly prominent in patients already on vitamin K antagonists.

BEDSIDE ECHOCARDIOGRAPHY IN THE EMERGENCY DEPARTMENT

If CS is suspected based on history, physical examination, and laboratory and routine diagnostic imaging studies, transthoracic echocardiography (TTE) is indicated.[18] Although bedside TTE in the ED may suffer from inherent technical limitations because of poor acoustic windows from patients who are difficult to position and those on mechanical ventilation, it may provide incremental diagnostic information.[19]

A comprehensive echocardiographic examination includes 2-dimensional (2D), M-mode and Doppler components. As ultrasound portability and availability have improved, some clinicians have advocated incorporating bedside echo into their initial assessment with hand-held devices such as the GE Vscan (**Fig. 2**).[20] While an adequate 2D and color flow Doppler examination can be performed, a complete echocardiographic assessment is not possible because continuous and pulse-wave Doppler functions and M-mode are not available. However, this may not be clinically significant; in the authors' experience, most causes of CS can be determined solely based on 2D and color Doppler examination.

Cardiac tamponade is a rapidly reversible, life-threatening condition most readily diagnosed by

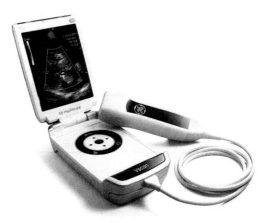

Fig. 2. GE Healthcare VScan. (*Courtesy of* GE Healthcare, Inc, Waukesha, WI, USA; with permission.)

echocardiogram. Echocardiographic signs of tamponade in the setting of a pericardial effusion include end-diastolic right atrial (RA) collapse (a highly sensitive sign) and RV collapse (less sensitive but more specific), inferior vena cava (IVC) dilation, and greater than 25% inspiratory variation in mitral inflow velocity measured by pulse-wave Doppler.[21,22] ED physicians trained in bedside echocardiography can diagnose pericardial effusions with excellent accuracy.[23] Echo-guided, bedside pericardiocentesis is safe and effective, and can be performed without the need for fluoroscopy.[24]

CS can be virtually excluded in the presence of normal or hyperkinetic ventricular function in the absence of a severe valvular lesion or cardiac tamponade, both of which are readily apparent on Doppler echocardiography. The presence of a reduced LV ejection fraction (LVEF) in the setting of shock does not establish a diagnosis of CS. It bears emphasis that while a hyperkinetic ventricle in the absence of other structural heart disease is effective at excluding the diagnosis of CS, the presence of LV dysfunction is not diagnostic. Furthermore, initiation of inotropic therapies before establishing a diagnosis of CS, based on a finding of reduced LVEF on TTE, may be deleterious.[25,26]

Evaluation for volume assessment using echo is most easily accomplished by measuring IVC diameter and percent IVC collapse with sniff (caval index). This method was demonstrated in one series of 83 patients, in whom IVC diameter and caval index were measured by TTE within 24 hours of invasive hemodynamic measurement. Forty-one of 48 patients with caval index less than 50% had RA pressure (RAP) higher than 10 mm Hg, whereas 30 of 35 patients with caval index greater than 50% had RA pressure less than 10 mm Hg.[27]

Emergency physicians may develop proficiency in point-of-care ultrasonography by experience during their residency or fellowship programs, or through commercially available courses.

INVASIVE HEMODYNAMIC MONITORING

Pulmonary artery catheterization (PAC) may be performed in critically ill patients to establish a diagnosis of shock, differentiate causes of shock, assess volume status, and assist with therapy. The role of PAC in the intensive care unit (ICU) has evolved over time. Following an initial period of enthusiasm and widespread use, concerns developed regarding safety and efficacy of PAC-guided therapy. More recent randomized controlled trials (RCTs) have questioned the benefits of routine PAC in critically ill patients. In 2 trials randomizing patients with acute lung injury to PAC-guided therapy versus standard care, no differences in morbidity or mortality were demonstrated.[28,29] Patients presenting with acute decompensated heart failure, but not CS, randomized to PAC-guided therapy versus standard care, showed no mortality difference or decreased hospitalizations for HF.[30] RCTs have not focused on patients with CS, although subgroup analysis of larger shock studies has suggested a trend toward increased complications without any benefit.[31,32]

Despite the lack of rigorous evidence, PAC is recommended by the American College of Cardiology/American Heart Association (class I, level of evidence C) for STEMI patients with hypotension not responsive to intravenous fluid or when fluids may be contraindicated, as well as for patients with a suspected mechanical complication of MI in whom an echocardiogram has not been performed.[33] The authors believe the most compelling indication for the use of PAC is to assist in the diagnosis of CS in the patient when the cause of shock is unclear. Therapies directed at vasodilatory or hypovolemic shock may be deleterious in the CS patient. Once a diagnosis is established, treatment is directed toward restoring tissue perfusion and normalizing filling pressures, and not toward achieving arbitrary hemodynamic parameters.

The use of CVP monitoring may be tempting to use in place of PAC to guide management of volume status. Limited evidence exists for this practice, and a recent meta-analysis demonstrated a poor correlation between CVP and circulating blood volume, and showed that CVP did not predict the hemodynamic response to fluid challenge.[34] An older study that compared CVP with PCWP by PAC in assessing hemodynamic response to fluid and in predicting the presence of pulmonary congestion in patients with acute MI also demonstrated a poor correlation between CVP and PCWP.[35] The authors believe that in CS, CVP may not accurately reflect LV end-diastolic pressure (LVEDP), and caution is advised when using this measurement to assess overall volume status.

CARDIOPULMONARY STABILIZATION

Patients with CS may suffer from hypoxemic or hypercapnic respiratory failure from respiratory muscle fatigue and alveolar edema. Guidelines recommend maintaining arterial oxygen saturation above 95%.[36] Animal studies have shown that up to 25% of arterial oxygen consumption comes from respiratory muscle use, and that mechanical ventilation decreases oxygen demand.[37] Patients with CS and respiratory failure may be supported with either noninvasive positive pressure ventilation (NIPPV) or endotracheal intubation.

There are multiple potential physiologic benefits to endotracheal intubation in CS. However, the decision to intubate and mechanically ventilate a patient is an individual one, which should be made by an experienced clinician. Mechanical ventilation may decrease intrapulmonary shunting and improve lung compliance by recruiting atelectatic lung regions, reducing respiratory muscle work, and decreasing preload and afterload. STEMI patients with pulmonary edema, in particular, may benefit from early intubation with mechanical ventilation.

In patients who present to the ED with acute cardiogenic pulmonary edema and do not require immediate intubation with mechanical ventilation, NIPPV, using either continuous positive airway pressure (CPAP) or bilevel positive airway pressure (BPAP), may provide benefits over nasal cannula. The 3CPO trial included 1069 patients with cardiogenic pulmonary edema randomized to CPAP, BPAP, or standard therapy in a 1:1:1 fashion, but excluded patients who required urgent intubation or PCI. Although this trial did demonstrate a decrease in subjective dyspnea, heart rate, acidosis, and hypercapnia with noninvasive positive pressure ventilation, the primary end points of the trial, short-term mortality and the need for endotracheal intubation, were not met.[38] Despite this finding, meta-analyses have demonstrated a benefit of reduced endotracheal intubation and decreased mortality in patients treated with NIPPV versus standard care.[39–44] For patients who can tolerate this therapy and do not require intubation, the authors have a low threshold for initiation of NIPPV.

MEDICAL MANAGEMENT OF CS

Patients without congestion presenting with shock and inadequate tissue perfusion may be challenged with intravenous fluids, unless physical examination suggests elevated right- and left-sided filling pressures, or invasive hemodynamic data confirm that loading conditions are adequate. However, in many CS patients treatment of pulmonary venous systemic congestion is a key goal. This approach is often challenging, and hypotension limits the utility of intravenous diuretics. PAC may clarify management decisions. Treatment with vasopressors and inotropes may facilitate diuresis, although this has not been demonstrated in large RCTs. In fact, despite ubiquitous use, rigorous evidence for diuretic strategies in patients with CS is limited.

RV infarction typically presents in the setting of inferior MI. Physical examination demonstrates the triad of distended neck veins, clear lungs, and hypotension. These patients are preload sensitive, and may require several liters of fluid to maintain adequate perfusion pressure.

Morphine has been used historically to treat respiratory distress and pulmonary edema in patients with acute decompensated HF, and is still recommended in the setting of severe discomfort or chest pain; however, the role for morphine in CS is unclear, as retrospective data have demonstrated worsened outcomes, including increased mortality, in recipients compared with nonrecipients.[45]

Vasodilators, including nitroglycerin and nitroprusside, are generally avoided in the setting of CS because of their propensity to cause hypotension. β-Blockers, calcium-channel blockers, and renin-angiotensin-aldosterone system (RAAS) blockers, such as angiotensin-converting enzyme inhibitors and angiotensin-receptor blockers, should also not be administered to patients with signs of CS because of their negative inotropic and BP-lowering effects. This rule also applies to patients with "preshock": those with signs of low CO but without significantly low BP. In the COMMIT-CCS2 trial, patients with acute MI (87% STEMI) were randomized to metoprolol (up to 15 mg intravenously, followed by 200 mg orally daily) or placebo. Patients who received metoprolol were less likely to suffer from reinfarction or ventricular fibrillation, but had a significant 1.1% increase in absolute risk of developing CS.[46]

The role of chronic HF therapy and vasodilators in CS is outlined in **Table 4**.

INOTROPIC AND VASOPRESSOR THERAPY FOR CS

Vasopressors and inotropes are often required in CS patients to sustain adequate BP and CO. Limited evidence exists regarding comparative efficacy of the various drugs. As a general rule, they should be used at the lowest doses possible to achieve the desired tissue perfusion end points, as side effects and complications are dose dependent, and higher doses have been associated with higher mortality.[47,48]

The largest RCT comparing vasopressors was the SOAP-2 trial, which compared dopamine and norepinephrine (which both possess vasopressor as well as inotropic properties) in a heterogeneous group of patients with shock. In the subgroup of these patients with CS, norepinephrine was associated with reduced mortality, and dopamine with a higher arrhythmia burden.[49] Vasopressin and

Table 4
Pharmacologic therapy for congestion and chronic HF in cardiogenic shock

Drug Class	Role	Examples	Mechanism	Notes
Diuretics	Remove volume and decrease pulmonary congestion	Furosemide	Inhibits sodium and chloride resorption in the loop of Henle and the proximal and distal convoluted tubule (loop diuretic)	May exacerbate hypotension, used with caution Careful monitoring of renal function and electrolytes is recommended
		Metolazone	Inhibits sodium resorption in the distal tubule (thiazide diuretic)	Similar adverse effects to furosemide May facilitate diuresis if used in conjunction with furosemide
Vasodilators	Decrease preload may improve pulmonary congestion Decreased afterload may improve CO	Nitroglycerin	Forms nitric oxide, which increases cGMP in smooth muscle cells, and leads to vasodilation (veins>arteries)	Administration limited by hypotensive effects, but may otherwise be useful to relieve pulmonary congestion
		Nitroprusside	Direct arterial vasodilator	Administration limited by hypotensive effects, but may otherwise be useful to improve cardiac output
		Hydralazine	Direct arterial vasodilator	Similar to nitroprusside, but may be less appropriate for unstable patients because of oral and intravenous bolus dosing
β-Blockers	Improve symptoms, reduce hospitalizations, and reduce mortality in chronic HF. No role in CS	Metoprolol Carvedilol Bisoprolol	Block β-adrenergic receptors (also some α effect from carvedilol)	Avoided because of hypotensive and negative inotropic effects in cardiogenic shock
RAAS blockers	Improve symptoms, reduce hospitalizations, and reduce mortality in chronic HF. No role in CS	Lisinopril Candesartan Spironolactone	Block steps along the renin-angiotensin-aldosterone axis	Contraindicated in CS because of hypotension, and renal dysfunction
Opiates	May improve chest pain and anxiety and relieve pulmonary congestion	Morphine Dilaudid Fentanyl	Relief of pain and anxiety decreases work of breathing, reduces sympathetic output, and vasodilates, leading to decreased filling pressures	May exacerbate hypotension May increase mortality in CS[45]

Abbreviation: cGMP, cyclic guanidine monophosphate.

dopamine have a role as second add-on agents for persistent hypotension. Phenylephrine, a pure α-agonist, is generally avoided, as it may significantly increase afterload and decrease the effectiveness of an already failing left ventricle.

Inotropes improve CO, but are proarrhythmic and, importantly, may exacerbate hypotension. The authors typically initiate therapy with dobutamine for patients in CS. In those patients who are on long-acting β-blockers as an outpatient, the authors may initiate therapy with milrinone, owing to its mechanism of action distal to the β1-adrenergic receptor. **Table 5** summarizes the mechanism of action and side effects of available inotropes.

REPERFUSION

For patients with CS complicating STEMI, the authors recommend emergent cardiac catheterization and anticoagulation in accordance with published guidelines.[47,50]

Emergent percutaneous or surgical revascularization reduces mortality in patients presenting with STEMI and CS. The landmark SHOCK trial compared percutaneous or surgical revascularization (n = 152) with initial medical stabilization (n = 150) in patients presenting within 12 hours of STEMI. At 30 days, there was a nonsignificant 9% absolute mortality reduction in the revascularization group (46.7% vs 56%, P = .11); however, at 6 months a significant 13% absolute mortality reduction was detected with revascularization (50.3% vs 63.1%, P = .027).[51]

If percutaneous or surgical revascularization is not available, or can only be provided after a long delay, thrombolysis may be considered if administered within 3 hours of onset of symptoms. One meta-analysis demonstrated an absolute 7% decrease in mortality in patients with STEMI and systolic BP lower than 100 mm Hg and pulse higher than 100 beats/min (54% vs 61%).[52] Thrombolytic therapy is clearly inferior to percutaneous revascularization for CS, and should be reserved for those patients who do not have access to PCI.[51,53–55]

INTRA-AORTIC BALLOON COUNTERPULSATION

Intra-aortic balloon pumps (IABPs) improve hemodynamics by decreasing afterload and augmenting diastolic pressure. A balloon is percutaneously placed in the descending thoracic aorta, and inflates during diastole and deflates during systole. Diastolic inflation displaces blood from the aorta, augmenting peripheral and coronary perfusion pressure.

IABP insertion is recommended for patients with CS due to acute MR and VSR, as a bridge to cardiac surgery.[56] It is also recommended for hemodynamically unstable patients following a large MI,[47,50] though the evidence of clinical benefit is far from robust. In a meta-analysis that included 7 RCTs (n = 1009), IABP placement in STEMI with CS treated did not result in an improvement in 30-day mortality or LV function, but did lead to significantly higher stroke and bleeding rates.[57] The largest RCT evaluating IABP use in MI (both STEMI and NSTEMI) complicated by CS was recently published, and demonstrated similar results to the aforementioned meta-analysis, though a lack of safety was not demonstrated. In this trial, 600 patients were randomized to IABP or no IABP in addition to standard care, including revascularization. There was no significant difference in the primary endpoint of 30-day mortality (39.7% vs 41.3%, P = 0.69) or the secondary endpoints of hemodynamic stabilization, intensive care unit length of stay, serum lactate levels, catecholamine requirements, or renal function. There were also no differences in complication rates, including major bleeding (3.3% vs 4.4%, P = 0.51), stroke (0.7% vs 1.7%, P = 0.28), sepsis (15.7% vs 20.5%, P = 0.15), or peripheral ischemia (4.3% vs 3.4%, P = 0.53). The authors, as well as an accompanying editorial, call for a revision of the published guidelines based on these results.[58,59]

MECHANICAL CIRCULATORY SUPPORT

Full MCS is considered in patients who demonstrate inadequate tissue perfusion despite therapy with mechanical ventilation, reperfusion, inotropes, and IABP. Options for these patients include extracorporeal membrane oxygenation (ECMO), percutaneous ventricular assist devices (VADs), and surgically placed VADs. Temporary MCS allows stabilization of organ function, with a goal of bridging the patient to myocardial recovery, surgical revascularization, or more permanent MCS.[60]

In ECMO, deoxygenated venous blood is removed from the body, passed through an artificial oxygenator, and returned to the venous system (VV-ECMO) or the arterial system (VA-ECMO). VV-ECMO is used for patients with refractory hypoxic respiratory failure solely for oxygenation, whereas VA-ECMO is used for patients with CS. Usually femoral venous blood is removed and returned to a femoral vein or artery (peripheral ECMO), though occasionally RA blood is removed and returned directly to the aorta (central ECMO). Both central and peripheral ECMO can be placed in the cardiac catheterization laboratory, typically with the assistance of a cardiothoracic surgeon.

Table 5
Inotropes and vasodilators for cardiogenic shock

Drug Class	Role	Examples	Mechanism	Notes
Inotropes	Improve cardiac output	Dobutamine	Cardiac β1, and peripheral α2 and β2 adrenoceptor agonist (inotrope/vasodilator)	Vasodilating effects may exacerbate hypotension
		Milrinone	Phosphodiesterase-3 inhibitor, potentiates cAMP; cardiac sarcoplasmic reticulum Ca^{2+}-ATPase activity	Use limited by long half-life and renal metabolism May be of use in patients on β-blockers
		Levosimendan	Increases sensitivity to Ca^{2+}	Not available in USA Found to be equivalent to dobutamine in acute decompensated HF in SURVIVE except lower initial BNP levels[67]
Vasopressors	Increase blood pressure	Norepinephrine	α1 and β1 adrenoceptor agonist (both vasopressor and inotropic properties)[68]	Decreased mortality in subset of SOAP-2 with CS[49]
		Dopamine	Doses 5–10 µg/kg/min: β1 receptor agonist Doses 10–20 µg/kg/min: α1 agonist (both vasopressor and inotropic properties)[69]	Increased arrhythmogenicity in SOAP-2[49]
		Epinephrine	α1, β1, and β2 agonist (both vasopressor and inotropic properties)	In limited RCT data, CS patients treated with epinephrine had higher lactate levels, increased arrhythmias, and higher heart rates compared with norepinephrine/dobutamine[70]
		Phenylephrine	Pure peripheral α agonist	Limited evidence is available, though should probably be avoided because purely increased afterload may decrease the effectiveness of an already failing left ventricle

Abbreviations: ATPase, adenosine triphosphatase; BNP, B-type natriuretic peptide; cAMP, cyclic adenosine monophosphate.

No RCT trial data exist for the use of ECMO in CS, although retrospective data have demonstrated that these patients have an overall poor prognosis, with a mortality rate of more than 60%, largely related to overall illness chronicity and severity.[61]

Percutaneous LVADs do not require a sternotomy, and hold promise for the treatment of CS complicating acute MI. The 2 most studied devices are the TandemHeart (CardiacAssist, Inc, Pittsburgh, PA, USA) and the Impella (Abiomed, Aachen, Germany). Neither device is approved by the Food and Drug Administration for intermediate-duration treatment of CS.

The TandemHeart (**Fig. 3**) removes blood from the left atrium by transseptal insertion, augments flow through a centrifugal pump, and returns the blood to a femoral artery. Two small randomized trials of patients with CS have compared the TandemHeart with IABP. Although both trials demonstrated a significant improvement in hemodynamics of patients randomized to the Tandem-Heart, neither demonstrated an improvement in survival (TandemHeart survival 57% and 53% vs IABP survival 55% and 64%). The TandemHeart was also associated with significantly more serious complications, which included hemorrhage and limb ischemia.[62,63]

The Impella is placed across the aortic valve via the femoral artery, and propels blood out of the left ventricle into the aorta with an axial pump. There is a 2.5 Impella and a 5.0 Impella. The 5.0 Impella generates greater flow, but requires a surgical cut down for placement. A small study randomized 25 patients to the Impella or IABP, and found a significant improvement in hemodynamics with

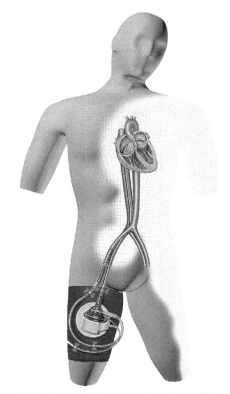

Fig. 3. TandemHeart System. (*Courtesy of* Cardiac-Assist, Inc, Pittsburgh, PA, USA; with permission.)

the Impella; however, similar to the TandemHeart, this did not translate into a mortality benefit (survival was 57% in both groups). As opposed to the TandemHeart, however, there was no difference in major complications between the 2 groups.[64]

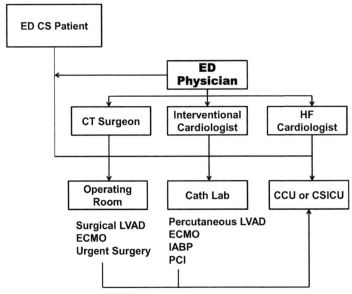

Fig. 4. Proposed "CS consult" algorithm.

The Levitronix CentriMag is another short-term VAD that may be used for LV, RV, or biventricular support for patients in CS as a bridge to recovery, transplant, or long-term VAD. This device is advantageous because of its ease of insertion and a pump system that prevents hemolysis owing to its levitating magnetic rotor. In observational data, profoundly ill patients have had a successful recovery, and additional research is ongoing.[65]

Limited success has been achieved in the placement of a long-term surgical VAD in the setting of acute CS. The authors' practice is to stabilize these patients with one of the aforementioned strategies, and then consider long-term LVAD for those who fail to recover. Multiple comorbidities in these acutely ill patients, including coagulopathy and renal insufficiency, often lead to higher rate of perioperative complications.

A NEW PARADIGM OF CS

The authors believe that the successful treatment of CS requires an interdisciplinary approach. Cardiology expertise is necessary in the treatment of all patients. In patients who fail to improve despite revascularization, IABP, and inotropic therapies, surgical consultation is mandatory. For patients in the community or tertiary care setting a "mobile cardiogenic shock team" concept is evolving. A mobile team from a quaternary care cardiovascular center, often including a perfusionist, surgeon, and trained professionals, travels to the patient's location, stabilizes the patient and offers the most effective therapy based on experience, then transports the patient back to the center.[66]

For patients already in an advanced care setting, a concept of a unified "CS consult," which would bring together the ED physician, interventional cardiologist, cardiovascular surgeon, and possibly an advanced HF cardiologist, may provide the most optimal care for such patients. This group would decide on the optimal therapy, location of therapy (catheterization laboratory vs operating room), and ultimate destination for the patient (CS ICU vs medical cardiac care unit). **Fig. 4** illustrates a proposed CS consult team algorithm.

PROGNOSIS

Although the mortality remains high for patients presenting to hospital with CS, significant progress has been made over the past 2 decades. Prompt diagnosis, expedient stabilization, initial medical management, and appropriate triage and consultation can drastically alter the course

of the disease. Observational series show that between 1995 and 2004, in-hospital mortality from CS has decreased from 60.3% to 47.9%, largely related to an increase in availability and expertise with PCI.[2] It is hoped that technological advances in MCS, as well as system improvements in the delivery of care, will allow further improvements in overall survival.

REFERENCES

1. Goldberg RJ, Spencer FA, Gore JM, et al. Thirty-year trends (1975 to 2005) in the magnitude of, management of, and hospital death rates associated with cardiogenic shock in patients with acute myocardial infarction: a population-based perspective. Circulation 2009;119(9):1211–9.
2. Babaev A, Frederick PD, Pasta DJ, et al. Trends in management and outcomes of patients with acute myocardial infarction complicated by cardiogenic shock. JAMA 2005;294(4):448–54.
3. Swan HJ, Forrester JS, Diamond G, et al. Hemodynamic spectrum of myocardial infarction and cardiogenic shock. A conceptual model. Circulation 1972;45(5):1097–110.
4. Forrester JS, Diamond G, Chatterjee K, et al. Medical therapy of acute myocardial infarction by application of hemodynamic subsets (first of two parts). N Engl J Med 1976;295(24):1356–62.
5. Brodie BR, Stuckey TD, Hansen C, et al. Comparison of late survival in patients with cardiogenic shock due to right ventricular infarction versus left ventricular pump failure following primary percutaneous coronary intervention for ST-elevation acute myocardial infarction. Am J Cardiol 2007;99(4):431–5.
6. Hasdai D, Harrington RA, Hochman JS, et al. Platelet glycoprotein IIb/IIIa blockade and outcome of cardiogenic shock complicating acute coronary syndromes without persistent ST-segment elevation. J Am Coll Cardiol 2000;36(3):685–92.
7. Holmes DR Jr, Berger PB, Hochman JS, et al. Cardiogenic shock in patients with acute ischemic syndromes with and without ST-segment elevation. Circulation 1999;100(20):2067–73.
8. Hochman JS, Buller CE, Sleeper LA, et al. Cardiogenic shock complicating acute myocardial infarction—etiologies, management and outcome: a report from the SHOCK Trial Registry. SHould we emergently revascularize Occluded Coronaries for cardiogenic shocK? J Am Coll Cardiol 2000;36(3 Suppl A):1063–70.
9. Holmes DR, Bates ER, Kleiman NS, et al. Contemporary reperfusion therapy for cardiogenic shock: the GUSTO-I trial experience. J Am Coll Cardiol 1995;26(3):668–74.
10. Vazquez R, Gheorghe C, Kaufman D, et al. Accuracy of bedside physical examination in distinguishing

categoriesofshock:apilotstudy.JHospMed2010;5(8): 471–4.

11. Deol GR, Collett N, Ashby A, et al. Ultrasound accurately reflects the jugular venous examination but underestimates central venous pressure. Chest 2011;139(1):95–100.

12. Nohria A, Tsang SW, Fang JC, et al. Clinical assessment identifies hemodynamic profiles that predict outcomes in patients admitted with heart failure. J Am Coll Cardiol 2003;41(10):1797–804.

13. Sleeper LA, Reynolds HR, White HD, et al. A severity scoring system for risk assessment of patients with cardiogenic shock: a report from the SHOCK Trial and Registry. Am Heart J 2010;160(3):443–50.

14. Sugiura T, Nagahama Y, Takehana K, et al. Prognostic significance of precordial ST-segment changes in acute inferior wall myocardial infarction. Chest 1997;111(4):1039–44.

15. Zehender M, Kasper W, Kauder E, et al. Right ventricular infarction as an independent predictor of prognosis after acute inferior myocardial infarction. N Engl J Med 1993;328(14):981–8.

16. Eisenberg MJ, de Romeral LM, Heidenreich PA, et al. The diagnosis of pericardial effusion and cardiac tamponade by 12-lead ECG: a technology assessment. Chest 1996;110(2):318–24.

17. Collins SP, Lindsell CJ, Storrow AB, et al, ADHERE Scientific Advisory Committee, Investigators and Study Group. Prevalence of negative chest radiography results in the emergency department patient with decompensated heart failure. Ann Emerg Med 2006;47(1):13–8.

18. Labovitz AJ, Noble VE, Bierig M, et al. Focused cardiac ultrasound in the emergent setting: a consensus statement of the American Society of Echocardiography and American College of Emergency Physicians. J Am Soc Echocardiogr 2010; 23(12):1225–30.

19. Jones AE, Tayal VS, Sullivan DM, et al. Randomized, controlled trial of immediate versus delayed goal-directed ultrasound to identify the cause of nontraumatic hypotension in emergency department patients. Crit Care Med 2004;32(8):1703–8.

20. GE Healthcare Product features—Vscan. 2012. Available at: https://vscan.gehealthcare.com/gallery/a-quick-look-at-vscan#/gallery/a-quick-look-at-vscan. Accessed January 30, 2012.

21. Reydel B, Spodick DH. Frequency and significance of chamber collapses during cardiac tamponade. Am Heart J 1990;119(5):1160–3.

22. Zhang S, Kerins DM, Byrd BF 3rd. Doppler echocardiography in cardiac tamponade and constrictive pericarditis. Echocardiography 1994;11(5): 507–21.

23. Mandavia DP, Hoffner RJ, Mahaney K, et al. Bedside echocardiography by emergency physicians. Ann Emerg Med 2001;38(4):377–82.

24. Tsang TS, Enriquez-Sarano M, Freeman WK, et al. Consecutive 1127 therapeutic echocardiographically guided pericardiocenteses: clinical profile, practice patterns, and outcomes spanning 21 years. Mayo Clin Proc 2002;77(5):429–36.

25. Moore CL, Rose GA, Tayal VS, et al. Determination of left ventricular function by emergency physician echocardiography of hypotensive patients. Acad Emerg Med 2002;9(3):186–93.

26. Randazzo MR, Snoey ER, Levitt MA, et al. Accuracy of emergency physician assessment of left ventricular ejection fraction and central venous pressure using echocardiography. Acad Emerg Med 2003; 10(9):973–7.

27. Kircher BJ, Himelman RB, Schiller NB. Noninvasive estimation of right atrial pressure from the inspiratory collapse of the inferior vena cava. Am J Cardiol 1990;66(4):493–6.

28. Richard C, Warszawski J, Anguel N, et al. Early use of the pulmonary artery catheter and outcomes in patients with shock and acute respiratory distress syndrome: a randomized controlled trial. JAMA 2003;290(20):2713–20.

29. National Heart, Lung, and Blood Institute Acute Respiratory Distress Syndrome (ARDS) Clinical Trials Network, Wheeler AP, Bernard GR, Thompson BT, et al. Pulmonary-artery versus central venous catheter to guide treatment of acute lung injury. N Engl J Med 2006;354(21):2213–24.

30. Binanay C, Califf RM, Hasselblad V, et al. Evaluation study of congestive heart failure and pulmonary artery catheterization effectiveness: the ESCAPE trial. JAMA 2005;294(13):1625–33.

31. Rhodes A, Cusack RJ, Newman PJ, et al. A randomised, controlled trial of the pulmonary artery catheter in critically ill patients. Intensive Care Med 2002;28(3):256–64.

32. Harvey S, Harrison DA, Singer M, et al. Assessment of the clinical effectiveness of pulmonary artery catheters in management of patients in intensive care (PAC-Man): a randomised controlled trial. Lancet 2005;366(9484):472–7.

33. Jessup M, Abraham WT, Casey DE, et al. 2009 focused update: ACCF/AHA Guidelines for the Diagnosis and Management of Heart Failure in Adults: a report of the American College of Cardiology Foundation/American Heart Association Task Force on Practice Guidelines: developed in collaboration with the International Society for Heart and Lung Transplantation. Circulation 2009;119(14):1977–2016.

34. Marik PE, Baram M, Vahid B. Does central venous pressure predict fluid responsiveness? A systematic review of the literature and the tale of seven mares. Chest 2008;134(1):172–8.

35. Forrester JS, Diamond G, McHugh TJ, et al. Filling pressures in the right and left sides of the heart in acute myocardial infarction. A reappraisal of

central-venous-pressure monitoring. N Engl J Med 1971;285(4):190–3.

36. Nieminen MS, Bohm M, Cowie MR, et al, ESC Committee for Practice Guideline (CPG). Executive summary of the guidelines on the diagnosis and treatment of acute heart failure: the Task Force on Acute Heart Failure of the European Society of Cardiology. Eur Heart J 2005;26(4):384–416.

37. Aubier M, Viires N, Syllie G, et al. Respiratory muscle contribution to lactic acidosis in low cardiac output. Am Rev Respir Dis 1982;126(4):648–52.

38. Gray A, Goodacre S, Newby DE, et al. Noninvasive ventilation in acute cardiogenic pulmonary edema. N Engl J Med 2008;359(2):142–51.

39. Collins SP, Mielniczuk LM, Whittingham HA, et al. The use of noninvasive ventilation in emergency department patients with acute cardiogenic pulmonary edema: a systematic review. Ann Emerg Med 2006;48(3):260–9.

40. Masip J, Roque M, Sanchez B, et al. Noninvasive ventilation in acute cardiogenic pulmonary edema: systematic review and meta-analysis. JAMA 2005; 294(24):3124–30.

41. Peter JV, Moran JL, Phillips-Hughes J, et al. Effect of non-invasive positive pressure ventilation (NIPPV) on mortality in patients with acute cardiogenic pulmonary oedema: a meta-analysis. Lancet 2006; 367(9517):1155–63.

42. Winck JC, Azevedo LF, Costa-Pereira A, et al. Efficacy and safety of non-invasive ventilation in the treatment of acute cardiogenic pulmonary edema—a systematic review and meta-analysis. Crit Care 2006;10(2):R69.

43. Vital FM, Saconato H, Ladeira MT, et al. Non-invasive positive pressure ventilation (CPAP or bilevel NPPV) for cardiogenic pulmonary edema. Cochrane Database Syst Rev 2008;(3):CD005351.

44. Weng CL, Zhao YT, Liu QH, et al. Meta-analysis: noninvasive ventilation in acute cardiogenic pulmonary edema [Erratum appears in Ann Intern Med 2010;153(1):67]. Ann Intern Med 2010;152(9): 590–600.

45. Peacock WF, Hollander JE, Diercks DB, et al. Morphine and outcomes in acute decompensated heart failure: an ADHERE analysis. Emerg Med J 2008;25(4):205–9.

46. Chen ZM, Pan HC, Chen YP, COMMIT (ClOpidogrel and Metoprolol in Myocardial Infarction Trial) collaborative group. Early intravenous then oral metoprolol in 45,852 patients with acute myocardial infarction: randomised placebo-controlled trial. Lancet 2005; 366(9497):1622–32.

47. Van de Werf F, Bax J, Betriu A, ESC Committee for Practice Guidelines (CPG). Management of acute myocardial infarction in patients presenting with persistent ST-segment elevation: the Task Force on the Management of ST-Segment Elevation Acute Myocardial Infarction of the European Society of Cardiology. Eur Heart J 2008;29(23):2909–45.

48. Valente S, Lazzeri C, Vecchio S, et al. Predictors of in-hospital mortality after percutaneous coronary intervention for cardiogenic shock. Int J Cardiol 2007;114(2):176–82.

49. De Backer D, Biston P, Devriendt J, et al. Comparison of dopamine and norepinephrine in the treatment of shock. N Engl J Med 2010;362(9):779–89.

50. Antman EM, Anbe DT, Armstrong PW, et al. ACC/AHA guidelines for the management of patients with ST-elevation myocardial infarction—executive summary. A report of the American College of Cardiology/American Heart Association Task Force on Practice Guidelines (Writing Committee to revise the 1999 guidelines for the management of patients with acute myocardial infarction). J Am Coll Cardiol 2004;44(3):671–719.

51. Hochman JS, Sleeper LA, Webb JG, et al. Early revascularization in acute myocardial infarction complicated by cardiogenic shock. SHOCK Investigators. SHould we emergently revascularize Occluded Coronaries for cardiogenic shocK. N Engl J Med 1999;341(9):625–34.

52. Indications for fibrinolytic therapy in suspected acute myocardial infarction: collaborative overview of early mortality and major morbidity results from all randomised trials of more than 1000 patients. Fibrinolytic Therapy Trialists' (FTT) Collaborative Group. Lancet 1994;343(8893):311–22.

53. Effectiveness of intravenous thrombolytic treatment in acute myocardial infarction. Gruppo Italiano per lo Studio della Streptochinasi nell'Infarto Miocardico (GISSI). Lancet 1986;1(8478):397–402.

54. Randomised trial of intravenous streptokinase, oral aspirin, both, or neither among 17,187 cases of suspected acute myocardial infarction: ISIS-2. ISIS-2 (Second International Study of Infarct Survival) Collaborative Group. Lancet 1988;2(8607):349–60.

55. Wilcox RG, von der Lippe G, Olsson CG, et al. Trial of tissue plasminogen activator for mortality reduction in acute myocardial infarction. Anglo-Scandinavian Study of Early Thrombolysis (ASSET). Lancet 1988;2(8610):525–30.

56. Gold HK, Leinbach RC, Sanders CA, et al. Intra-aortic balloon pumping for ventricular septal defect or mitral regurgitation complicating acute myocardial infarction. Circulation 1973;47(6):1191–6.

57. Sjauw KD, Engstrom AE, Vis MM, et al. A systematic review and meta-analysis of intra-aortic balloon pump therapy in ST-elevation myocardial infarction: should we change the guidelines? Eur Heart J 2009;30(4):459–68.

58. Thiele H, Zeymer U, Neumann FJ, et al. Intraaortic Balloon Support for Myocardial Infarction with Cardiogenic Shock. N Engl J Med 2012; August 26, 2012. [Epub ahead of print].

59. O'Connor CM, Rogers JG. Evidence for Overturning the Guidelines in Cardiogenic Shock. N Engl J Med 2012; August 26, 2012. [Epub ahead of print].

60. Cove ME, MacLaren G. Clinical review: mechanical circulatory support for cardiogenic shock complicating acute myocardial infarction. Crit Care 2010; 14(5):235.

61. Bermudez CA, Rocha RV, Toyoda Y, et al. Extracorporeal membrane oxygenation for advanced refractory shock in acute and chronic cardiomyopathy. Ann Thorac Surg 2011;92(6):2125–31.

62. Thiele H, Sick P, Boudriot E, et al. Randomized comparison of intra-aortic balloon support with a percutaneous left ventricular assist device in patients with revascularized acute myocardial infarction complicated by cardiogenic shock. Eur Heart J 2005;26(13):1276–83.

63. Burkhoff D, Cohen H, Brunckhorst C, et al. A randomized multicenter clinical study to evaluate the safety and efficacy of the TandemHeart percutaneous ventricular assist device versus conventional therapy with intraaortic balloon pumping for treatment of cardiogenic shock. Am Heart J 2006; 152(3):469.e1–8.

64. Seyfarth M, Sibbing D, Bauer I, et al. A randomized clinical trial to evaluate the safety and efficacy of a percutaneous left ventricular assist device versus intra-aortic balloon pumping for treatment of cardiogenic shock caused by myocardial infarction. J Am Coll Cardiol 2008;52(19):1584–8.

65. John R, Liao K, Lietz K, et al. Experience with the Levitronix CentriMag circulatory support system as a bridge to decision in patients with refractory acute cardiogenic shock and multisystem organ failure. J Thorac Cardiovasc Surg 2007;134(2):351–8.

66. Jaroszewski DE, Kleisli T, Staley L, et al. A traveling team concept to expedite the transfer and management of unstable patients in cardiopulmonary shock. J Heart Lung Transplant 2011;30(6):618–23.

67. Mebazaa A, Nieminen MS, Packer M, et al. Levosimendan vs dobutamine for patients with acute decompensated heart failure: the SURVIVE Randomized Trial. JAMA 2007;297(17):1883–91.

68. Practice parameters for hemodynamic support of sepsis in adult patients in sepsis. Task Force of the American College of Critical Care Medicine, Society of Critical Care Medicine. Crit Care Med 1999;27(3): 639–60.

69. Lollgen H, Drexler H. Use of inotropes in the critical care setting. Crit Care Med 1990;18(1 Pt 2):S56–60.

70. Levy B, Perez P, Perny J, et al. Comparison of norepinephrine-dobutamine to epinephrine for hemodynamics, lactate metabolism, and organ function variables in cardiogenic shock. A prospective, randomized pilot study. Crit Care Med 2011;39(3): 450–5.

Acute Decompensated Heart Failure

Jennifer R. Brown, MD[a], Stephen S. Gottlieb, MD[b],*

KEYWORDS

- Acute decompensated heart failure • Heart failure • ADHF • Heart failure hospitalization

KEY POINTS

- Acute decompensated heart failure (ADHF) is the most common cause of cardiovascular hospital admission; 1 in 4 patients with heart failure is readmitted within 30 days of being discharged, and ADHF consumes 1% to 2% of the total health care resources.
- The most effective approach for preventing heart failure hospitalizations is a combination of improvement in management of these patients while they are in the hospital and comprehensive post hospitalization care.
- Decreasing the length of hospitalization can increase readmission rate, so optimization of inpatient and outpatient care is essential, including ensuring adequate diuresis before discharge, optimization of medical treatment for heart failure during the hospitalization, thorough patient education before discharge, and close outpatient follow-up.

Acute decompensated heart failure (ADHF) is characterized by the heart's inability to keep up with the metabolic demands of the body without increasing cardiac pressures. The clinical syndrome is characterized by the development of acute dyspnea, often associated with the rapid accumulation of pulmonary edema. ADHF can result from systolic or diastolic dysfunction or from changes in loading conditions. The causes of a cardiomyopathy are diverse, including coronary atherosclerosis, hypertension, valvular disease, idiopathic dilated cardiomyopathy, toxins, metabolic disorders, and myocarditis; however, an acute exacerbation of heart failure is usually a result of dietary indiscretion, medication noncompliance, inadequate dosing of medication, failure to seek care, or a combination of all these.

The management of chronic heart failure is known and well accepted. We know from multiple studies that beta-adrenergic-blockers, angiotensin-converting enzyme (ACE) inhibitors and aldosterone antagonists offer a survival benefit in patients with reduced left ventricular (LV) function. We know that diuretics make patients feel better, but offer minimal effect on mortality. We know that patients who go home with inotropes have worse outcomes. We know that defibrillators reduce the incidence of sudden cardiac death and that, in certain patients, cardiac resynchronization therapy can improve LV function, quality of life, and survival.

But what do we know about the management of ADHF? The truth is, very little. And this is alarming given that ADHF is the leading cause for cardiac admission to the hospital, and, even more concerning, that 1 in 4 patients with heart failure is readmitted within 30 days of being discharged.[1] The economic impact that heart failure has on our country's health system is undeniable and yet we have not developed a successful approach for keeping these patients out of the hospital. Current therapy of ADHF revolves around relief of symptoms and amelioration of pathophysiologic and hemodynamic imbalances; yet, data suggest that there are ways to improve long-term

[a] Division of Cardiology, Department of Medicine, Emory University School of Medicine, 1365 Clifton Road, NE Atlanta, GA 30322, USA; [b] Division of Cardiology, Department of Medicine, University of Maryland School of Medicine, 110 North Paca Street, Baltimore, MD 21201, USA
* Corresponding author.
E-mail address: sgottlie@medicine.umaryland.edu

Cardiol Clin 30 (2012) 665–671
http://dx.doi.org/10.1016/j.ccl.2012.07.006
0733-8651/12/$ – see front matter Published by Elsevier Inc.

cardiology.theclinics.com

outcomes. In this article, we discuss the role, in the acute setting, of diuretics, ultrafiltration, vasodilator therapy, neurohormonal blockade, inotropes, and mechanical support for treatment of ADHF. Just as importantly, we need to consider prognosis, discharge planning and optimization of outpatient care.

THE ROLE OF DIURETICS

Diuresis provides a reduction of intracardiac filling pressures, thereby reducing pulmonary pressures and improving patients' symptoms. They have never been shown in the long-term to improve morbidity or mortality, and, in fact, some data suggest that diuretics may be deleterious when used long term. Nevertheless, adequate diuresis is clearly essential for acute improvement in symptoms. Loop diuretics are the most commonly used in ADHF because of their superior efficacy and rapid onset compared with other diuretics. Intravenous diuretics are usually given initially, as patients with significant volume overload may have intestinal edema delaying their oral absorption. It is recommended that the lowest possible dose of diuretic thought to be effective be given first, as the goal is to precipitate symptom relief while minimizing potential side effects, such as electrolyte disturbances, hypotension, and hypokalemia. Bolus doses have been the historical standard of care. If optimal results are not seen, the dosage, as well as the frequency, can be increased until goal diuresis is met. Continuous intravenous infusion can also be administered. Studies comparing intermittent intravenous administration of furosemide compared with continuous infusion suggest that either regimen works, with the total dose being most important.[2] Nevertheless, inadequate diuresis and fear of using necessary high doses are common problems in clinical practice.

Individual loop diuretics differ in their pharmacokinetic properties. Furosemide's bioavailability after oral administration is variable and approximately 50%, whereas bumetanide and torsemide both have bioavailabilities closer to 90%. In patients with decompensated heart failure and simultaneous renal insufficiency, higher doses of diuretics are often needed to provoke a therapeutic response. Doses of 200 mg of intravenous furosemide may be necessary. Combination of diuretics may also be helpful. In some patients, renal insufficiency may improve with diuresis because of decreased intra-abdominal pressure. Often, however, increased diuresis may worsen the renal insufficiency without eliciting the needed diuretic response. Such patients may need more aggressive therapy.

Another challenging question in the hospital setting is when to transition to oral diuretics. This is usually done when the symptoms of fluid overload have resolved and the patient is close to a euvolemic state. Too often patients are transitioned to oral diuretics and discharged when they are still considerably volume overloaded; this is likely one reason for the high rehospitalization rate in this patient population. When a patient is approaching euvolemia, it is appropriate to consider switching to oral diuretics, but the dosage must be carefully considered. Patients should be monitored for at least 24 hours after the transition to demonstrate effective response to the oral regimen before discharge, and close follow-up should be arranged to ensure rapid fluid accumulation does not occur.

ULTRAFILTRATION

When diuretic resistance develops, ultrafiltration is an alternative approach for effective fluid removal. In the Ultrafiltration vs IV Diuretics for Patients Hospitalized for Acute Decompensated CHF (UNLOAD) trial, 200 patients hospitalized with ADHF were randomly assigned to receive ultrafiltration or standard care (including intravenous diuretics).[3] At 48 hours, patients assigned to ultrafiltration had significantly greater fluid loss than those in the standard care arm; however, the change in renal function was no better, with patients often demonstrating increased creatinine when good fluid loss was achieved. At 90 days, patients assigned to ultrafiltration had significantly fewer heart failure rehospitalizations than patients assigned to standard care, perhaps because of the larger fluid loss. Whether increased diuretic doses in the standard of care group would have achieved the same results is unknown. Ultrafiltration is reserved for patients who do not achieve an adequate response to an aggressive diuretic regimen. The sickest patients, however, may develop renal dysfunction with the necessary fluid removal.

VASODILATOR THERAPY

In the setting of decompensated heart failure, there may be a role for vasodilator therapy to aid with decongestion. Vasodilators result in decreased afterload, decreased preload, and a reduced pulmonary capillary wedge pressure. Vasodilators may be given orally or intravenously. In the acute setting, intravenous agents, such as nitroglycerin, nitroprusside, or nesiritide, are often used. Oral agents, such as the combination of hydralazine and isosorbide mononitrate or isosorbide dinitrate, may also be used.

Intravenous nitroglycerin is primarily a venodilator and therefore results in decreased preload and decreased left-sided filling pressures. It may also lower blood pressure. It is an effective agent for the acute reduction in symptoms in the setting of ADHF; however, dose escalation is often limited by hypotension and headache.

Nitroprusside is another option for intravenous vasodilation, and, in particular, should be considered when reduced afterload is needed. For this reason, nitroprusside can be particularly useful in the setting of ADHF secondary to hypertensive emergency, acute aortic or mitral regurgitation, or acute septal rupture. Nitroprusside requires continuous blood pressure monitoring, usually with an arterial line and should not be used for more than 48 to 72 hours, as thiocyanate toxicity may develop. Additionally, nitroprusside should be used with extreme caution, if at all, in patients with liver or renal disease.

Nesiritide is a third option for intravenous vasodilator therapy in ADHF. Nesiritide is recombinant B-type natriuretic peptide (BNP), and has been shown to decrease the pulmonary capillary wedge pressure and perhaps improve acute symptoms in patients with decompensated heart failure.[4] Nesiritide has been shown to have no long-term benefit. The Acute Study of Clinical Effectiveness of Nesiritide in Decompensated Heart Failure Trial (ASCEND-HF) randomized patients with ADHF to receive standard therapy and either a continuous intravenous infusion of nesiritide or placebo. The results showed no significant difference in the prespecified end point of dyspnea, and at 1 month the rate of death and hospital readmission for heart failure was not statistically different[5]; however, the investigators also found no evidence of an increase in mortality or renal injury.

Careful consideration must be taken before starting these agents and, in particular, close attention to blood pressure is needed. Hypotension must be avoided to ensure that adequate renal perfusion is maintained. The effects of a vasodilator on blood pressure are unpredictable, with increased cardiac output often minimizing the blood pressure effects. Although vasodilators improve hemodynamics in the short term, there is no good evidence to suggest they provide any long-term benefit. Retrospective studies suggest improved outcomes in patients who receive vasodilators as compared with inotropes, but this may be because of selection bias or adverse effects of inotropes.

INOTROPIC THERAPY

Inotropic agents increase cardiac contractility, thereby improving cardiac output and may be indicated in ADHF when low output and poor organ perfusion are suspected; however, whereas inotropes may be beneficial in improving hemodynamics in ADHF, the use of inotropes is associated with a number of adverse cardiovascular events, and may worsen patient outcomes in the long term (**Fig. 1**).[6] Limitations and adverse effects of inotropic therapy include tachyarrhythmias, ischemia, hypotension, and, with chronic use, increased pathologic ventricular remodeling.

Intravenous inotropes should therefore be considered only in the management of ADHF when other therapies, such as diuretics and vasodilators, have been ineffective. Whenever possible,

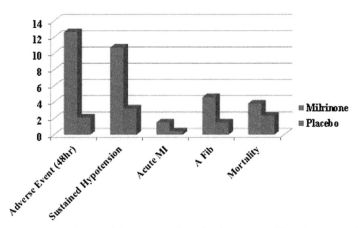

Fig. 1. In OPTIME-HF, patients receiving milrinone were found to have a significantly increased adverse event rate by 48 hours as compared with placebo. (*Data from* Cuffe MS, Califf RM, Adams KF Jr, et al. Outcomes of a Prospective Trial of Intravenous Milrinone for Exacerbations of Chronic Heart Failure (OPTIME-CHF) Investigators. Short-term intravenous milrinone for acute exacerbation of chronic heart failure: a randomized controlled trial. JAMA 2002;287(12):1541–7.)

inotropic support should be short term, although inotropes may need to be continued in patients with severe advanced heart failure who are awaiting heart transplantation or are being considered for mechanical circulatory support. Despite their limitations and no controlled studies, inotropes still play an essential role in the resuscitation of a select patient population.

NEUROHORMONAL BLOCKADE

A decline in cardiac output leads to activation of various neurohormonal cascades as compensatory processes. This includes activation of the sympathetic nervous system and the renin-angiotensin-aldosterone axis. Increased concentrations of catecholamines, angiotensin II, vasopressin, atrial/brain natriuretic peptides, and endothelin are seen. Although the short-term results of these processes often are helpful, the long-term consequences are more problematic. The proper use of neurohormonal blocking agents in the acute setting is thus difficult, with need to consider both short-term and long-term consequences.

There are minimal data about how to manage beta-blockers in patients with ADHF. Discontinuing beta-blockers in these patients may improve hemodynamics in the short term, but the withdrawal of beta-blocker therapy may permit more rapid ventricular remodeling and worsen long-term prognosis. The goal should therefore be to continue as much beta-blocker as possible while stabilizing the patient as rapidly as possible.

Thus, patients who come into the hospital with ADHF should remain on some dosage of beta-blocker if they are not in cardiogenic shock. If the exacerbation is mild, with fluid overload being the main issue, the home dosage of beta blocker can be maintained. (However, make sure that the patient is truly taking the prescribed dosage at home!) If the exacerbation is more severe, then it is reasonable to consider cutting the dosage in half until perfusion is improved. The sickest patients may need withdrawal of beta blockade. Patients with ADHF, who have either not been on beta-blocker therapy or who have not been compliant with beta-blockers, should not be restarted on beta-blocker therapy acutely. Low-dose initiation may be considered just before discharge in stable reliable patients.

Long-term use of any medication is improved if started in the hospital. For this reason, once the patient has been optimized from a hemodynamic standpoint, beta-blockers can be started at a low dose and titrated up very slowly (usually every 2 weeks), as an outpatient. Obviously more caution should be used in patients requiring inotropic therapy, and those with symptomatic hypotension, bradycardia, or recent cardiogenic shock.

ACE inhibitors were the first drugs shown to improve outcomes in patients with advanced heart failure. They have been shown to improve survival when started in patients hospitalized with refractory heart failure.[7] The Cooperative North Scandinavian Enalapril Survival Study provides the basis for initiating therapy with ACE inhibitors during initial treatment of advanced heart failure while the patient is in the hospital. Angiotensin receptor blockers (ARB) can be used in patients who develop a cough or angioedema with ACE inhibitors.

Agents should be initiated at a low dose in patients with low blood pressure. In patients who are being aggressively diuresed, there is a risk of renal dysfunction and therefore the initiation of an ACE inhibitor can be delayed until the patient is euvolemic. It is also important to remember when initiating these medications that patients may experience an early rise in creatinine levels, to approximately 25% above their baseline. The serum creatinine concentration is likely to stabilize after 4 weeks of therapy, and this rise is expected and should not be a reason for discontinuing the drug. Renal dysfunction may be acutely impaired in the setting of aggressive diuresis, and if ACE inhibitors or ARBs are held acutely, they should be restarted when the creatinine returns to baseline.

Patients with advanced heart failure should also be treated with aldosterone antagonists because these agents have been shown to improve survival in patients receiving ACE inhibitors or ARBs.[8] They have little acute hemodynamic effect, and can safely be started early in most patients. In clinical practice, early treatment may aid with diuresis, prevent hypokalemia, and permit the long-term effects to occur sooner.

Mechanical Circulatory Support

In the sickest patients, usually those presenting in cardiogenic shock, adequate perfusion cannot be maintained with the previously described therapies and mechanical circulatory support is needed. Occasionally patients will present to the hospital very unstable and in need of emergent cardiopulmonary resuscitation. In these select patients, an initial period of support with extracorporeal membrane oxygenation is an effective strategy to allow triage and stabilization. As these patients are stabilized, and the medical team gets to know the patient a little better, the patient's prognosis can be assessed and long-term support (such as an LV assist device) can be considered if medical therapy is not successful. On the other hand, patients who present in more chronic low-output heart failure and have failed medical therapy, including diuretics and inotropes, with refractory poor perfusion and often end-organ failure, should be considered for a longer-term implantable ventricular assist device, as either destination therapy or as a bridge to transplantation. More often than not, patients are transferred to tertiary care centers for consideration of mechanical support after they have developed significant sequelae of chronic low-output heart failure, making them at higher risk for surgery and poor outcomes. Patients will likely do better if referred earlier in these circumstances.

PROGNOSIS

Many important therapeutic tools have been implemented over the past 20 years that have significantly improved the prognosis and quality of life for patients with heart failure. These include neurohormonal antagonists, implantable cardioverter-defibrillators, and cardiac resynchronization therapy, as well as advances in mechanical support and heart transplantation. Despite these advances, many patients with heart failure still remain impaired with respect to functional status and quality of life, and experience an accelerated course until death.

Advanced chronic heart failure is still associated with a 1-year mortality rate as high as 51%.[9] Multiple biomarkers in heart failure have been shown to be predictors of mortality in patients with ADHF. Hospitalization for heart failure represents an important event in the life of a cardiac patient. It is associated with a high in-hospital mortality of 15.8%, and 32.0% are readmitted within 1 year.[10] In a pooled analysis of 1256 patients with ADHF, a troponin of more than 0.03 was found to be an independent predictor of mortality, with a 3.4-fold higher risk for death at 76 days (**Fig. 2**).[11]

Worsening renal function in heart failure has also been associated with adverse outcomes. Worsening renal function is common in decompensated heart failure and is associated with higher mortality. Moreover, hyponatremia, anemia, and poor nutritional status have also been associated with worse outcomes in patients with advanced heart failure. Recognizing higher-risk patients earlier in the hospitalization is essential to improving outcomes in this sick patient population.

DISCHARGE PLANNING AND OUTPATIENT CARE

The most important aspect of acute care may be arranging close and careful follow-up. Thought should be given to the cause of decompensation for each

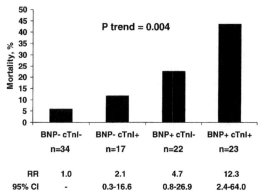

Fig. 2. Cardiac troponin I used in conjunction with BNP improves prognostic value. Those with higher troponin and BNP concentrations have higher rates of mortality. (*From* Horwich TB, Patel J, MacLellan WR, et al. Cardiac troponin I is associated with impaired hemodynamics, progressive left ventricular dysfunction, and increased mortality rates in advanced heart failure. Circulation 2003;108:833–8; with permission.)

individual patient, and a plan to avoid recurrence should be put in place so that future hospital admissions can be prevented. Education on managing their disease at home, medication management, and nutrition are paramount. Patients and their families need to understand the dietary and fluid restrictions and have an opportunity to speak with a nutritionist while in the hospital to make sure that all of their questions have been answered. Patients need to understand the importance of weighing themselves daily, and keeping a written record of these daily weights at home, to help their cardiologists keep them out of the hospital. Patients should be counseled that if they gain more than 3 pounds in 1 day or 5 pounds in 1 week, that they should call their cardiologist immediately for instructions regarding diuretic titration. This close communication with patients and frequent outpatient visits are imperative to reducing the rates of rehospitalization in this sick population. Along these same lines, an appointment should be made for the patient with his or her cardiologist no more than 2 weeks after discharge from the hospital.

Studies show that various home-monitoring interventions can be beneficial[12]; however, the aspects that are important are not clear. Patients in such programs tend to receive more evidence-based medicines, have earlier detection of decompensation or fluid overload, and may receive consultations from nutritionists, pharmacists, or social workers in addition to their follow-up. The randomized results have been uncertain and have not clearly shown which aspects of follow-up care are most beneficial. Some studies have shown improved survival, but no decrease in hospitalization.[13,14] Negative studies are often associated with close medical follow-up in all patients (including the comparison group).[15] Although the most important attributes of close follow-up care are not known, there is no doubt that close and knowledgeable follow-up care is essential.

When seen in the outpatient setting, a continuing effort has to be placed on medical optimization. Patients' drug regimens should be pushed to reach target dosages. Medical care providers may be too concerned about asymptomatic "hypotension" and not titrate to proven dosages. Similarly, patients who appear to be "stable" are often not given effective dosages of medicines that improve long-term prognosis.

These patients need to be seen frequently, so that aggressive diuresis can continue in the outpatient setting and so that they can continue to receive much-needed dietary counseling. It has clearly been shown that frequent communication between the patient and the caretaker improves outcomes. Additionally, the patients need to understand that if their regimens are adjusted by physicians outside of their cardiology team, they need to notify their cardiologist right away.

It is also very important to realize, both in the acute setting and chronically, that patients who are difficult to manage should be considered for referral to a tertiary care center. There are many options for patients with advanced heart failure, including mechanical assist devices and transplantation, which have dramatically improved the outcomes in these patients in the long term. These patients should be referred before damage to the kidneys or other organs has been prolonged. Renal insufficiency and prolonged hepatic congestion, leading to cirrhosis, increase the risk of mechanical support and transplantation, so it is better to err on the side of referring too early.

SUMMARY

Congestive heart failure is the most common cause of cardiovascular hospital admission. Not only is chronic heart failure a major cause of morbidity and mortality in the general population, but it also consumes 1% to 2% of the total health care resources.[16] The total costs for congestive heart failure care have increased considerably over the past 10 years. The most effective approach for preventing heart failure hospitalizations is a combination of improvement in management of these patients while they are in the hospital and comprehensive post hospitalization care. Decreasing the length of hospitalization can increase readmission rate, so optimization of inpatient and outpatient care is essential. This should include ensuring adequate diuresis before discharge, optimization of medical treatment for heart failure during the hospitalization, thorough patient education before discharge, and close outpatient follow-up.

REFERENCES

1. Ross JS, Chen J, Lin ZQ, et al. Recent national trends in readmission rates after heart failure hospitalization. Circ Heart Fail 2010;3(1):97–103.
2. Felker MG, Lee KL, Bull DA, et al. Diuretic strategies in patients with acute decompensated heart failure. N Engl J Med 2011;364:797–805.
3. Costanzo MR, Guglin ME, Saltzberg MT, et al, UNLOAD Trial Investigators. Ultrafiltration versus intravenous diuretics for patients hospitalized for acute decompensated heart failure. J Am Coll Cardiol 2007;49:675–83.
4. Young JB, Abraham WT, Warner-Stevenson L, et al. Results of the VMAC trial: vasodilation in the management of acute congestive heart failure. Circulation 2000;102:2794.
5. O'Connor CM, Starling RC, Hernandez AF, et al. Effect of nesiritide in patients with acute decompensated heart failure. N Engl J Med 2011;365: 32–43.
6. Cuffe MS, Califf RM, Adams KF Jr, et al, Outcomes of a Prospective Trial of Intravenous Milrinone for Exacerbations of Chronic Heart Failure (OPTIME-CHF) Investigators. Short-term intravenous milrinone for acute exacerbation of chronic heart failure: a randomized controlled trial. JAMA 2002;287(12):1541–7.
7. The CONSENSUS Trial Study Group. Effects of enalapril on mortality in severe congestive heart failure: results of the Cooperative North Scandinavian Enalapril Survival Study (CONSENSUS). N Engl J Med 1987;316:1429–35.
8. Zannad F, McMurray JJ, Krum H, et al. Eplerenone in patients with systolic heart failure and mild symptoms. N Engl J Med 2011;364:11–21.
9. Levy D, Kenchaiah S, Larson MG, et al. Long-term trends in the incidence of and survival with heart failure. N Engl J Med 2002;347:1397.
10. Tsuyuki RT, Shibata MC, Nilsson C, et al. Contemporary burden of illness of congestive heart failure in Canada. Can J Cardiol 2003;19:436–8.
11. Horwich TB, Patel J, MacLellan WR, et al. Cardiac troponin I is associated with impaired hemodynamics, progressive left ventricular dysfunction, and increased mortality rates in advanced heart failure. Circulation 2003;108:833–8.
12. McAlister F, Stewart S, Ferrua S, et al. Multidisciplinary strategies for the management of heart failure patients at high risk for admission. A systematic review of randomized trials. J Am Coll Cardiol 2004;44:810–9.

13. Cleland JG, Louis AA, Rigby AS, et al. Noninvasive home telemonitoring for patients with heart failure at high risk of recurrent admission and death. J Am Coll Cardiol 2005;45:1654–64.

14. Goldberg L, Piette J, Walsh M, et al. Randomized trial of a daily electronic home monitoring system in patients with advanced heart failure: the Weight Monitoring in Heart Failure (WHARF) trial. Am Heart J 2003;146:705–12.

15. Jaarsma T, van der Wal M, Lesman-Leegte I, et al. Effect of moderate or intensive disease management program on outcome in patients with heart failure. Coordinating Study Evaluating Outcomes of Advising and Counseling in Heart Failure (COACH). Arch Intern Med 2008;168:316–24.

16. Berry C, Murdoch DR, McMurray JJ. Economics of chronic heart failure. Eur J Heart Fail 2001;3(3): 283–91.

Management of Implantable Assisted Circulation Devices
Emergency Issues

Thomas Klein, MD[a], Miriam S. Jacob, MD[b],*

KEYWORDS

- Heart failure • Ventricular assist device • Mechanical circulatory support

KEY POINTS

- The number of end-stage heart failure patients who are refractory to medical therapy continues to expand.
- Transplant is a limited resource that has led to expansion of the use of long-term mechanical circulatory support.
- Emergency departments in the United States will increasingly encounter patients with left ventricular assist devices, and will need to be equipped to deal with their associated complications.
- Common complications of left ventricular assist device include bleeding, thrombosis, mechanical obstruction, infection, right ventricular failure, and arrhythmias.
- Knowledge of basic technical aspects of left ventricular assist devices is essential to provide care and correctly diagnose problems that may arise.

INTRODUCTION

Despite the advances in medical therapy for systolic heart failure (HF) in the past 20 years, the prevalence of this disease continues to increase. A recent American Heart Association (AHA) publication estimated the prevalence of HF in the United States at 5.7 million people,[1] with the incidence in patients more than 65 years of age approaching 1%. Several studies have documented a continued upward trend in the size of the HF population.[2,3] The proportion of patients with chronic advanced disease refractory to medical therapy has been estimated at up to 5% of the HF population,[4] with a 6-month mortality approaching 80%.[5–7] The donor population for heart transplantation remains small, and can accommodate only a small fraction of these patients; this

number has plateaued at about 2000 transplants per year performed in the United States.[8]

In selected patients with advanced HF, ventricular assist devices (VADs) have become an option as either bridge to transplant (BTT) or destination therapy (DT), and provide a significant survival advantage to optimal medical therapy, as documented in the landmark Randomized Evaluation of Mechanical Assistance for the Treatment of Congestive Heart (REMATCH) trial in 2001.[7] The pool of community-dwelling patients with VADs continues to expand, and an accelerating rate of implantation has been documented after US Food and Drug Administration (FDA) approval of the continuous-flow (CF) left ventricular assist device (LVAD) for DT in January, 2010. Almost 600 LVADs were implanted between January and

The authors have nothing to disclose.
[a] Division of Cardiology, University of Maryland School of Medicine, 110 South Paca Street, Baltimore, MD 21202, USA; [b] Division of Cardiology, Department of Medicine, University of Maryland School of Medicine, University of Maryland, 110 South Paca Street 7th Floor, Baltimore, MD 21202, USA
* Corresponding author.
E-mail address: mjacob@medicine.umaryland.edu

June, 2010, versus fewer than 400 during the same time period 1 year earlier (**Fig. 1**).[9]

Despite their documented survival benefit, these devices carry a considerable complication rate. Patients increasingly present to emergency departments (EDs) throughout the United States with a variety of complications caused by VADs, which must be recognized and managed. This article provides an overview of the types of VADs and the diagnosis and up-front management of emergent complications.

TYPES OF VADS

The 2 main varieties of VADs are pulsatile flow (PF) and CF. CF devices are subdivided into axial-flow and centrifugal-flow pumps. PF LVADs were first approved for use in the United States by the FDA in 1994, and are still in use; however, CF LVADs account for more than 98% of those currently implanted.[9]

PF VADs consist of 2 conduits attached to a volume-displacement pump. The inflow conduit is implanted into the apex of the left ventricle (LV), and delivers blood to the volume-displacement chamber, which is generally implanted in a pocket between the abdominal wall and peritoneum. A plate within the volume-displacement chamber expands and compresses the chamber by moving up and down, powered by an attached electric motor. Expansion of the chamber during diastole creates a negative-pressure chamber that draws blood from the left ventricle, whereas compression shifts blood back to the peripheral vasculature.

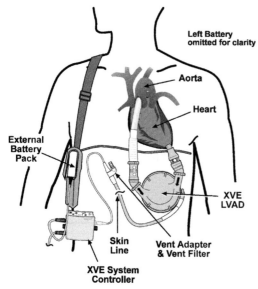

Fig. 1. Thoratec HeartMate XVE. (*Reprinted* with the permission of Thoratec Corporation, Pleasanton, California.)

Power is supplied to the motor by a driveline that tunnels through the skin of the upper abdomen. Direction of blood flow is maintained by inflow and outflow valves at both sides of the volume-displacement chamber. An outflow conduit carries blood to the ascending aorta. The percutaneous driveline also includes a conduit that allows pneumatic decompression or manual hand pumping in case of emergency.

Examples of PF VADs include the Novacor device (World Heart Inc, Salt Lake City, UT), Thoratec Paracorporeal Ventricular Assist Device (PVAD) and Implantable Ventricular Assist Device (IVAD), HeartMate IP1000, HeartMate VE, and HeartMate XVE (all manufactured by Thoratec Corporation, Pleasanton, CA, see **Fig. 1**). The HeartMate XVE has been most extensively studied for use as DT, and was evaluated in the REMATCH trial,[7] in which 129 patients with stage D HF not eligible for transplant were randomized to medical therapy or to receive the HeartMate XVE as destination therapy. Those who received the VAD had improved survival (25% 1-year mortality, vs 52% in the medical therapy group) and improved quality of life, despite an increased risk of complications. Based on the results of this and other trials, the HeartMate XVE is FDA approved for use as BTT and DT.

PF VADs have multiple limitations. The pumps are bulky and audible, involve a highly invasive surgery at initial implantation, have stringent body surface area (BSA) requirements for recipients (BSA>1.5 m²), and require a large-diameter percutaneous conduit.[10,11] In addition, device durability has been an issue; 63% of patients randomized to receive a HeartMate XVE in the REMATCH trial who survived to 2 years required replacement for infection or device malfunction.[7,12]

CF VADs include axial-flow and centrifugal-flow pumps. These pumps maintain circulation without pulsatile flow. Axial-flow pumps propel blood forward with a rotor made up of helical blades, known as an impeller, which rotates along a central shaft, akin to a corkscrew. Similar to the volume-displacement VAD, the device includes an inflow and an outflow conduit. Electrical power is fed to the pump through a percutaneous driveline that uses electromagnetic induction to drive blood forward. Centrifugal-flow VADs include a smooth-surfaced, conical impeller, which draws blood to its apex and then forward and toward the outer edge of the pump, and then is accelerated perpendicular to the axis of the impeller by a spinning rotor to an outflow cannula. New-generation CF VADs have been built to minimize the mechanical interactions of moving parts, thereby increasing device longevity.

The HeartMate II Left Ventricular Assist System (LVAS; Thoratec Corporation, **Fig. 2**), the DeBakey VAD (MicroMed Cardiovascular, Houston, TX), the Jarvik 2000 FlowMaker (Jarvik Heart, New York City, NY), and the INCOR (Berlin Heart AG, Berlin, Germany) are examples of axial-flow VADs. The HeartMate II was approved by the FDA in April, 2008,[13] for bridge to transplantation based on a trial in which 75% of the 133 patients enrolled had either been transplanted, had recovered cardiac function, or were still eligible for transplant at 180 days.[14] The HeartMate II was compared with the HeartMate XVE in a randomized, controlled trial published in 2009, in which 134 patients ineligible for transplant were randomized to 1 of the 2 therapies.[15] Those assigned to the CF pump had increased 2-year survival (58% vs 24%, $P = .008$) and were free of disabling stroke or reoperation at 2 years (46% vs 11%, $P<.001$). Based on the results of this trial, Thoratec obtained premarket approval in January 2010 for use of the HeartMate II for DT.[16]

The HeartWare HVAD (HeartWare International, Inc, Framingham, MA; **Fig. 3**), the DuraHeart (Terumo Cardiovascular Systems, Ann Arbor, MI), the VentrAssist (Ventracor, Chatswood, New South Wales, Australia), the CorAide (Arrow International, Reading, PA), the HeartQuest (MedQuest Products, Inc, Salt Lake City, UT), the HeartMate III (Thoratec Corporation), and the WorldHeart

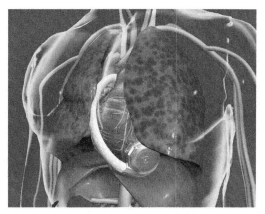

Fig. 3. HeartWare HVAD. (*Courtesy of* HeartWare, Inc, Framingham, MA; with permission. CAUTION: Investigational device. Limited by United States law to investigational use.)

Levacor (WorldHeart Corporation, Salt Lake City, UT) are examples of centrifugal pumps. All of these are currently awaiting FDA approval or are being implanted in clinical trials.

CF pumps have been found to have fewer device-related complications than volume-displacement pumps. In the HeartMate II trial,[15] significantly fewer patients required pump replacement or developed infectious complications. However, both groups in this trial had significantly improved quality of life, as measured by New York Heart Association (NYHA) class, 6-minute walk distance, and 2 standardized questionnaires.

COMPLICATIONS
Hematologic

Bleeding and thrombosis are frequently encountered complications of a VAD. Varying degrees of anticoagulation are required to balance these 2 entities. Bleeding may occur at the time of implantation and as a consequence of anticoagulation. Thrombosis can occur within the VAD pump or conduits and lead to dysfunction of the VAD or peripheral embolization to the brain, other organs, or the limbs. The HeartMate XVE was designed to have a textured, rather than a smooth, internal surface, which leads to the formation of a fibrin-cellular matrix that is nonthrombogenic.[17] This feature enables patients to remain off anticoagulation with the device in place, using only aspirin. On this regimen, in the REMATCH trial, the rate of thromboembolic events was not significantly increased in the HeartMate XVE group (which did not receive systemic anticoagulation) compared with the medical therapy group.[7] The overall risk of thromboembolism on this regimen is approximately 2% to 14%.[7,17,18]

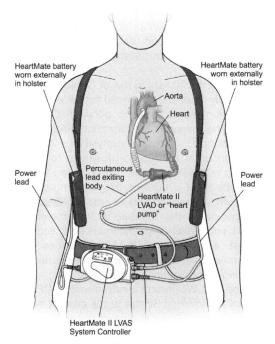

Fig. 2. Thoratec HeartMate II. (*Reprinted* with the permission of Thoratec Corporation, Pleasanton, California.)

Despite their numerous benefits compared with PF VADs, CF VADs carry a risk of pump thrombosis and thromboembolism, and require systemic anticoagulation. Initial trial data suggested that the optimal anticoagulant regimen included warfarin, with goal International Normalization Ratio (INR) 2.5 to 3.5, in addition to aspirin and dipyrimidole[14]; however, subsequent data suggest that a lower INR may be optimal to balance the risk of bleeding and thrombosis.[19] The present recommended antithrombotic regimen consists of warfarin, with a goal INR of 1.5 to 2.5 depending on the device, as well as aspirin 81 mg daily. The risk of thromboembolism of CF VADs on this regimen is low, and approximates that of PF VADs. Compared directly with the HeartMate XVE, (with an INR between 2 and 3), the HeartMate II led to 0.02 pump thrombosis events/patient year risk (vs. none in the HeartMate XVE group) and 0.06 ischemic stroke events/patient year (vs. 0.1 events/patient year for the HeartMate XVE group), a nonsignificant difference.[15]

The incidence of heparin-induced thrombocytopenia (HIT) may be increased in patients with VADs, and a high index of suspicion should be maintained in patients with thromboembolic events, especially cerebral ischemia. These patients are exposed to heparin for prolonged durations throughout their perioperative and postoperative courses, and the risks of developing heparin-induced immunization and clinical HIT are 65% and 10%, respectively.[20]

Pump thrombosis is a life-threatening event that requires expedient recognition and management (**Fig. 4**). Echocardiography is invaluable in making the diagnosis, in which thrombus can be visualized in the left ventricle, at the entrance of a cannula, or in other cardiac chambers. The traditional treatment has been pump replacement; however, this surgery may be associated with significant morbidity and mortality.[21] The use of successful intracavitary thrombolysis and glycoprotein IIb/IIIa inhibitors has also been reported, although data are limited.[22–25] Peripheral thromboembolism is treated with embolectomy, and may require more extensive surgical intervention.

Bleeding that is clinically relevant in PF and CF VADs is one of the most important adverse events to occur with these devices. In the REMATCH trial, 42% of VAD recipients had a bleeding episode within 6 months of implantation.[7] One series of 281 patients implanted with the axial-flow device showed that bleeding was the most common complication encountered in the first 30 days after implantation, documenting 72 bleeding events requiring surgery and 190 bleeding events requiring transfusion of more than 2 units of packed red blood cells.[21] Bleeding episodes may present with an obvious source such as epistaxis, genitourinary bleeding, gastrointestinal (GI) bleeding, or intracranial hemorrhage, or may be obscure. Although both PF and CF VADs have been found to have increased (and comparable) rates of major bleeding, either requiring blood transfusions or surgery,[15] CF VADs lead to more GI bleeding. This outcome was documented in a retrospective series of 55 patients who received CF devices and 46 patients who received pulsatile devices, in which there were 0.63 GI bleeds (defined as requiring at least 2 units of packed red blood cells/patient year) and 0.068 GI bleeds per patient year ($P = .0004$), respectively.[26]

Although the increased risk of GI bleeding may be partially caused by the need for systemic anticoagulation, an association between CF VADs and GI arteriovenous malformations (AVMs) has been found.[27] The pathophysiology of this phenomenon is thought to be similar to that of patients with severe aortic stenosis and type IIa von Willebrand syndrome (Heyde syndrome),[28] in which increased shear stress leads to a decrease in the number of high-molecular-weight von Willebrand multimers that promote platelet aggregation.[29,30] Multiple series have now shown that, although not all patients develop bleeding complications after VAD, all patients develop von Willebrand syndrome after CF VAD implantation.[29,31,32] Similar to the case of severe aortic stenosis, if the source of shear stress (ie, VAD or severely stenotic aortic valve) is removed or corrected, von Willebrand syndrome resolves.[28,32]

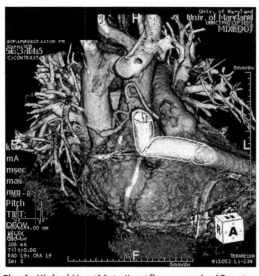

Fig. 4. Kinked HeartMate II outflow cannula. (*Courtesy* of Erika Feller, MD, University of Maryland Medical Center.)

Initial management of bleeding in the setting of a VAD consists of resuscitation with packed red blood cells. In severe bleeding or life-threatening situations, coagulopathy can be corrected with fresh frozen plasma. Endoscopic or surgical therapy may be required to manage refractory GI bleeding, and surgical therapy may be required for retroperitoneal or intracranial hemorrhage. Recombinant factor VII has been used for life-threatening bleeding in these patients, but may be associated with increased thrombotic complications and must be used with extreme caution.[33,34]

Hemolysis is caused by increased stress on erythrocytes caused by shear forces, flow acceleration, and interaction with artificial surfaces.[35] It may present as hematuria (with dark-colored urine), jaundice, or may present subacutely with typical symptoms of anemia (ie, shortness of breath, fatigue). Blood tests may reveal anemia, increased free plasma hemoglobin, decreased haptoglobin, increased bilirubin, and increased LDH.

The incidence of hemolysis has decreased as CF VADs have come to replace PF VADs. PF VADs have significant incidence of hemolysis, which may be caused by damage to erythrocytes during suction and chamber filling, and through interaction with the inflow and outflow valves. One small study that measured laboratory abnormalities consistent with hemolysis showed minimal hemolysis in centrifugal VADs, some hemolysis in axial-flow VADs, but significant hemolysis, with almost no detectable haptoglobin in PF VADs.[36]

The presence of hemolysis in a VAD warrants an investigation for coexisting disorders, because hemolysis may be associated with outflow cannula kinking or malposition, HIT, hypercoagulable states, or pump thrombosis.[37] Imaging, especially computed tomography (CT) and echocardiography, is useful to rule out mechanical defects involving inflow or outflow conduits or thrombi. Lowering the speed of the pump or adjusting cannula position may be required if deemed to be contributing to hemolysis.

Hypotension

Low blood pressure in a patient with a VAD may be caused by several different processes, including bleeding (discussed earlier), cannula or mechanical obstruction (including thrombosis, discussed earlier), right ventricular (RV) failure, dehydration, and sepsis. Standard HF medications are continued after placement of a VAD to minimize neurohormonal maladaptive mechanisms (renin-angiotensin-aldosterone and sympathetic systems) for a goal mean blood pressure of 60 to 90 mm Hg and to maximize the chance of myocardial recovery.

Blood pressures lower than a mean of 60 mm Hg or a sudden decrease from previously stable blood pressures may signify a new pathologic process.[38]

Evaluation of a patient with a VAD with hypotension begins with documenting system-provided performance parameters, including speed, power, pulsatility index (PI), and estimated flow. Often the trend in these values is more helpful than absolute numbers. Flow and power should correlate in the presence of normal device function. Power is directly measured by the device, and flow is estimated based on power and pump speed. If power is increased, not related to increased flow, the device may overestimate flow. This phenomenon may occur in the case of thrombus on the rotor. An occlusion in the path of flow may lead to a decrease in power and a corresponding decrease in flow. The PI reflects the relative increase in flow with ventricular contraction. Increased pump support leads to decreased PI, whereas improved LV function leads to increased PI. A decrease in PI without a change in pump speed may be a sign of decreased circulating volume. An increase in PI may reflect improved myocardial function, infusion of inotropes, increased sympathetic tone, or increased volume status. Pump speed is adjusted by VAD specialists to achieve optimal cardiac index and LV size without septal shift and with occasional aortic valve opening.

Cannula obstruction, kinking (see **Fig. 4**), or malposition (**Fig. 5**) may be suspected based on the aforementioned VAD performance parameters. Further evaluation may be undertaken with imaging. Echocardiography is used to determine inflow and outflow cannula velocities. If transthoracic imaging

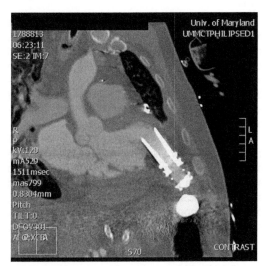

Fig. 5. Malpositioned inflow cannula facing left ventricular lateral free wall. (*Courtesy of* Erika Feller, MD, University of Maryland Medical Center.)

is suboptimal, transesophageal studies may be necessary. The inflow cannula may be visualized on echocardiography facing one of the walls, leading to partial obstruction and high velocities. Chest radiography may allow visualization of pump and cannula placement and cannula kinking or twisting. CT scanning may allow similar, but more accurate, visualization, and may also identify thrombus, but does not allow visualization of the titanium portion of the VAD. MRI may not be performed in the presence of a VAD because of VAD incompatibility with magnetic fields. Heart catheterization (left and/or right) may also be useful in the evaluation of a patient with suspected cannula obstruction or kinking to assess hemodynamics and graft patency with left ventriculography if necessary.

Adequate RV function is essential to effective LVAD therapy in that, without a functional RV, the LV does not receive the preload it needs to maintain cardiac output. RV failure after LVAD implantation is common, as was shown by an analysis of the Heart-Mate II BTT trial, which showed that 6% of patients required right ventricular assist device (RVAD) support after LVAD implantation, 7% required extended inotropes, and 7% required late inotropes for RV dysfunction.[39] Other series have documented post-VAD RV failure in 5% to 18% of patients, which is most commonly managed with extended inotropes, but does require RVAD implantation in refractory or severe cases.[15,40] Post-VAD RV failure is associated with significantly increased mortality.[15,39,40] In patients with preoperative RV dysfunction, LVAD implantation has been shown to improve RV function and right-sided hemodynamics. This improvement may be caused by favorable changes in RV architecture after unloading the LV.[40]

RV dysfunction may be suspected from the presence of hypotension with signs of RV failure, including peripheral edema, ascites, increased jugular venous pressure, hepatic dysfunction from congestion, and renal dysfunction. Echocardiography may show a dilated, dysfunctional RV with tricuspid regurgitation. Invasive hemodynamic studies may also be considered.

In CF VADs, frequent suction events may occur in the setting of RV failure when there is inadequate preload to the LV to accommodate a given pump speed. Suction events occur in other pathologic states as well, such as dehydration, hypovolemia, or cardiac tamponade. Malpositioning of the inflow cannula in the LV may predispose a patient to suction events. When the system detects a suction event, the pump speed decreases to a preset level (usually 400–800 rpm less than the fixed speed setting), and then gradually increases speed back to the fixed setting when suction is no longer

present. This decrease in speed decreases flow, and is displayed as a decrease in estimated flow.

Dehydration may lead to hypotension in patients with VADs, especially those on high doses of diuretics. PI may be decreased, and suction events occur commonly (discussed earlier). Management consists of fluid status management (decreasing diuretic doses and possibly administering additional intravenous fluids) and decreasing pump speed to minimize suction events.

Infection

A high index of suspicion for infection and sepsis should be maintained in any patient with a VAD presenting with hypotension. Transcutaneous energy transfer, a concept in which power may be supplied to an implanted device battery through the skin, is under development but is not yet commercially available. Until this is available, the percutaneous driveline continues to be a potential portal of infection that can remain for the life of the VAD.

Infectious complications were the most common cause of death in the REMATCH trial of PF VADs, accounting for 41% of deaths. In this trial, 42% of patients at 1 year and 52% of patients at 2 years developed sepsis, which corresponded with an increased mortality. Patients who developed sepsis had significantly worsened mortality compared with patients who did not (61% vs 40% at 1 year and 92% vs 62% at 2 years, $P<.06$), although percutaneous site or pocket infection did not affect survival.[41] In CF VADs, freedom from sepsis was found to be improved. In the HeartMate II BTT study, 20% of patients developed sepsis, and 20% of deaths were attributed to sepsis at 6 months.[14] In the HeartMate II DT trial, sepsis developed at 2 years in 36% of patients with CF VADs versus 44% in patients with PF VADs ($P<.001$).[15]

Local infection is also common in patients with VADs. A series of 133 LVADs (86 CF) showed that 36% of patients with CF VADs and 60% of patients with PF VADs developed driveline or pocket infections. Most of these infections occurred more than 90 days after VAD implantation.[42] Blood stream infections and driveline infections in patients with VADs are most commonly caused by *Staphylococcus aureus*; however, other common sources of infection are *Corynebacterium* species, *Pseudomonas aeruginosa*, methicillin-resistant *S aureus* (MRSA), *Candida* species, and *Enterococcus faecalis*.[42–45] Patients with driveline erythema or discharge, fevers, or leukocytosis should have blood and wound cultures performed immediately. Patients who are hemodynamically unstable are treated with broad-spectrum antibiotics, and therapy should be tailored to culture results when possible. Infectious disease consultants should be involved early in the disease course. CT scanning of the chest and abdomen should be considered in the setting of infection to rule out abscess or fluid collection. Surgical consultation is warranted, because local device-related infection may necessitate extensive surgical debridement or even exploration of the entire system.

Ventricular Arrhythmias

Patients with VADs are prone to ventricular tachyarrhythmias for many reasons, including underlying cardiomyopathy, electrolyte abnormalities, ischemic myocardium, RV failure, and myocardial irritation around the inflow cannula. The incidence of these arrhythmias has been reported to be 30% to 50% in small series.[46,47] Although these arrhythmias may be well tolerated in the short term (i.e. minutes to hours), their intermediate-term to long-term presence can lead to RV dysfunction, suction events, and hypotension. Suction events can also lead to tachyarrhythmias.[48] This phenomenon may result from excessive ventricular unloading, and may resolve with treatment of the suction event (i.e. with decreasing pump speeds).

Evaluation for treatment of the underlying cause of ventricular arrhythmia should be pursued when possible. Electrolytes should be checked and an evaluation for myocardial ischemia or acute infarction should be considered if appropriate. Patients with VADs and acute coronary syndromes are treated the same as those without, and coronary angiography is safe in these patients, as long as passing catheters through the pump is avoided. Echocardiographic evaluation should be performed if suction events are present, and volume repletion should be performed if necessary. An invasive hemodynamic study may be considered if RV failure is suspected.

Ventricular tachyarrhythmias should be treated promptly, even if they are hemodynamically tolerated. Preoperative β-blockers and antiarrhythmic medications are continued after the implantation of LVADs. Patients who have implantable cardioverter-defibrillators (ICDs) in place have been found to have improved survival compared with those without, and ICD generators should be changed when their battery life runs low.[49] Although most patients receiving VADs already have ICDs in place at the time of VAD implantation, first-time ICD implantation should also be strongly considered in patients with LVADs and ventricular tachyarrhythmias.[46,47,50,51]

Technical Issues

As described earlier, a VAD consists of an intracorporeal pump connected to an extracorporeal power source and a controller with a cable. Patients and their families are trained before hospital discharge in technical aspects of the device, including battery exchanges, driveline exit site care, significance of possible alarms, and management of emergencies. They are supplied with cards to be displayed prominently in their places of residence and to be carried on their persons to provide management information for emergency responders. In addition, many hospitals hold workshops on emergent VAD complications for local emergency responders.

The cable cannot be easily replaced, but is exposed to daily mechanical stress in the extracorporeal environment. Cable damage may be caused by chronic twisting or bending, or may be damaged deliberately. This damage occurs at a frequency of approximately 0.06 events per patient year.[52–56] However, the only option for patients with significant cable damage is device exchange.

If a VAD ceases to work for any reason that cannot be immediately fixed (ie, battery exchange), the patient must be transferred expeditiously to the nearest hospital. Although some patients may survive for the short term without the VAD, some patients require urgent pump replacement. In patients who develop immediate life-threatening cardiogenic shock on cessation of normal VAD functioning, venoarterial extracorporeal membrane oxygenation may be considered for transport and as a bridge to VAD replacement.

When PF VADs cease functioning, the inflow and outflow valves prevent backflow of blood from the aorta; however, CF VADs possess no such valves, and the cessation of function is accompanied by regurgitant blood through the VAD from the aorta. A stagnant pump does not allow blood to flow freely from aorta to LV or, conversely, from the LV to the aorta. This problem may be significant for patients with a degree of LV outflow tract or aortic valve obstruction.

For the HeartMate II, if a pump stop is caused by complete power loss, a continuous alarm sounds, and no indicator lights are visible on the controller. If the pump stop is not caused by a loss of power, an alarm sounds, and is accompanied by an illuminated red heart on the controller. In this situation, on the power module or power base unit, the pump power is zero, the flow and speed are not displayed, and a pump stop indicator is displayed. If all connections to the controller are in place and the pump is stopped, pressing the Test Select or Alarm Reset button restarts the pump.

SUMMARY

As the prevalence of systolic HF increases, the population of patients in need of advanced therapies becomes larger. As the number of transplants performed each year plateaus, the prevalence of community-dwelling patients with VADs increases. A broad range of physicians, including emergency physicians, general cardiologists, and generalists, will be exposed to these patients, and must be informed on the disease processes and complications specific to these devices. With an understanding of up-front evaluation and management, these patients may be triaged and stabilized, and will benefit before referral for definitive care by a VAD specialist.

REFERENCES

1. Roger VL, Go AS, Lloyd-Jones DM, et al. Heart disease and stroke statistics–2011 update: a report from the American Heart Association. Circulation 2011;123(4):e18–209.
2. McCullough PA, Philbin EF, Spertus JA, et al. Resource Utilization Among Congestive Heart Failure (REACH) Study. Confirmation of a heart failure epidemic: findings from the Resource Utilization Among Congestive Heart Failure (REACH) study. J Am Coll Cardiol 2002;39(1):60–9.
3. Barker WH, Mullooly JP, Getchell W. Changing incidence and survival for heart failure in a well-defined older population, 1970–1974 and 1990–1994. Circulation 2006;113(6):799–805.
4. Costanzo MR, Mills RM, Wynne J. Characteristics of "Stage D" heart failure: insights from the Acute Decompensated Heart Failure National Registry Longitudinal Module (ADHERE LM). Am Heart J 2008; 155(2):339–47.
5. Hershberger RE, Nauman D, Walker TL, et al. Care processes and clinical outcomes of continuous outpatient support with inotropes (COSI) in patients with refractory endstage heart failure. J Card Fail 2003;9(3):180–7.
6. Rogers JG, Butler J, Lansman SL, et al. Chronic mechanical circulatory support for inotrope-dependent heart failure patients who are not transplant candidates: results of the INTrEPID Trial. J Am Coll Cardiol 2007;50(8):741–7.
7. Rose EA, Gelijns AC, Moskowitz AJ, et al, Randomized Evaluation of Mechanical Assistance for the Treatment of Congestive Heart Failure (REMATCH) Study Group. Long-term use of a left ventricular assist device for end-stage heart failure. N Engl J Med 2001;345(20):1435–43.
8. Stehlik J, Edwards LB, Kucheryavaya AY, et al. The Registry of the International Society for Heart and Lung Transplantation: twenty-seventh official adult heart transplant report–2010. J Heart Lung Transplant 2010;29(10):1089–103.
9. Kirklin JK, Naftel DC, Kormos RL, et al. Third INTERMACS Annual Report: the evolution of destination therapy in the United States. J Heart Lung Transplant 2011;30(2):115–23.
10. Frazier OH, Rose EA, Oz MC, et al. Multicenter clinical evaluation of the HeartMate vented electric left ventricular assist system in patients awaiting heart transplantation. J Thorac Cardiovasc Surg 2001; 122(6):1186–95.
11. El-Banayosy A, Arusoglu L, Kizner L, et al. Novacor left ventricular assist system versus Heartmate vented electric left ventricular assist system as a long-term mechanical circulatory support device in bridging patients: a prospective study. J Thorac Cardiovasc Surg 2000;119(3):581–7.
12. Dembitsky WP, Tector AJ, Park S, et al. Left ventricular assist device performance with long-term circulatory support: lessons from the REMATCH trial. Ann Thorac Surg 2004;78(6):2123–9.
13. FDA. Thoratec HeartMate II LVAS – P060040. Available at: http://www.fda.gov/MedicalDevices/Productsand MedicalProcedures/DeviceApprovalsandClearances/ Recently-ApprovedDevices/ucm074231.htm. Accessed February 24, 2012.
14. Miller LW, Pagani FD, Russell SD, et al. Use of a continuous-flow device in patients awaiting heart transplantation. N Engl J Med 2007;357(9): 885–96.
15. Slaughter MS, Rogers JG, Milano CA, et al. Advanced heart failure treated with continuous-flow left ventricular assist device. N Engl J Med 2009; 361(23):2241–51.
16. FDA. FDA approves left ventricular assist system for severe heart failure patients. Available at: http://www. fda.gov/newsevents/newsroom/pressannouncements/ ucm198172.htm. Accessed February 24, 2012.
17. Sun BC, Catanese KA, Spanier TB, et al. 100 long-term implantable left ventricular assist devices: the Columbia Presbyterian interim experience. Ann Thorac Surg 1999;68(2):688–94.
18. McCarthy PM, Smedira NO, Vargo RL, et al. One hundred patients with the HeartMate left ventricular assist device: evolving concepts and technology. J Thorac Cardiovasc Surg 1998;115(4): 904–12.
19. Boyle AJ, Russell SD, Teuteberg JJ, et al. Low thromboembolism and pump thrombosis with the HeartMate II left ventricular assist device: analysis of outpatient anti-coagulation. J Heart Lung Transplant 2009;28(9):881–7.
20. Warkentin TE, Greinacher A, Koster A. Heparin-induced thrombocytopenia in patients with ventricular assist devices: are new prevention strategies required? Ann Thorac Surg 2009; 87(5):1633–40.

21. Pagani FD, Miller LW, Russell SD, et al. Extended mechanical circulatory support with a continuous-flow rotary left ventricular assist device. J Am Coll Cardiol 2009;54(4):312–21.

22. Kiernan MS, Pham DT, DeNofrio D, et al. Management of HeartWare left ventricular assist device thrombosis using intracavitary thrombolytics. J Thorac Cardiovasc Surg 2011;142(3):712–4.

23. Delgado R 3rd, Frazier OH, Myers TJ, et al. Direct thrombolytic therapy for intraventricular thrombosis in patients with the Jarvik 2000 left ventricular assist device. J Heart Lung Transplant 2005; 24(2):231–3.

24. Rothenburger M, Wilhelm MJ, Hammel D, et al. Treatment of thrombus formation associated with the MicroMed DeBakey VAD using recombinant tissue plasminogen activator. Circulation 2002; 106(12 Suppl 1):189–92.

25. Thomas MD, Wood C, Lovett M, et al. Successful treatment of rotary pump thrombus with the glyco-protein IIb/IIIa inhibitor tirofiban. J Heart Lung Transplant 2008;27(8):925–7.

26. Crow S, John R, Boyle A, et al. Gastrointestinal bleeding rates in recipients of nonpulsatile and pulsatile left ventricular assist devices. J Thorac Cardiovasc Surg 2009;137(1):208–15.

27. Letsou GV, Shah N, Gregoric ID, et al. Gastrointestinal bleeding from arteriovenous malformations in patients supported by the Jarvik 2000 axial-flow left ventricular assist device. J Heart Lung Transplant 2005;24(1):105–9.

28. Vincentelli A, Susen S, Le Tourneau T, et al. Acquired von Willebrand syndrome in aortic stenosis. N Engl J Med 2003;349(4):343–9.

29. Uriel N, Pak SW, Jorde UP, et al. Acquired von Willebrand syndrome after continuous-flow mechanical device support contributes to a high prevalence of bleeding during long-term support and at the time of transplantation. J Am Coll Cardiol 2010;56(15): 1207–13.

30. Geisen U, Heilmann C, Beyersdorf F, et al. Non-surgical bleeding in patients with ventricular assist devices could be explained by acquired von Willebrand disease. Eur J Cardiothorac Surg 2008; 33(4):679–84.

31. Crow S, Chen D, Milano C, et al. Acquired von Willebrand syndrome in continuous-flow ventricular assist device recipients. Ann Thorac Surg 2010; 90(4):1263–9.

32. Meyer AL, Malehsa D, Bara C, et al. Acquired von Willebrand syndrome in patients with an axial flow left ventricular assist device. Circ Heart Fail 2010; 3(6):675–81.

33. Gandhi MJ, Pierce RA, Zhang L, et al. Use of activated recombinant factor VII for severe coagulopathy post ventricular assist device or orthotopic heart transplant. J Cardiothorac Surg 2007;2:32.

34. Apostolidou I, Sweeney MF, Missov E, et al. Acute left atrial thrombus after recombinant factor VIIa administration during left ventricular assist device implantation in a patient with heparin-induced thrombocytopenia. Anesth Analg 2008;106(2): 404–8.

35. Yasuda T, Shimokasa K, Funakubo A, et al. An investigation of blood flow behavior and hemolysis in artificial organs. ASAIO J 2000;46(5):527–31.

36. Heilmann C, Geisen U, Benk C, et al. Haemolysis in patients with ventricular assist devices: major differences between systems. Eur J Cardiothorac Surg 2009;36(3):580–4.

37. Bhamidipati CM, Ailawadi G, Bergin J, et al. Early thrombus in a HeartMate II left ventricular assist device: a potential cause of hemolysis and diagnostic dilemma. J Thorac Cardiovasc Surg 2010; 140(1):e7–8.

38. Jessup M, Abraham WT, Casey DE, et al. 2009 focused update: ACCF/AHA Guidelines for the Diagnosis and Management of Heart Failure in Adults: a report of the American College of Cardiology Foundation/American Heart Association Task Force on Practice Guidelines: developed in collaboration with the International Society for Heart and Lung Transplantation. Circulation 2009;119(14):1977–2016.

39. Kormos RL, Teuteberg JJ, Pagani FD, et al. Right ventricular failure in patients with the HeartMate II continuous-flow left ventricular assist device: incidence, risk factors, and effect on outcomes. J Thorac Cardiovasc Surg 2010;139(5):1316–24.

40. Lee S, Kamdar F, Madlon-Kay R, et al. Effects of the HeartMate II continuous-flow left ventricular assist device on right ventricular function. J Heart Lung Transplant 2010;29(2):209–15.

41. Holman WL, Park SJ, Long JW, et al. Infection in permanent circulatory support: experience from the REMATCH trial. J Heart Lung Transplant 2004; 23(12):1359–65.

42. Schaffer JM, Allen JG, Weiss ES, et al. Infectious complications after pulsatile-flow and continuous-flow left ventricular assist device implantation. J Heart Lung Transplant 2011;30(2):164–74.

43. Gordon RJ, Quagliarello B, Lowy FD. Ventricular assist device-related infections. Lancet Infect Dis 2006;6(7):426–37.

44. Simon D, Fischer S, Grossman A, et al. Left ventricular assist device-related infection: treatment and outcome. Clin Infect Dis 2005;40(8):1108–15.

45. Topkara VK, Kondareddy S, Malik F, et al. Infectious complications in patients with left ventricular assist device: etiology and outcomes in the continuous-flow era. Ann Thorac Surg 2010;90(4):1270–7.

46. Oswald H, Schultz-Wildelau C, Gardiwal A, et al. Implantable defibrillator therapy for ventricular tachyarrhythmia in left ventricular assist device patients. Eur J Heart Fail 2010;12(6):593–9.

47. Andersen M, Videbaek R, Boesgaard S, et al. Incidence of ventricular arrhythmias in patients on long-term support with a continuous-flow assist device (HeartMate II). J Heart Lung Transplant 2009;28(7):733–5.

48. Vollkron M, Voitl P, Ta J, et al. Suction events during left ventricular support and ventricular arrhythmias. J Heart Lung Transplant 2007;26(8):819–25.

49. Cantillon DJ, Tarakji KG, Kumbhani DJ, et al. Improved survival among ventricular assist device recipients with a concomitant implantable cardioverter-defibrillator. Heart Rhythm 2010;7(4):466–71.

50. Bedi M, Kormos R, Winowich S, et al. Ventricular arrhythmias during left ventricular assist device support. Am J Cardiol 2007;99(8):1151–3.

51. Refaat M, Chemaly E, Lebeche D, et al. Ventricular arrhythmias after left ventricular assist device implantation. Pacing Clin Electrophysiol 2008;31(10):1246–52.

52. Birks EJ, Tansley PD, Yacoub MH, et al. Incidence and clinical management of life-threatening left ventricular assist device failure. J Heart Lung Transplant 2004;23(8):964–9.

53. Chrysant GS, Horstmanshof DA, Snyder T, et al. Successful percutaneous management of acute left ventricular assist device stoppage. ASAIO J 2010;56(5):483–5.

54. Pelenghi S, Colombo T, Montorsi E, et al. Failure and off-pump replacement of Incor LVAD system. ASAIO J 2009;55(1):121–2.

55. Slaughter MS. Long-term continuous flow left ventricular assist device support and end-organ function: prospects for destination therapy. J Card Surg 2010;25(4):490–4.

56. Slaughter MS, Tsui SS, El-Banayosy A, et al. Results of a multicenter clinical trial with the Thoratec Implantable Ventricular Assist Device. J Thorac Cardiovasc Surg 2007;133(6):1573–80.

Index

Note: Page numbers of article titles are in **boldface** type.

A

Ablation
  of AF
    in AF management, 584–585
  of atrial flutter
    in AF management, 585
  for rate control of AF
    in AF management, 585
ACS. *See* Acute coronary syndrome (ACS)
Acute coronary syndrome (ACS), **617–627**
  AF in
    acute management of, 574
  chest pain due to, 502–504
    EDOU care for
      evidence for, 503
      future directions in, 503–504
      patient selection for, 502–503
  described, 617–618
  evaluation of
    cardiac biomarkers in, 621–622
    chest radiography in, 621
    ECG in, 620–621
    imaging in, 620–622
    patient history in, 619–620
    physical examination in, 620
    risk factors for, 618–619
  treatment of, 622–624
    anticoagulants in, 623–624
    aspirin in, 622–623
    β-blockers in, 624
    disposition after, 624
    future directions in, 625
    GP IIB/IIIA inhibitors in, 624
    nitrates in, 623
    STEMI–related, 622
    thienopyridines in, 623
Acute decompensated heart failure (ADHF),
  665–671
  described, 665–666
  discharge planning related to, 669–670
  diuretics for, 666
  inotropic therapy for, 667–668
  mechanical circulatory support for, 668–669
  neurohormonal blockade for, 668
  outpatient care for, 669–670
  prognosis of, 669
  ultrafiltration for, 666
  vasodilator therapy for, 666–667
Acute heart failure

in clinical evaluation of hypertension crisis in ED, 538
Acute heart failure syndrome
  EDOU evaluation of, 512–517
    evidence for, 513–517
    future directions in, 517
Acute renal insufficiency
  in clinical evaluation of hypertension crisis in ED, 539
ADHF. *See* Acute decompensated heart failure (ADHF)
Adrenal insufficiency
  steroids and, 644
AF. *See* Atrial fibrillation (AF)
Amiodarone
  in AF management, 578, 582
Aneurysm(s)
  ventricular
    previous infarction with
      mimicking STEMI, 605–606
Angina
  Prinzmetal
    mimicking STEMI, 606
Antiarrhythmic medications
  in rate control
    in AF management, 578
Anticoagulants
  in ACS management, 623–624
Antiplatelet therapy
  in AF management, 584
Aortic dissection
  blunt aortic injury and, 552–553
  in clinical evaluation of hypertension crisis in ED, 538–539
Aortic pseudoaneurysm
  blunt aortic injury and, 553
Aortic rupture
  blunt aortic injury and, 551–552
Apical ballooning syndrome, 607
Arrhythmias
  cardiac
    syncope due to, 559
  ventricular
    VADs and, 679
Aspirin
  in ACS management, 622–623
Atrial dysrhythmias
  blunt cardiac injury and, 545–546
Atrial fibrillation (AF)

http://dx.doi.org/10.1016/S0733-8651(12)00108-7
0733-8651/12/$ – see front matter © 2012 Elsevier Inc. All rights reserved.

cardiology.theclinics.com

United States Postal Service

Statement of Ownership, Management, and Circulation
(All Periodicals Publications Except Requestor Publications)

1. Publication Title	2. Publication Number	3. Filing Date
Cardiology Clinics	0 0 0 - 7 0 1	9/14/12

4. Issue Frequency	5. Number of Issues Published Annually	6. Annual Subscription Price
Feb, May, Aug, Nov	4	$305.00

7. Complete Mailing Address of Known Office of Publication (Not printer) (Street, city, county, state, and ZIP+4®)

Elsevier Inc.
360 Park Avenue South
New York, NY 10010-1710

Contact Person
Stephen R. Bushing

Telephone (Include area code)
215-239-3688

8. Complete Mailing Address of Headquarters or General Business Office of Publisher (Not printer)

Elsevier Inc., 360 Park Avenue South, New York, NY 10010-1710

9. Full Names and Complete Mailing Addresses of Publisher, Editor, and Managing Editor (Do not leave blank)

Publisher (Name and complete mailing address)

Kim Murphy, Elsevier, Inc., 1600 John F. Kennedy Blvd. Suite 1800, Philadelphia, PA 19103-2899

Editor (Name and complete mailing address)

Barbara Cohen-Kligerman, Elsevier, Inc., 1600 John F. Kennedy Blvd. Suite 1800, Philadelphia, PA 19103-2899

Managing Editor (Name and complete mailing address)

Barbara Cohen-Kligerman, Elsevier, Inc., 1600 John F. Kennedy Blvd. Suite 1800, Philadelphia, PA 19103-2899

10. Owner (Do not leave blank. If the publication is owned by a corporation, give the name and address of the corporation immediately followed by the names and addresses of all stockholders owning or holding 1 percent or more of the total amount of stock. If not owned by a corporation, give the names and addresses of the individual owners. If owned by a partnership or other unincorporated firm, give its name and address as well as those of each individual owner. If the publication is published by a nonprofit organization, give its name and address.)

Full Name	Complete Mailing Address
Wholly owned subsidiary of	1600 John F. Kennedy Blvd., Ste. 1800
Reed/Elsevier, US holdings	Philadelphia, PA 19103-2899

11. Known Bondholders, Mortgagees, and Other Security Holders Owning or Holding 1 Percent or More of Total Amount of Bonds, Mortgages, or Other Securities. If none, check box ☐ None

Full Name	Complete Mailing Address
N/A	

12. Tax Status (For completion by nonprofit organizations authorized to mail at nonprofit rates) (Check one)
The purpose, function, and nonprofit status of this organization and the exempt status for federal income tax purposes:
☐ Has Not Changed During Preceding 12 Months
☐ Has Changed During Preceding 12 Months (Publisher must submit explanation of change with this statement)

PS Form 3526, September 2007 (Page 1 of 3 (Instructions Page 3)) PSN 7530-01-000-9931 PRIVACY NOTICE: See our Privacy policy in www.usps.com

---

13. Publication Title		14. Issue Date for Circulation Data Below
Cardiology Clinics		August 2012

15. Extent and Nature of Circulation			Average No. Copies Each Issue During Preceding 12 Months	No. Copies of Single Issue Published Nearest to Filing Date
a. Total Number of Copies (Net press run)			917	739
b. Paid Circulation (By Mail and Outside the Mail)	(1)	Mailed Outside-County Paid Subscriptions Stated on PS Form 3541 (Include paid distribution above nominal rate, advertiser's proof copies, and exchange copies)	427	373
	(2)	Mailed In-County Paid Subscriptions Stated on PS Form 3541 (Include paid distribution above nominal rate, advertiser's proof copies, and exchange copies)		
	(3)	Paid Distribution Outside the Mails Including Sales Through Dealers and Carriers, Street Vendors, Counter Sales, and Other Paid Distribution Outside USPS®	190	199
	(4)	Paid Distribution by Other Classes Mailed Through the USPS (e.g. First-Class Mail®)		
c. Total Paid Distribution (Sum of 15b (1), (2), (3), and (4))		▶	617	572
d. Free or Nominal Rate Distribution (By Mail and Outside the Mail)	(1)	Free or Nominal Rate Outside-County Copies Included on PS Form 3541	64	66
	(2)	Free or Nominal Rate In-County Copies Included on PS Form 3541		
	(3)	Free or Nominal Rate Copies Mailed at Other Classes Through the USPS (e.g. First-Class Mail)		
	(4)	Free or Nominal Rate Distribution Outside the Mail (Carriers or other means)		
e. Total Free or Nominal Rate Distribution (Sum of 15d (1), (2), (3) and (4))		▶	64	66
f. Total Distribution (Sum of 15c and 15e)		▶	681	638
g. Copies not Distributed (See instructions to publishers #4 (page 83))		▶	236	101
h. Total (Sum of 15f and g)		▶	917	739
i. Percent Paid (15c divided by 15f times 100)		▶	90.60%	89.66%

16. Publication of Statement of Ownership

If the publication is a general publication, publication of this statement is required. Will be printed ☐ Publication not required
in the November 2012 issue of this publication.

17. Signature and Title of Editor, Publisher, Business Manager, or Owner

Stephen R. Bushing [signature]

Date
September 14, 2012

Stephen R. Bushing – Inventory Distribution Coordinator

I certify that all information furnished on this form is true and complete. I understand that anyone who furnishes false or misleading information on this form or who omits material or information requested on the form may be subject to criminal sanctions (including fines and imprisonment) and/or civil sanctions (including civil penalties).

PS Form 3526, September 2007 (Page 2 of 3)

Moving?

Make sure your subscription moves with you!

To notify us of your new address, find your **Clinics Account Number** (located on your mailing label above your name), and contact customer service at:

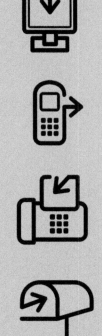

Email: journalscustomerservice-usa@elsevier.com

800-654-2452 (subscribers in the U.S. & Canada)
314-447-8871 (subscribers outside of the U.S. & Canada)

Fax number: 314-447-8029

Elsevier Health Sciences Division
Subscription Customer Service
3251 Riverport Lane
Maryland Heights, MO 63043

Printed and bound by CPI Group (UK) Ltd, Croydon, CR0 4YY

03/10/2024

01040344-0014